Toward Sustainable Transitions in Healthcare Systems

Health systems have long been considered key determinants of well-being within modern societies, a valuable resource which has faced a series of reform initiatives throughout the past decades. These reforms have been used to manage the cost of development, measure the tenability of health systems in globalizing economies and promote the increasing importance of health problems related to lifestyle and living conditions, yet they have failed to provide a true resolution to the persistent economical and logistical problems facing modern-day health systems.

This rich, interdisciplinary work explores the hypothesis that many of these problems cannot be adequately addressed without structural changes to our health systems, and examines the embedded features of our health systems that underlie contemporary challenges as well as how, and under what conditions, our health systems can be made more sustainable. Combining and building upon theoretical approaches from transition and innovation studies for analysing health system deficits, *Toward Sustainable Transitions in Healthcare Systems* raises fundamental questions about how new research, new needs and exogenous trends are transforming current health systems.

Providing an original and substantial analysis of the complex structural features of the health innovation system, this book will be of interest to students and practitioners of the politics of health, social epidemiology, medical sociology and those with an interest in transition theory.

Jacqueline E.W. Broerse is Professor of Innovation and Communication in the Health and Life Sciences, and Director of the Athena Institute at Vrije Universiteit Amsterdam.

John Grin is Professor of Policy Science, with a focus on System Innovation, at the Department of Political Science at the University of Amsterdam.

Toward Sustainable Transitions in Healthcare Systems

Edited by Jacqueline E.W. Broerse and John Grin

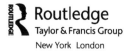

Routledge
Taylor & Francis Group
New York London

First published 2017 by Routledge

711 Third Avenue, New YorK, NY 10017

2 ParK SQuare, Milton ParK, Abingdon, Oxfordshire OX14 4RN

Routledge is an imprint of the Taylor & Francis Group, an informa business

First issued in paperbacK 2018

British Library Cataloguing in Publication Data
A catalogue record for this book is available from the British Library

Library of Congress Cataloging in Publication Data
Title: Toward sustainable transitions in healthcare systems.
Description: New York, NY : Routledge, 2017. | Series: Routledge studies in sustainability transitions | "Selection and editorial matter, Jacqueline Broerse and John Grin; individual chapters, the contributors"–Copyright statement, t.p. verso.
Identifiers: LCCN 2016043182| ISBN 9780415888417 (hbk) | ISBN 9781315232133 (ebk)
Subjects: LCSH: Health care reform. | Health planning.
Classification: LCC RA394 .T69 2017 | DDC 362.1/0425–dc23
LC record available at https://lccn.loc.gov/2016043182

ISBN: 978-0-415-88841-7 (hbk)
ISBN: 978-0-367-02699-8 (pbk)

Typeset in Bembo
by Wearset Ltd, Boldon, Tyne and Wear

Contents

Figures

Tables

Contributors

Editors

Jacqueline E.W. Broerse is a full Professor of Innovation and Communication in the Health and Life Sciences. She is Director of the Athena Institute, Vrije Universiteit Amsterdam. She holds a Master's degree in Biomedical Sciences (cum laude). In 1998 she obtained her PhD degree on the development of an interactive approach to include users in research agenda-setting processes on biotechnology. Her current research is focused on methodology development for and implementation of multi-stakeholder innovation processes, reflexive monitoring and evaluation of interventions, and system innovations, in order to contribute to a better embedding of new interventions in society (globally). Many of her research projects are in the health sector. She has been involved as adviser and facilitator in various interactive policy-making trajectories of the Dutch Ministry of Health, Welfare and Sports. She is program coordinator of the Erasmus Mundus Joint Degree Program on Transdisciplinary Solutions to Global Health Challenges and program director of the research Master's in Global Health; she also coordinates and lectures in various courses on health policy and health system innovation. She is a board member of the Dutch National Research School in Science, Technology and Modern Culture (WTMC).

John Grin is a full Professor of Policy Science, especially system innovation, in the Department of Political Science, University of Amsterdam. A physicist by training (BSc, 1983; MSc, 1986), he obtained his PhD in 1990 at Vrije Universiteit Amsterdam by defending a thesis on technology assessment in the area of military technology and international security. Next, he worked on these issues for another two years at Vrije Universiteit and Princeton University. In 1992 he joined the University of Amsterdam. The constant throughout his career has been an interest in the relationships between science, technology, society and politics. He is particularly interested in understanding the "politics" of knowledge and technology and ways to analyze them, as well as the question of how knowledge and technology may be made to help resolve rather than create social problems.

In addition to system innovations and transitions, his research interests include policy analysis and design (including technology assessment), policy implementation, policy learning and novel modes of democratic governance. Empirically, much of his work focuses on agrofood, healthcare, and water management. He was co-director and co-founder of the Dutch Knowledge Network on System Innovations, specifically responsible for the KSI sub-program on governance studies, as well as for its interface between research and practice. He coordinates a postgraduate course for practitioners engaged in system innovation.

Contributors

Paul Baart is Director of the Dutch Center Work Health (Centrum Werk Gezondheid) and Managing Director of the International Institute for Health Management and Quality (IHMQ). He studied social sciences at the Groningen University and organizational change management at SIOO. Following a career in the mental health sector and innovative projects, also in the health sector, he became Director of the Dutch Center for Workplace Health Promotion (Centrum GBW) and Director of SKB, an expert center on occupational health. He is active in international and European programs on work and health. The Dutch Center Work Health is an associated member of the European Network for Workplace Health Promotion (ENWHP).

Ingrid Bakker was a postdoc in issues of health and society at Wageningen University between 2007 and 2010. She has an MSc in Psychology and Epidemiology. Her PhD project at Vrije Universiteit Amsterdam was devoted to stress-related mental disorders, sick leave, and general practice. Currently she is a policy adviser with the Dutch Ministry of Social Affairs and Employment.

Eric Berkers is Senior Researcher with the Foundation for the History of Technology at Eindhoven University of Technology. He graduated as an economic and social historian, with specializations in business history and the history of technology. He received his PhD at Delft University of Technology for research about the history of Dutch water management. He participated in national research projects in the fields of the history of technology in the Netherlands in the nineteenth and twentieth century (TIN-19 and TIN-20) and the history of Dutch business in the twentieth century (BINT). Within the latter, his focus was on innovations in small and medium-sized firms. Furthermore, he published about the development of knowledge infrastructures in the Netherlands in different domains, such as energy, water management, geodesy, horticulture, food and healthcare. One of his current research topics is transitions in healthcare due to the production and use of information technology since the 1950s.

Williem I. (Pim) de Boer is currently Senior Grant Advisor at VUmc and a consultant at HuMedSci Consultancy. He has an MSc in biology (University of Utrecht) and a PhD degree in the field of pathology (Erasmus University Rotterdam). He worked for more than ten years as executive director of research at the Lung Foundation. His aim is to contribute to the improved quality of life of patients and to find solutions via (bio)medical research and state-of-the-art education, specifically involving patients' needs, ideas and experiences.

David Clements worked in the area of health policy, communications and knowledge exchange for over 15 years. He is currently Executive Director of the Healthcare Innovation Secretariat at the federal Department of Health in Ottawa, Canada. He is also an adjunct professor in the Department of Health Sciences at Carleton University, Ottawa. He has worked for a number of federal and provincial government agencies and NGOs, including the Canadian Institute for Health Information (CIHI), the Canadian Health Services Research Foundation (CHSRF), and the Canadian Agency for Drugs and Technology in Health (CADTH). He is also an associate with the Ottawa-based Centre for Excellence in Communications, where he teaches science communication. Holding a Master's degree from the School of Policy Studies at Queen's University, he is currently pursuing a doctorate in innovation studies at Vrije Universiteit Amsterdam.

Janneke E. Elberse is Research and Program Coordinator at the Dutch Cancer Society. She has a double Master's degree in Molecular Sciences and Science and Technology Studies. From 2007 until 2013 she was researcher at the Athena Institute, Vrije Universiteit Amsterdam. In 2012 she obtained her PhD degree for research in the area of enhancing patient involvement in decision-making on health research. A point of departure for her research was transition theory and a change toward a more needs-oriented research system. By using different case studies, she tried to understand and overcome obstacles for active patient involvement within the health research system. At the Dutch Cancer Society, she is involved in innovating the culture, structure and practice to optimize the acilitation and financing of oncological health research, with an emphasis on enhancing the process from "bench to bedside."

Dirk Essink is a postdoc researcher and lecturer at the Athena Institute, Vrije Universiteit Amsterdam. He completed his Master's degree in Health Sciences (cum laude) with a specialization in international public health (2008). In 2012, he obtained a PhD degree from Vrije Universiteit by defending a thesis on the role of change agents in sustainable health system innovation. His current research focuses on system innovation and stakeholder/public engagement in research, policy, and care practice. He is involved in various Dutch and international projects that aim to gain an insight into effective strategies, interventions, and conditions in order to realize sustainable systems innovation, focusing on end-user and stakeholder involvement. He coordinates the Master's specialization in International Public Health of the Master's program in Management, Policy-analysis, and Entrepreneurship in Health and Life Sciences, and coordinates and lectures in a wide variety of courses on such issues as health policy and system, infectious diseases, and research methods for needs assessment.

Jorge Garcés is a full Professor at the University of Valencia and Prince of Asturias Distinguished Visiting Professor at Georgetown University (Washington, DC, USA). He is also Director of the Polibienestar Research Institute, a specialized center in public policy research and consultancy using an interdisciplinary methodological approach. His research has focused on comparative social policy in Europe, with an emphasis on aging and social innovation as well as on the increase of the efficiency and effectiveness of long-term care policies in Europe. He has been a main researcher or member of research teams in nearly 100 projects and research contracts with European, regional, and local administrations. He has participated as an expert in the Commission of Social Policy of the Spanish Parliament and in different committees organized by the European Commission. In 2009 he was awarded a doctorate honoris causa by the University of San Pedro, Peru, and in 2013 by the University of Encarnación, Paraguay.

Fjalar J. de Haan is Lecturer – Sustainability Transitions at the Melbourne School of Design and an associate of the Melbourne Sustainable Society Institute, both at the University of Melbourne. Being a theoretician, he is of the opinion that "theory is technology, tools for understanding." He is also an advocate, and practitioner, of computational and mathematical modeling approaches to the field of sustainability transitions. One of his main theoretical contributions is the "multi-pattern approach" and the constellation concept, which facilitate systematic transitions analysis, increased comparability of case studies, and provide a basis for analyses with modeling approaches. He obtained his PhD in Transitions Studies at the Dutch Research Institute for Transitions and also holds an MSc in theoretical physics (non-linear dynamics and pattern formation) from Leiden University.

Erica ter Haar-van Twillert conducted research into the impact of innovative projects in Dutch healthcare for finding solutions to existing persistent problems and expected future challenges. Her empirical research includes projects which use communication technologies to develop new (better) ways of treatment and care (telecare). She holds a Master's degree in social sciences, policy, and politics. In the past she worked as an occupational therapist in several fields of Dutch healthcare. Currently she is a policy adviser concerning societal support.

Maria Koelen chairs the Health and Society Group of the Department of Social Sciences, Wageningen University. She studied social psychology and research methodology (University of Groningen) and obtained her PhD at Wageningen Agricultural University (1988). Her research focuses on the combined influence of the social and physical environment on people's lifestyle, their health, and quality of life. Specific areas are community-based health promotion, and methods in health promotion research. She is a member of the IUHPE Global Working Group on Salutogenesis (GWGS), and member of the course team of the European Training Consortium in Public Health and Health Promotion.

Jord Neuteboom graduated from Wageningen University in landscape planning, communication sciences, and business management. He has extensive experience in the development of policies and programs in the fields of environmental policy, agriculture, and energy. He served as manager of transition management programs on energy efficiency in Central European countries (Novem, the Netherlands) and as marketing and communication manager in the field of nature conservation (NGO Natuurmonumenten). For several years he was process manager of healthcare at the Dutch Research Institute for Transitions (DRIFT, Erasmus University Rotterdam). He is currently leading the transition management consultancy firm Viatore, which aims at personal transformations and societal transitions. As a transition management practitioner he has been providing assistance to start-up companies, societal initiatives and NGOs, entrepreneurs, sector organizations, insurance companies, and governmental organizations in several domains of healthcare.

Tamara Raaijmakers is Program Manager in the field of workplace health. Her background is in human movement sciences at Vrije Universiteit Amsterdam, labor and health serving as her specialty. She is currently working for the Dutch Center Work Health, which concentrates on the coordination and introduction of programs in the field of work and health, performing practice-oriented research and stimulating professionalization by developing guidelines, working methods, and the organization of international exchanges. She is also an auditor for the International Institute for Health Management and Quality (IHMQ).

Roel van Raak has a BSc and an MSc in Systems Engineering, Policy Analysis and Management from Delft Technical University. He also worked at this university and UNESCO-IHE before he joined DRIFT in February 2005. In 2010, he completed his PhD project, devoted to integrating various conceptual frameworks and scales in transition studies for policy purposes applied to the Dutch healthcare system. He is currently working at DRIFT as a senior researcher and adviser. His research interests are in connecting transition modeling to transition management and applying theory to (policy) practice. He has been active in various sectors, with a focus on water (management) and especially healthcare, both as a university researcher and commercial consultant.

Francisco Ródenas has a PhD in Sociology. Currently, he works as a researcher at the Polibienestar Research Institute and as a lecturer at the Faculty of Social Science, University of Valencia, Spain, where he teaches undergraduate and postgraduate courses on research in social welfare systems and health and social care, and is Director of the Master's in Social Welfare: Family Intervention. He leads a research line on efficiency and quality of health and social systems for long-term care. He has participated in eight European R&D projects, has directed various R&D projects in Spain funded by the Ministry of Education, and participated in over 30 research projects and research contracts from government and the private sector.

Tjerk Jan Schuitmaker is Assistant Professor at the Athena Institute, Vrije Universiteit Amsterdam, where he teaches a wide range of courses in the Master's program and the Honors program. As a researcher he is interested in persistent problems and system innovations. He currently works with regional partnerships of healthcare professionals in obstetrics on improving the quality and continuity of (pre)natal care. Furthermore, he investigates the implementation of new technologies that support a transition to a bio-based economy. His dissertation is about persistent problems in the Dutch healthcare system. He conducted this research at the AISSR, University of Amsterdam, as part of the KSI network, dealing with sustainability transitions.

Lenneke Vaandrager is Associate Professor and Research Coordinator of the Health and Society Group in the Department of Social Sciences, Wageningen University, the Netherlands. Her main research interests are workplace health promotion and health and the natural environment. Most of her work is inspired by systems thinking and salutogenesis. She has a PhD in Communication and Organizational Change. She is Chair of the Implementation Committee of the Dutch ZonMw Research Funding Program on Participation and Health (research on sustainable healthy working lives), coordinator of the European Training Consortium in Public Health and Health Promotion (ETC-PHHP, formed by ten public health institutions), and a member the IUHPE Global Working Group on Salutogenesis (GWGS). In her former job she was program co-ordinator of the Department of Work and Health at the Netherlands Institute of Health Promotion (NIGZ).

Suzanne Van den Bosch is a researcher, adviser and trainer for her own consultancy SUSi. She holds a Master's degree in Innovation Management (specialization sustainable development). In 2010 she obtained a PhD in transition management at the Dutch Research Institute for Transitions, Erasmus University Rotterdam. Her PhD research included transition experiments in mobility, the Learning for Sustainable Development Program, and the Transition Program in Long-term Care. Subsequently she worked as a consultant for Viatore. She established SUSi in 2012. She worked for the Pioneers into Practice Program of the Climate-KIC in Emilia Romagna (Italy), the Transition Academy, and the STG/Health Management Forum Foundation (Dutch network for future research, strategy development, and healthcare innovation). She also conducted various research and monitoring activities for the Dutch program "In for care!", an initiative of the Dutch Ministry of Health, Welfare and Sports and Vilans (Center of Expertise for Long-term Care). Her current research focuses on the scaling up of successful transition experiments in healthcare.

1 Introduction

John Grin and Jacqueline E.W. Broerse

> The way health systems are designed, managed and financed affects people's lives and livelihoods. The difference between a well-performing health system and one that is failing can be measured in death, disability, impoverishment, humiliation and despair.
>
> (Gro Brundtland, WHO, 2000: vii)

1.1 Health and health systems: trends, problems and responses

Health systems are key determinants of health in modern societies. In 1948 the World Health Organization (WHO) defined health as "a state of complete physical, mental and social well-being and not merely the absence of disease or infirmity." The 1986 Ottawa Charter for Health Promotion[1] states that "health is a resource for everyday life, not the objective of living. Health is a positive concept emphasizing social and personal resources, as well as physical capacities." Health *systems* were subsequently defined to include:

> all actors, institutions and resources that undertake health actions – where the primary intent of a health action is to improve health. It is broader than personal medical and non-personal health services. It incorporates selected inter-sectoral actions in which the stewards of the health system take responsibility to advocate for health improvements outside their direct control, such as regulations to reduce fatalities from traffic accidents.
>
> (Murray and Evans, 2003: 7–8)

Taken together, these WHO definitions of health and health systems underline that health is a resource and a condition for living productive lives. They also point to the widely shared conviction among policy-makers that health systems are crucial for realizing health.

Nevertheless, health systems are hard pressed in meeting their goals, even in the advanced welfare states of Western Europe and North America on which this book focuses. To be sure, virtually all infectious diseases have been brought under control, while significant progress in areas such as cancer and cardiovascular disease have led to notable increases in years of life lived in good health. But at the same time – partly as the flip side of their very successes, partly due to pressure on health systems – we see the (future) emergence of numerous complex problems. This book explores the hypothesis that many of these problems cannot be adequately addressed without structural changes to our health systems. More specifically, its chapters examine the embedded features of our health systems that underlie contemporary challenges as well as how, and under what conditions, health systems can be made more sustainable.

"System reforms" of health systems have been attempted by many welfare states since the economic crises of the late 1970s. Such reforms, however, are not what we are hinting at. Their focus has been on *containing costs* and, to a lesser extent, to improving accessibility; even their proponents generally agree that they have, at best, only been partly successful. The following section elaborates upon our hypothesis that many of the problems faced by health systems, as well as the flaws in attempts to resolve them, are rooted in their structural features. In transition studies, complex problems that endure – due to the same features of the system underlying problems as well as solution pathways and mechanisms – are referred to as "persistent problems." Any resolution is thus bound to involve mutually reinforcing innovative practices as well as structural adaptation (Grin et al., 2010: 2–4).

These processes of profound change are called "transitions." Transitions are long-term, complex structural changes in societal systems in which radical shifts occur from one system, or configuration, to another (Geels and Schot, 2010). Transitions include changes in institutionalized identities, social relations and "self-evident" assumptions, and typically involve multiple actors from government, the private sector, science and civil society (Grin, 2010). Although breakthroughs can occur relatively quickly, transitions stretch over periods of one or two generations (Rotmans et al., 2001). This book therefore does not offer quick fixes. Nevertheless, case studies of earlier transitions and the mechanisms of their successes and failures in the emerging field of transition studies[2] have yielded insights into how radically innovative practices and structural changes can reinforce each other over time, eventually yielding a transition (Grin, 2006, 2010: 265–284; Geels and Schot, 2010: 47–51).

This book will investigate whether and how the transition perspective helps us identify more promising ways to understand and address the problems confronting contemporary health systems. Through the conceptual framework of transition studies, it seeks to: (1) better understand the embedded features in the foundations of our health systems that underlie complex problems, and (2) find ways to innovate health systems to more sustainably address these problems. The following section provides an overview of modern health systems, the problems facing them, and their attempted solutions. Drawing upon key insights from transition studies, we will then further outline the book's design.

1.2 Modern health systems, their challenges and attempted solutions

Many of the problems facing modern health systems, we argue, are embedded in their foundational features, while the difficulties encountered in addressing persistent problems often reveal how these features reproduce themselves. Nevertheless, pursuing analysis on the generic level of modern health systems is a risky undertaking that needs to be preceded by at least three disclaimers. First, while we believe that our analysis of problems and their causes is relevant across a wide range of health systems, we acknowledge diversity between and within systems, and in how and how far our claims hold. Second, we do not reify particular structural features and suggest that they determine practices; we instead adhere to what Giddens (1984) has called the "duality of structure," where structures are both the medium and outcomes of action. It is agency within practices that yields diversity. Third, we do not claim that our analysis is anything close to comprehensive. Our aim is to render plausible our hypothesis – the starting point of our analysis – and to tie our argument to wider discussions about health, healthcare and health systems.

Infectious diseases

Modern health systems have a proven track record in combatting infectious diseases, in some cases having eradicated them. But the work is far from over as new challenges emerge, partially due to, and more often complicated by, the global mobility of people and pathogens. HIV/AIDS and Ebola are two cases in point. Another is how climate change is increasing the incidence of Leishmaniasis in Europe (Ready, 2010) with the sand fly, its vector, following rising temperatures. Such challenges require changes in how we organize prevention, surveillance and care for emerging diseases.

Since the seventeenth century, the medical profession has come to rely on what Toulmin (2001) describes as "applied biology": medicine typically relies on applying to a particular case universal knowledge of a supposedly universal body, understood from the quintessentially modern perspective that we can control nature on the basis of universal principles. Disease is then understood as an abnormal state caused by outside pathogens or (hereditary) internal malfunction, to be remedied through interventions based on this knowledge (e.g. surgery or medicinal correction of hormone levels), prevented by intervening in the pathogenic process (e.g. antibiotics), or by denying access to pathogens (e.g. through sanitary or job safety measures). This approach has obviously been successful. Modern medicine has realized a significant part of the dream that accompanied its birth during the early Enlightenment when Francis Bacon (1626: 449) proclaimed that Newtonian science would enable medicine to go beyond the two aims stressed by the ancient Greeks, namely remedying disease and promoting health. It would, he claimed, now also become possible to prolong life.

This modern vision has guided the development of medical science as well as relationships among medical practitioners, researchers, government, industry and patients. Health maintenance is primarily understood as the responsibility of the health system which – in line with the WHO definitions cited above – is to enable people to live productive lives. This has typically translated into a relatively strict functional differentiation between the health system and other societal systems, such as the energy system and the educational system. A key feature of health systems in advanced welfare states (e.g. Patel and Rushefsky, 1999) is the central role of both medical rationality and medical professionals. The modernization of the medical profession was accompanied by a process of "protoprofessionalization" (De Swaan, 1996) – the internalization of professional rationality by members of the general public who now name and address their diseases and health in professional medical terms, and rely on professional advice and intervention to maintain and restore health. The flip side of this reliance on formal medical knowledge is the tendency to de-emphasize local conditions and tacit knowledge, generating in healthcare what Scott (1998: 302) has observed elsewhere: the "logic of homogenisation and virtual elimination of local knowledge." This is also reflected in priority-setting for medical technology, where medical interventions are seen as much more important determinants of health and disease than patients' life conditions, lifestyles and agency (Van der Wilt, 1995).

A crucial consequence is that modern health systems tend to intertwine public knowledge institutions, the medical profession and industry, yielding a well-oiled machine that produces a *continuous new supply of aids and appliances* for diagnosis, medicine and treatment. These factors together tend to fuel *supply-driven development*, further encouraged by the dominant policy mechanisms of "innovation support," "drug admission" and "reimbursement."

The emphasis on modernization and associate, reductionist conventional medical rationality in both clinical practice and the organization of health (research) systems has systemically embedded problem-solving paradigms that do not acknowledge the complex and interconnected nature of (problems in) health systems. In the words of Plsek and Greenhalgh (2001: 625):

> The traditional ways of "getting our heads round the problem" are no longer appropriate. Newton's "clockwork universe", in which big problems can be broken down into smaller ones, analysed, and solved by rational deduction, has strongly influenced both the practice of medicine and the leadership of organisations.... But the machine metaphor lets us down badly when no part of the equation is constant, independent, or predictable.

Complex challenges often lead to persistent problems. One set of problems concerns the perverse effects of dominant practices, which can undermine their own effectiveness. A well-known example is the overuse of antibiotics, which together with poor compliance among patients triggers resistance in microbials (Levy and Marshall, 2004). The most obvious solutions – reduced prescription and use, patient compliance with treatment regimes, and the development of new antibiotics – are difficult to implement due to the economic interests of pharmacies and the livestock industry (where antibiotics are used to promote growth), demand from patients (belief in antibiotics as silver bullets), the willingness of physicians to fulfill patient demands, difficulties in realizing compliance (lack of awareness), and lack of incentives for the pharmaceutical industry to develop new antibiotics. Below we will elaborate more on the perverse effects of dominant practices in health systems.

Non-communicable diseases

So-called non-communicable diseases (NCDs) – diseases that are non-infectious and non-transmissible among people – have entered the limelight over the past few decades. This class of afflictions comprises both chronic diseases that progress slowly and diseases that appear suddenly. Examples include diabetes, Alzheimer's, auto-immune diseases, chronic obstructive pulmonary disease, cancer, cardiovascular diseases and obesity. NCDs were designated as "one of the major challenges for sustainable development in the twenty-first century"[3] at the United Nations Rio+20 conference in 2012, and are also included in the agenda of the Sustainable Development Goals (2016). According to the WHO,[4] NCDs now account for nearly two-thirds of global mortality, and more in Europe and the USA. Figure 1.1 shows both the successes of modern health systems in combatting infectious diseases and the

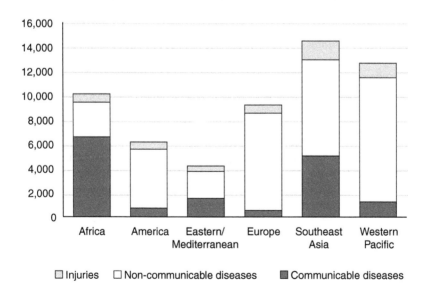

Figure 1.1 Causes of death by region: communicable diseases, non-communicable diseases and injuries[5]

increasing prevalence of NCDs. This is partly a consequence of that success and partly due to other facts, not least changing lifestyles and the structural landscape trends underlying that shift (including urbanization, individualization. and changing practices and structures in industrialized food production).

The pathology of NCDs is usually complex: in addition to (hereditary) physical defects, life conditions (toxic substances, radiation), lifestyle (poor nutrition, lack of physical activity, smoking and stress) and patient agency are mutually interacting causal factors (Balbus et al., 2013; Horton, 2013). While NCDs may be partly addressed through standard research, policy and health-care practices that focus on cure, the most effective approach is prevention by controlling risk factors in circumstances and lifestyles, and promoting patient agency. And though a wide range of prevention efforts have been tried, their success is often limited, as existing health systems are geared more toward cure than prevention.

Echoing Beck's (1992) notion of risk society, risk factors may be seen as the dark side of established practices in other domains: stress at work, toxic substances from industrial and transportation emissions in the environment, dietary patterns associated with urban lifestyles, and so on. Appeals to adapt eating, drinking and exercise habits, or to maintain lower stress levels in the workplace, may well threaten "normal" practices. As prevention efforts often reverse the relationship between health and other social realms, they violate the culturally embedded expectation that (health) professionals are responsible for ensuring health so that people can lead productive lives.

Conventional medical rationality is still far from fully grasping the complex interactions among physical disorders, life conditions and lifestyles, and patient agency. The promotion of healthy lifestyles in many countries is even at odds with acceptable relations between health professionals and their (proto-professionalized) patients. Thus the capacity of health knowledge infrastructures to develop and support measures to remedy or prevent NCDs remains limited; when innovative prevention practices emerge, their effectiveness often cannot be proven according to the structurally embedded standards of "evidence-based medicine (EBM)," upon which decisions on admission and reimbursement are usually based. EBM theoretically and methodologically reflects the assumptions of conventional medical rationality, and is thus well tailored to relatively mono-causal afflictions such as infectious diseases but a simplification at best for more complex pathologies with interacting dimensions, as in NCDs. Based on the case studies that follow, we will return to this issue in the concluding chapter of this volume.

Increasing demand for long-term care

Another problem facing health systems in advanced welfare states is the increasing demand for long-term care. This is at least as much due to the increasing prevalence of NCDs as it is to the graying of the population. As reported by the OECD (2005; see Figure 1.2), the correlation between the

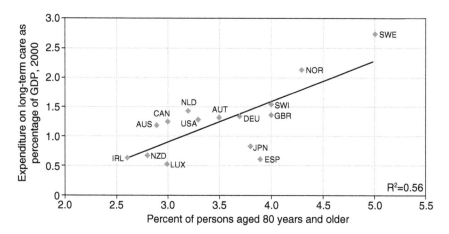

Figure 1.2 The correlation between the demand for care and aging

Source: OECD (2005: 5).

demand for care and aging is weak. In part, this is because today's comparatively healthy elderly population have fewer care needs than their predecessors (see e.g. Muszyńska and Rau, 2012). Nevertheless, demographic trends remain crucial – not only as they partially inform the demand for care, but because they reduce the share of the population that will generate income and provide (professional and informal) care to meet this demand. In the Netherlands, the old-age dependency ratio[6] is expected to rise from 20 percent in 2000 to 43 percent in 2050 (Meier and Werding, 2010). Similar patterns exist for the EU as a whole, where the old-age dependency ratio is expected to double to nearly 55 percent in 2050, in the USA (from 18 to 35 percent) and in Japan (from 35 to 70 percent).[7]

Demographic trends provide another set of challenges for modern health systems, with the growing demand for care and changing old-age dependency ratios dramatically increasing the financial burden. In virtually all OECD countries,[8] there is a gap between the demand for care and available personnel (OECD, 2011), a problem often exacerbated by cost-cutting measures and the introduction of new public management, which have undermined job satisfaction in the sector. In addition, as argued, for instance, by the Institute of Medicine (2011) and by Triantafillou et al. (2010: 22), the very notion of "being taken care of" in standardized ways decreasingly fits contemporary lifestyles shaped by individualization, cultural and economic globalization (Beck and Beck Gernsheim, 2002), and neoliberalization (Newman and Tonkens, 2011).

Here again, key features of the health system may be a part of the problem. In many welfare states, care has become highly professionalized and institutionalized, though with significant variation between countries. Expectations placed on the welfare state have grown, while individuals' and communities' sense of agency and responsibility has declined (Olson, 1994; Leichsenring et al., 2013). Paradoxically, this is accompanied by citizens rejecting patronization by the state and healthcare professionals, as well as the emergence of novel practices of (virtual) community care, informal care, new professionalism and so on.

Yet, innovative practices often remain plagued by problems rooted in health systems (Nies et al., 2013). Care often focuses on patients with NCDs; practices here thus face the same kinds of problems discussed above for NCDs. Informal caregivers in the future may also be in shorter supply due to changing old-age dependency ratios and gender and family relations (e.g. the share of broken marriages has increased). In addition, the meager social appreciation of care work that accompanies the dominance of reductionist conventional medical rationality and new public management shapes the image of informal care. Healthy citizens expect to be able to focus on their working lives and leisure. All of these factors together already imply a significant burden for informal caregivers, especially for women who provide the lion's share of informal and community care (Triantafillou et al., 2010: 55ff.).

Increasing costs

The rising cost of healthcare is the problem that has received the most political attention. The percentage of GDP spent on health increased significantly between 1980 and 2010 in nearly all EU countries (see Figure 1.3), with health spending in EU countries growing by an annual average of 4.6 percent per capita between 2000 and 2009.

Due to growing concerns over financial tenability, many reforms have focused on cost containment. In 2010, for the first time since 1975, health spending in Europe declined – by 0.6 percent per capita. This is partly due to the effect of different cost containment policies. These typically include restricting reimbursement of medical treatment (among others by stimulating the use of cheap generics over brand medication), giving room to health insurance companies to bargain with health providers for reduced prices, and providing hospitals with a limited own budget. Less common (tellingly), but recently emerging (Schippers, 2016) in, for instance, the Netherlands are possibilities to bargain (collectively) with pharmaceutical companies for price reductions. In a very different way, the financial crisis played a role in this, with significant spending reductions in countries like Ireland and Greece as extreme cases. While increasing uncertainty over the availability of future resources for healthcare may help create room for systemic change, hitherto blunt austerity motives seem to drive the process.[9]

But these successes in cost containment seem to be short-lived. Although for several decades only small steps in drug improvement were witnessed (the so-called "me-too" products), recently a new category of medicines, based on biotechnologies, are reaching the market often for unmet needs (e.g. lung cancer, cystic fibrosis and hepatitis-C). The good news is that patients are

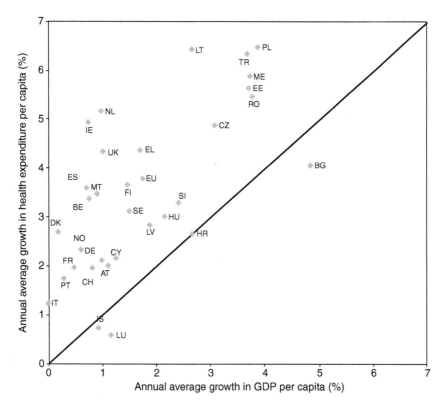

Figure 1.3 Annual average growth in health expenditure and GDP per capita, in real terms, 2000–2010 (or nearest year)

cured or live longer with improved quality of life. This comes at considerable cost, however. Using public innovation subsidies and market protection mechanisms to their advantage, pharmaceutical companies are labeling these new biologicals as personalized medicines or orphan drugs, which enables them to set so-called societally value prices,[10] The prices of these new, innovative, monopolistic personalized medicines can be extremely high, up to as much as 500,000 euros per patient per year (Godman et al., 2015). Governments around the globe thus find themselves in a continuous rat race with other stakeholders in the system in which cost containment and profit maximization continuously try to catch up with each other.

While budgetary problems continue to be a major focus of governments in welfare states, concerns about the quality, appropriateness and accessibility of health services remain as well, despite increasing investments in care, knowledge and available technology (Dirkzwager and Verhaak, 2007; Jankauskienė and Jankauskaitė, 2011). Questions arise on what kind of care one is entitled to, and what "good care" is. Should we conduct invasive medical procedures on the very elderly? Which drugs are really needed and how much are we willing to pay for them? Whose decision is this to make? Discussions over which kinds of care can be removed from reimbursement packages are now the order of the day. And despite the aim of equitable distribution of costs and benefits in health systems, less privileged socio-economic groups continue to live less in perceived good health.

Over the past decades, discontent with the functioning of health systems has led to advanced welfare states pursuing a wide range of health system reforms, defined as purposeful changes to the structure of the health system (Roberts et al., 2004; Mills and Ranson, 2012). Due to growing concerns over financial sustainability, reforms have tended to focus on finances and organizational structures (Martineau and Buchan, 2000). And reflecting the global tendency of neoliberalization, policies have emphasized reliance on the private sector and market mechanisms (also within the public sector) as the ultimate solution for challenges facing health systems (Figueras, 2003). Evidence of the effects of such reforms is scarce due to poor monitoring and evaluation, while the number of variables makes causality difficult to determine. But in most cases evidence indicates that costs have not really been tamed, quality concerns have not been solved, the poor are not benefiting, and reforms have had unintended effects such as reduced equity (see Gwatkin, 2001; Whitehead et al., 2001; Stambolovic, 2003; Pollock, 2005; WHO, 2007; De Savigny and Adam, 2009; Mills and Ranson, 2012). In addition, reforms at the system level have usually only focused on one concern (funding, quality, access, etc.).

We argue that these reforms have generally not resulted in the hoped-for changes because they were not radical enough to change the health system's underlying features: to the extent that structures were changed, this mainly involved market-conforming measures, while dominant culture (the way of thinking) has been addressed insufficiently (Essink, 2012). Underlying features include the supply-driven nature of the health system – which cannot be remedied by casting patients as consumers (knowledge asymmetry and the protoprofessionalism of patients mean that they cannot easily become critical consumers of healthcare). Casting health institutions as competing businesses is no solution either – lack of transparency on quality and price, and lack of choice in health providers and treatments mean there is often no genuine competition. The strategy of casting health insurers as "consumers" in the health system – often advocated by policy-makers as the next best route – is constrained by the profit-focused interests of health insurers. In the meantime, each stakeholder blames the others for the failure of cost containment.

Transformative experiments, usually more radical in their set-up, have also had limited success because the dominant structure and culture of the system yield inertia (Grin, 2004; Moret-Hartman et al., 2007), i.e. innovative practices cannot draw upon the incumbent regime and thus often suffer a lack of resources outside experimental settings, which inhibits scaling up (Essink, 2012: 101–122), as we will further explain in the next section.

The previous discussion has aimed to shed light on some of the key issues confronting health systems and the attempts to address them. We have argued that both the problems themselves and many of the bottlenecks encountered in trying to resolve them have systemic roots. In transition studies, these issues represent "persistent" problems.

1.3 Central notions from transition theory and system innovation studies

The persistence of problems may be understood through the notion of "co-evolution," inspired by evolutionary sociology and evolutionary economics (Perez, 1983; Callon, 1991; Nelson, 1994; Kemp et al., 2007). In transition research, co-evolution refers to, first, how individual societal subsystems (such as the health system) evolve in interaction with other societal subsystems (e.g. the food system). It also refers to the mutual shaping, as they evolve, of dominant structures and practices (Grin, 2006; Voß et al., 2006) in the dialectical sense of structuration theory (Giddens, 1984). Structures and practices co-evolve around, and are thus shaped by, the central issues of a particular historical period. If a novel issue later emerges, it is far from certain that these practices and structures are optimally suited for, or even capable of, dealing with them. In such cases, the issue will appear as a persistent problem.

A key concept in understanding both the persistence of problems and their resolution through a transition is the "multi-level perspective" (MLP), which studies transitions as the interaction of processes at three different scale levels: landscape developments (long-term, exogenous trends), a patchwork of regimes (dominant structure, culture and practice) and niche experiments (innovative practices) (see Figure 1.4). The multi-level perspective provides a descriptive ordering framework that also has explanatory value (Schot, 1998; Rip and Kemp, 1998; Geels, 2002; Van Driel and Schot, 2005; Smith et al., 2010). In a sense, it refers to wider insights from social theory (e.g. Giddens, 1984; Bourdieu, 1990) and history (e.g. Braudel, 1976) that changing practices, structural change and exogenous tendencies unfold parallel to each other and sometimes interact to produce non-incremental changes in practices and structures (Grin, 2008). Its central claim is that regime shifts occur through interlinkage and interaction among multiple developments on the three levels. More recently, scholars have found that transitions require:

- the *creation of niches*, locations that are protected from the influence of existing regimes (Hoogma, 2000; Raven, 2005).
- *strategic action* in the sense of creating linkages to overcome and, despite the existing regime and its path dependencies, connect dynamics at all three levels (Smith and Stirling, 2007; Schot and Geels, 2007; Roep et al., 2003).

Conversely, the MLP may also serve to explain the barriers encountered in experiments when these are *not* (sufficiently) linked to dynamics at the regime

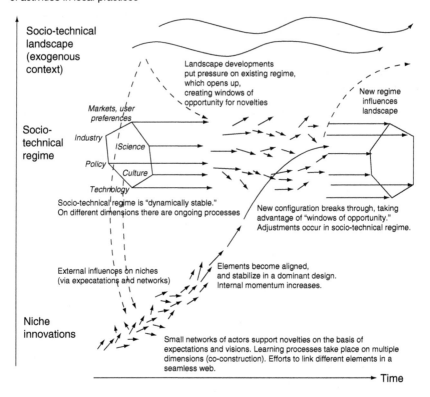

Figure 1.4 Multi-level perspective on transitions

Source: Geels and Schot (2010: 25).

and landscape levels. This was one of the key insights originally based on the MLP in one of its founding formulations (Rip and Kemp, 1998) – one which continues to inform empirical studies that relate flaws in experiments to features of the incumbent regime (Roep et al., 2003; Grin, 2004; Grin et al., 2004; Bos and Grin, 2008; Lauridsen and Jørgensen, 2010; Cohen, 2010). This latter insight also informs the book's underlying hypothesis as well as the case studies in Part II, where we analyze how barriers encountered in experiments may be used to identify problematic system features and how these are reproduced within experiments. This will help us "diagnose" contemporary health systems and to identify some of their common problems.

MLP has inspired significant empirical and conceptual research on the dynamics of transition. This has led to the identification of a variety of ideal-typical transition trajectories (Geels and Schot, 2007). In parallel, another strand of transition literature based on complex adaptive systems theory has identified similar trajectories (Rotmans and Loorbach, 2010). While it would be mistaken to use these for "blueprint planning" to realize these trajectories, they may help agents involved in transitions make sense of the situations in which they find themselves (Elzen et al., 2004; Grin, 2008). More prescriptive notions have been developed in transition studies to support the development and realization of transition strategies, including transition management, strategic niche management and dual track governance.

Although transitions can probably neither be controlled nor steered, they can be influenced in their direction and speed (Rotmans, 2005). "Transition management" addresses complex societal problems through the guiding vision of sustainable development and joint learning among multiple stakeholders, comprising a cyclical process of development at different levels and in different domains. A central instrument of transition management is the "transition arena": an experimental setting at the niche level where interested actors develop new insights through the processes of social learning. This process is understood as an iterative process of four steps, comprising (1) joint definitions of problems, (2) shared visioning and joint action planning, (3) design and implementation of various transition experiments, and (4) monitoring and evaluating the transition process, and learning lessons.

In "strategic niche management" (SNM), radical socio-technical changes are understood as processes promoted within niches which gradually develop into wider changes including regime transformation. SNM, an offspring from the literature on constructive technology assessment (Rip and Schot, 1996), is both a research model and a governance approach; we discuss it in its latter capacity. Raven (2005: 51), on the basis of an excellent overview of the SNM literature, argues that:

> [P]revious SNM work has focused too much on internal niche dynamics, *i.e.* how voicing and shaping of expectations, networks dynamics and learning processes account for niche development ... [with regimes assumed stable, and showed] too little interest in niche–regime interaction.

Raven therefore proposes to extend SNM with the multi-level perspective to better understand regime transformation. It is no longer assumed that an otherwise stable regime will change through processes of niche development, niche accumulation and so on; for this, niche experiments must be connected to regime instabilities and other regime dynamics, as well as to landscape trends. The processes that take place at the niche level are described as strategic niche management (Geels, 2005; Hoogma et al., 2002; Kemp et al., 1998). Strategic niche management may be used both as a research model and a policy tool (Raven, 2005). Here again, recent work has shown that attention to politics is crucial.

In these prescriptive notions, *learning* is crucial in promoting "reframing," i.e. developing novel, shared perceptions of problems and innovative directions for sustainable solutions (see e.g. Roep et al., 2003; Grin et al., 2004; Loeber, 2004; Raven, 2005). Such learning does not take place detached from practice, but is intertwined with actors' actions and interactions (Schön, 1983; Grin and Van de Graaf, 1996; Broerse and Bunders, 2000; Loeber, 2004; Grin and Loeber, 2007). To develop this actor perspective, Grin (2010: 233) turns to the notion of "reflexive monitoring."

> In reflexive monitoring, agents consciously reflect on the intended and unintended consequences of their own actions. They do so in relation to the structural conditions in which they find themselves, taking into account the potential of change in structural context, both through their conduct and through exogenous trends. Reflexive monitoring therefore is what we consider the heart of governance efforts of *Re*-structuration.

Thus innovation becomes eventually consolidated in societal practices. In most cases this also assumes changes in underlying concepts, or second order learning (Loeber et al., 2007).

A more recent strand of work on transitions and system innovation, under the heading of "reflexive governance" (Grin et al., 2004; Voß et al., 2006; Hendriks and Grin, 2007; Avelino et al., forthcoming), seeks to further understand such politics.

Reflexive governance here refers to forms of governance in which the structural embedment of both governance practices and the practices being governed become the object of scrutiny. One key issue pertains to processes of "power," which have only recently received serious attention in transition studies (Avelino and Rotmans, 2009; Grin, 2010). A key insight is that agents, in exercising power, draw upon structure. As transitions include structural transformation, transition dynamic and powering should be understood as essentially intertwined. In the worst case scenario, actors may successfully draw upon incumbent structure to resist a transition, or novel practices may experience lack of support from incumbent structures. The challenge for agents engaged in a transition then becomes to bring about a constructive, iterative interaction between the innovative practices they are engaged in and transforming structures. Hoffman (2013; Hoffman and Loeber, 2016) have developed a relational perspective on powering, depicting the work involved as creatively connecting practices to each other and their structural context.

Another key question of politics concerns the relation between transitions and deep socio-material structures. Transitions are seen as coherent changes of practices and the (discursive, institutional and material) structures in which they are embedded; or, in somewhat different words, a transition is the reorientation of the co-evolution of practices and their structural embedment. What counts as structure here is contingent – in the same sense as Giddens' understanding of a system as the whole of (a set of) practices and the structural elements they draw upon, thus reproducing or transforming them. It is a key debate within social science to what extent it is important to see deeper (especially material) structures as a key determinant of practices and the structural elements upon which they draw (Marsh, 2010).

In this volume, we focus on the more tangible influence of discourses, institutions and material infrastructures and objects. The way in which these structural elements of health systems have been shaped by underlying structures is largely left out of consideration, although trends at the "landscape" level, such as globalization or individualization, may be justifiably seen as changes in such structures. We believe, however, that the influence of deeper structures is mediated by these more intermediate structures of both the health system and "adjacent" systems (e.g. social security, food policy or welfare), and also that this works bidirectionally, i.e. that a transition in, for example, the health system may to some extent co-shape adjacent systems and thus the ways in which deeper structures affect society as well (see also Avelino et al., 2016).

1.4 Sustainable health systems

We propose the notion of sustainable healthcare as a second, more normative, sensitizing framework. Calls for equitable reform show that not only the financial sustainability of health systems but also other values are at stake (Gwatkin, 2001). Toebes (1999) has identified four values most often mentioned in international declarations on health: affordability, accessibility, acceptability and quality of healthcare. Essink et al. (2010) argue that balancing these core values in health system reform – with its one-sided focus on finances – is necessary to address problems resulting from this partial "tinkering." Frenk (1992), Berman (1995) and Sowada (2003) have likewise argued that reforms should be based on a vision of the health sector as a whole, a process that entails trade-offs and the balancing of objectives.

A (long-term) vision or normative orientation toward change is considered a basic requirement in transition theory (Rotmans et al., 2001). A vision provides a clear direction for change and aligns the different actors. In transition theory, sustainable development is a long-term, multi-level and multi-actor process (Loorbach, 2007). According to Loorbach (2007: 23):

> [T]he call for sustainable development from a transitions perspective is a plea to transform societal systems that struggle with complex and persistent problems structurally. Since regular and traditional solutions result in optimization of existing structures, fundamental and innovative approaches are needed. A link between transitions and sustainable development therefore speaks for itself.

Attempts to institutionalize sustainable development in other policy domains such as energy, the environment and agriculture have nevertheless revealed the difficulties of balancing conflicting values and interests. In practice, furthering sustainable development – achieving a better balance between people, planet and profit – is a learning process that involves iterative cycles of actions for change. Sustainable development is thus an open-ended orientation toward change (Grin et al., 2010) that lends itself to deliberative, participatory governance (Grin, 2006). As a concept informing the management of transitions in health systems, we focus on the idea of "unbalanced" systems where core values need to be rethought and balanced in a guiding vision.

The concept of sustainable development has rarely featured in health system reform. Although pleas for balancing core values are found throughout the literature, Essink et al. (2010) found only one instance of health system reform explicitly guided by the concept of sustainability. Their study also traced the concept's emergence to the advent of the "health field" approach coined by Lalonde (1974), which emphasized people's responsibility for their own health, the environment's impact on health and the importance of healthy communities. All this makes the step toward sustainability a logical one. Although there is as yet no evidence that sustainable development is a fruitful vision to guide health system reform, it is worth exploring further.

1.5 Central aims, research questions and outline of the book

This book examines the hypothesis that the current, complex problems facing our health systems are rooted in their core features. This transition studies perspective is to help us to (1) better understand the embedded features in the foundations of our health systems that underlie complex problems, and (2) find ways to innovate health systems to more sustainably address these problems. The following research questions are central:

- How did system innovations and transitions emerge in the health domain in the past, and how do the insights presented here shed light on the origin of persistent problems currently encountered?
- What visions of sustainable healthcare are, implicitly or explicitly, articulated in the contemporary innovations discussed in this book?
- What may we learn from the successes and, especially, failures of these contemporary innovations in the nature of these problems and the features in health systems on which the development of sustainable healthcare critically depends?
- What do the answers to these questions, as well as earlier insights from transition studies, suggest about strategies for remedying persistent problems through structural change in health systems?

Part I presents historical studies on health system changes from a system innovation and transition perspective. In Chapter 2, Eric Berkers begins with a discussion of contemporary changes in health systems and their persistent problems before turning to the Dutch case where a regime centered on evidence, technology, cure and the hospital has come under increasing pressure since the 1970s. Challenges to affordability and the quality and acceptability of care are illustrated through developments in mental healthcare, gynecology, pharmaceutical care, and a range of legal and financial instruments to control the supply side of the health system. The Dutch case also shows how the dominant health regime has been in a constant process of reconfiguration, trying to meet pressures from the landscape as well as its own negative side-effects. In Chapter 3, Roel van Raak and Fjalar de Haan examine the historical roots of three main features of the modern Dutch health system: its emphasis on curative measures, professionalization and specialization, and its focus on the patient's body and physical health. These foundational features have created a supply-dominated system in which patients are (or at least feel like) the objects of treatment.

Part II examines recent innovative practices in which innovations were implemented at the niche level of the health system. In Chapter 4, Tjerk Jan Schuitmaker and Erica ter Haar-van Twillert analyze the Dutch health system by focusing on its main problem-producing and reproducing features, such as standardization, protoprofessionalization, specialization and evidence-based medicine. These features, however, are precisely the strongholds of the current system, which bias certain solution pathways. The chapter focuses on two innovative practices that have aimed to reduce costs and increase the quality of care: one for patients with medically unexplained physical symptoms (MUPS), another for providing psychotherapy through the internet.

In Chapter 5, Lenneke Vaandrager and co-authors examine the reorientation of health promotion in the workplace. Traditionally, health and work are seen as functionally differentiated domains. To the extent that health is an issue in the work domain, it is a matter of occupational health services and prevention workers, while themes like employability, development and vitality, stemming from human resource management, are not included. Recent strategies, which emphasize the participation and responsibility of employees, have shifted their focus from individuals to organizations, from reducing costs associated with risk factors to investment in skills and empowerment, and from disease to health. This chapter analyzes practices that seek to bridge the boundary between occupational health and human resource management from the perspective of salutogenesis, whereby it is not the sources of disease that serve as a point of departure (as in the pathogenesis model) but those of health. The solutogenic model thus focuses on factors that support human health and well-being, rather than on factors that cause disease; it specifically addresses the relationship between health, stress and coping. Three case studies are used as an illustration. Salutogenesis may be seen as one interesting elaboration of sustainable healthcare. Unsurprisingly, like the innovations in other chapters, workplace health promotion also faces structurally embedded resistance and inertia.

In Chapter 6, Francisco Ródenas and Jorge Garcés present an innovative social and healthcare model – the so-called "Sustainable Socio-Health Model"

– that responds to three problems commonly experienced by (especially Southern) European welfare states: the rise in demand for services, the increasing dependency of the growing aging population on others and the crisis of informal support. Achieving social sustainability entails the reformulation of regulatory, care, economic, administrative, cultural and normative frameworks so that society can respond to the needs of long-term care without compromising the welfare of future generations. The chapter describes how the new model for long-term care was implemented in a Spanish pilot project and discusses its achievements and shortcomings as a transition experiment.

In Chapter 7, Suzanne Van den Bosch and Jord Neuteboom assess the Dutch Transition Program in Long-term Care, initiated in 2006 by the Ministry of Health, Welfare and Sports and care sector organizations to change how long-term care is provided in the Netherlands. Focusing on transition management, the program involves innovative experiments centered on end users and a commitment to learning for the entire care sector. The authors describe and analyze the set-up of the program, its main instruments and initial findings.

In Chapter 8, Erica ter Haar-van Twillert and Suzanne Van den Bosch examine two projects in the Transition Program in Long-term Care in greater detail. The first, "ACT-Youth Rotterdam," targets youths with complex social and psychiatric problems, which cannot be solved by existing healthcare institutions. The second, a pilot program on "video care for the elderly and chronically ill," involves ten care institutes. The chapter compares these two projects – their approaches, their relationship with the broader Transition Program, the resistance and barriers they encountered and the strategies pursued to overcome them. This yields insight into the structural factors that tend to reproduce themselves in pilot projects, the relationship between healthcare provision and patient agency, and the difficulties of determining what constitutes adequate evidence as a basis for decision-making.

In Chapter 9, David Clements and Dirk Essink show that problems in the Canadian health system – rising costs, dramatic variations in the quantity and quality of services received by patients, the supply of healthcare professionals, and the realization that increasing supply does not guarantee better access – remain largely unaffected by recent experiments involving financial incentives and local collaborations. Many Canadians have thus concluded that the health system itself is unsustainable. Alongside the overview of persistent problems in Canadian healthcare and attempts to address them, the authors assess the government's Executive Training for Research Application (EXTRA) program, which may be seen as a Transition Program "avant la letter." The EXTRA program aims to make the Canadian health system more sustainable by developing the competencies of selected health professionals to apply, contextualize and generate knowledge (or evidence) and to collaborate across healthcare professions, both through training and intervention projects. This, it is argued, will foster a culture of "evidence-informed decision-making" (EIDM) that will improve health system performance. Analyzing the experience of the EXTRA program in implementing the concept of IEDM, the authors derive lessons regarding the management of system innovation and vice versa, with a specific focus on whether and how to train and support change agents.

In Chapter 10, Janneke Elbersc and co-authors focus on the Dutch health *research* system. Decision-making in health research is traditionally the domain of a small group of scientists while the role of consumers (i.e. patients) is restricted to being the objects of study and the ultimate beneficiaries. It appears that outcomes commonly measured to determine the effectiveness of new products do not always (fully) reflect the needs of patients. Like the health system in general, the health research system is supply-driven, biasing the kinds of knowledge it produces. Interdisciplinary concerns (such as co-morbidity) and less sexy low-tech issues (such as ingrown toenails) are rarely addressed. The chapter analyzes processes of change towards a more "needs-oriented health research system" by discussing several experiments regarding the involvement of patients in decision-making processes on health research from a multi-level perspective, discussing trends at the landscape level, niche experiments and resistance from the regime. The chapter also discusses systemic instruments that may be used to overcome barriers.

In Part III, Chapter 11 synthesizes the findings of Parts I and II, analyzing the theoretical and methodical lessons for transitions and system innovation, as well as the merits and limits of strategies pursued to date. It discusses how experiments may be set up more effectively, as well as how learning in and from practice can be better organized.

Notes

1 Ottawa Charter for Health Promotion, First International Conference on Health Promotion, November 21, 1986 – WHO/HPR/HEP/95.1, page 1. Available at www.naspa.org/2012_Chicago_Hdts_1(1).pdf.

2 See e.g. Elzen et al. 2004; Geels 2005; the journal *Environmental Innovation and Sustainability Transitions*, and special issues of major international journals in various disciplines: Timmermans et al. (2014); Geels et al. (2008); Voß et al. (2009); Berkhout et al. (2009); Smith et al. (2010). Earlier volumes in this Routledge Sustainability Transitions series present an overview of theoretical achievements (Grin et al., 2010) as well as empirical findings in the domains of mobility (Geels et al., 2012), energy (Verbong and Loorbach, 2012) and food (Spaargaren et al., 2012).

3 *The Future We Want*. New York: United Nations (2012).

4 Available at www.who.int/gho/ncd/mortality_morbidity/ncd_total_text/en/index.html.

5 Based on "Cause-specific Mortality, 2008: WHO Sub-regions by Country." Available at http://apps.who.int/gho/data/node.main.888?lang=en.

6 Old-age dependency ratio: people aged above 65 compared to those aged 15 to 64.

7 "Old Age Dependency Ratios," *The Economist*, May 9, 2009.

8 OECD stands for Organization for Economic Co-operation and Development. OECD has 34 member countries each of them may be characterized as a welfare state; most are European countries but Australia, Canada, Chile, Japan, Mexico, New Zealand and USA are also members.

9 Available at www.euro.who.int/__data/assets/pdf_file/0005/162959/Eurohealth_Vol-18_No-1_web.pdf.

10 Prices may be set on the basis of costs to develop and produce a drug (including R&D costs, developments that fail, etc.), on the basis of the added value of the drug in the treatment of patients, or on the basis of the estimation of what a society is willing to pay.

Part I

Historical studies on health system changes

2 Contested health system, 1970 to the present

Eric Berkers

2.1 A regime under pressure

Medicalization of society: shifting connotations from Erasmus to Illich

"There is literally no part of life, that can be managed without help from medicine" wrote Desiderius Erasmus in the early sixteenth century (Erasmus, 1518). To him this meant an active policy by rulers to secure the physical well-being of citizens. Gyms, public baths, legal instructions for building homes, dredging of swamps, and control over food and drinks had all to be taken care of by the legislators in the interest of healthy, powerful and "proportionally developed" citizens. Almost at the same time Thomas More published his ideas of a modern health system. In his *Utopia*, well-equipped hospitals ("they may pass for little towns"), skilled physicians and dedicated nurses take care of the sick in such a way "so there is scarce one in a whole town that, if he should fall ill, would not choose rather to go thither than lie sick at home" (More, 1516). A century later, Francis Bacon, who is often regarded as a founding father of modern medicine, expressed his vision on how society should deal with illness and people who suffer from it (Bacon, 1626). The views of these three leading philosophers suggest a strong discontent with how things were organized in their own times, or, rather, with how they were not organized at all.

The work of the twentieth-century priest-philosopher Ivan Illich is also marked by broad social criticism, as well as a focus on the way in which society deals with illness and patients. In his *Medical Nemesis* (1976), Illich gave a whole different meaning to Erasmus' "medicalization" of life, claiming that all social relationships were influenced by a dependency on professional healthcare. In the view of Illich, this was an undesirable situation and he therefore saw no reason to praise modern medicine. On the contrary, the medical apparatus should be seen as dangerous, as it was gradually turning into a major threat to health itself: "In welfare states the increase of medicine has reached sickening dimensions" (Illich, 1975). In an immediate sense, an increasing number of people became ill because of bad, ineffective, unsafe and even toxic treatments (clinical iatrogenesis). Furthermore, life in general grew increasingly medicalized, as all kinds of "problems" of modern individuals were subjected to medical intervention. In a way, Illich argued, diseases were created, and the pharmaceutical industry and physicians were the only ones to benefit (social iatrogenesis). To this he added the loss of ability of modern man to deal with events such as death, pain and illness in a non-medicalized way (cultural iatrogenesis). This way, society created the new priests of a monolithic world religion: medical professionals (Illich, 1975; Smith, 2003).

If discontent with contemporary healthcare gave rise to medical utopias during the Renaissance, it led to harsh criticism around 1970. There the similarities seem to end. After all, by 1970 much had been accomplished in healthcare that had been desired for centuries. Determinants for health had radically improved. The increase of the average life expectancy at birth had doubled since the Renaissance. Perinatal and maternal mortality, for a long time epidemic, had become an exception, and deadly infectious and parasitic diseases like tuberculosis and typhoid were disappearing rapidly in the Western world. Furthermore, this decrease of lethal parasitic and infectious diseases allowed Western medicine to focus on new areas during the twentieth century. New challenges were taken up successfully, leading to numerous breakthroughs in medicine and a formerly unknown growth of the medical domain, in particular in the years between 1940 and 1970 (Le Fanu, 2000). At the same time the modern medical infrastructure became accessible to an ever-larger segment of the population thanks to new legislation. Important for the Netherlands was the *Ziekenfondsbesluit* of 1941, a compulsory healthcare insurance measure for workers and those with little financial means.

In other words, the scientific understanding of the body as rooted in the Renaissance, in combination with the emergence of socially responsible governments in the nineteenth century, culminated in hitherto unknown levels of health and healthcare in the twentieth century. "They who die young," as some concluded in the early 1970s, "are most of all victims of accidents, violence and suicide" (Illich, 1975; Wolleswinkel-Van den Bosch, 1998). As James le Fanu (2000), a British medical publicist and medical doctor, put it:

> The history of medicine in the fifty years since the end of the Second World War ranks as one of the most impressive epochs of human achievement ... developments, have been of immeasurable benefit, freeing people from the fear of illness and untimely death, and significantly ameliorating the chronic disabilities of ageing.

Which features of the modern health system, including its assumed success, in fact prompted the severe criticism of Illich and others in the early 1970s?

A regime centered around evidence, technology, cure and the hospital

In the above-mentioned medical utopias from the Renaissance, medical science, healthcare devices and technology, and the hospital served as prominent elements. They were all emphasized in a short documentary film showing "a day in the life" of Sheffield Royal Hospital in 1932,[1] and which added one more element: a focus on cure. While during the Renaissance and long afterwards a primary goal of medicine was to take good care of patients, by the 1930s hospitals had turned into institutes that were chiefly geared to curing the sick. Next to showing dedicated nurses – some of them involved in training their younger colleagues – and the almost hotel-like facilities for patients, including copious meals and hygienic laundry services, the movie highlights the curative capabilities of the specialists and their modern technological devices.

Clearly, this film celebrates the glory of a recently established, modern medical regime. Since the second half of the nineteenth century, things had changed at the landscape level. Urbanization, industrialization, new ways of transport and workers' emancipation had put pressure on the accessibility of the medical system. In the film we see people from all ranks and files – the old, the young, the well-dressed and wealthy citizens, as well as workers suffering from workplace-related injuries – attend the hospital to be treated. Furthermore, the film both implicitly and explicitly shows that there was a decline of many epidemic diseases, for social-economic reasons, while it underscores the role at the time of new basic-technologies like "Roentgen" and electricity, and the new significance of a focus on curing patients. The importance of the hospital laboratory is emphasized as well, as is true of new ways of diagnosis and therapy, sometimes in an experimental setting. Finally, it highlights the scientific training of the specialized physicians as a success factor of modern healthcare.

Technology plays an important role in the movie. This is hardly surprising, because it was a "resource" for professionalizing and specializing medicine (Stanton, 1999). In 1949 its importance in the Netherlands was noticed. Technology "created the possibility to record what long was un-recordable … gave chances to determine what seemed un-determinable; [made] accessible [those] parts of the body that were presumed un-accessible during life" (Reiser, 1984; Ten Doesschate, 1949).

In essence, the documentary thematized that the modern hospital configuration, along with technology, had entered the medical domain. Such hospitals soon became the geographical locus of medical care and cure, the place where agents of healthcare, patients and technology met. Medical technology centralized healthcare, and specialization allowed for routine, standardized procedures and a continuous monitoring of patients (Howell, 1995; Stanton, 1999). In hospitals, "separate medical interventions of diverse people" were linked through medical records (Reiser, 1984). In particular the close interconnection between technology, the hospital and medical records would contribute to a radically modernized medical practice after World War Two.

In the Netherlands, the number of hospital beds almost quadrupled between 1920 and 1970, a period in which the population almost doubled. Although the number of general practitioners "only" doubled in this period, thus keeping pace with the population's growth, the number of medical specialists saw a six-fold increase (CBS, n.d.). This transition toward centralization, specialization and use of technology in medicine was also fed by "the tendency to examine many patients in an economical Taylor-way system," as had already been observed in 1949 (Ten Doesschate, 1949).

According to the above-mentioned optimistic film, cure is a matter of science, technology and time. As the Renaissance medical utopia became fully realized in the first half of the twentieth century – including school doctors, hygienic education, water and sewer systems, preventive screening and so on – scientific and technological developments and their protagonists started to promise more: the elimination of many illnesses and a spectacular rise of life expectancy. With it, a rational-reductionist view became dominant in the health system, meaning that *illness* and the *doctor* and his tools (science and technology) became the central elements.

The various Western medical "utopias" had a considerable degree of similarity in their outcome: cure-oriented, driven by specialists, knowledge and technology, and with a strong emphasis on the hospital as the place of medical action. This foundation of the Western health system became contested in the 1970s.

The 1970s as turning point

In 1978 the World Health Organization (WHO) spread an alarming message, claiming that:

> [M]ost conventional healthcare systems are becoming *increasingly complex* and have *doubtful social relevance*. They have been *distorted by dictates of medical technology* and by *misguided efforts of a medical industry* providing medical consumer goods to society. Even some of the most affluent countries have come to realize the *disparity between the high care costs and low health benefits* to these systems.
>
> (WHO, 1978: 38, emphasis added)

During that same year, Colin Dollery, Professor of Clinical Pharmacology, published a book in which he also expressed concerns about the state of the health system. It was called *The End of an Age of Optimism*. Furthermore, it seemed that by the late 1970s medical students and young doctors were less interested in doing medical research than in the 1960s, as was observed by the president of the Association of American Physicians in 1979 (Wyngaarden, 1979). As was noted in *Nature*, dramatically decreasing average annual introductions of "new chemical entities" in, for example, drugs in the 1970s (dropping from 70 in the 1960s to 20) was another instance of the writing on the wall. Modern healthcare seemed to lose much of its prestige and its luster. Perhaps the booming 1950s and 1960s did not mark the start of a bright future for modern medicine, but rather its peak (Steward and Wibberley, 1980; Le Fanu, 2000). To cite Le Fanu (2000) once more:

> [J]ust as medicine's dramatic upward spiral started quite suddenly after the war, it was, by the close of the 1970s, almost equally suddenly coming to an end.… The relentless rise of the post-war years was coming to an end.

Prominent actors *within* the modern healthcare regime focused in their observations on innovativeness and measurable success of the regime. This self-reflection, introspection or even a professional identity crisis may be interpreted as a reaction to *external* socio-economic and cultural developments at the landscape level, which put pressure on many socio-technical regimes at the time. The healthcare regime was no exception.

In Dutch society, a redefinition of long-lasting socio-cultural values was at stake, due to processes of secularization, individualization and emancipation. In the Netherlands, the process of *ontzuiling*, or "de-pillarization," implied that the political representatives of large segments of the population, divided along beliefs and ideologies, lost grip on their parties as well as on political influence, also when it came to healthcare policies. Second, it became painfully clear that global economic developments encroached deeply into the domestic policy domain and in the achievements of the Western welfare states. And although the Dutch national government since the 1960s could draw a large income from its natural gas, which enabled many investments, "limits to growth" became a political fact. In the 1960s and 1970s fundamental questions were raised in the Western world. With regard to healthcare, it was discussed whether it was all really progress that was being paid for. Actors from outside the regime, such as politicians, philosophers, social and behavioral scientists, and empowered consumers/patients, began to question the dominant modern healthcare regime. To what extent was the above-mentioned "progress" a result of the health system as it functioned in the West? Was this system as desirable as some results seemed to prove? Was the remedy, including some of its side-effects (such as the high cost, society's medicalization, the huge power allotted to medical specialists) not worse than the disease?

Framed in the specific core values of good healthcare (see this volume's Introduction), the quality of modern healthcare was seen as very overrated. Furthermore, a growing number of critics believed that the modern health system was no longer acceptable. To complicate matters, the economic downturn of the early 1970s soon fueled concerns about the affordability and accessibility of the system.

In sections 2.2 and 2.3 below I will look more closely into the nature of the criticism of the Dutch healthcare regime as put forward from the 1970s onward. In what ways and to what extent were its targets rooted in the regime? Because healthcare is a very broad domain, I will explore this question by discussing several telling examples of the types of criticism mentioned above.

2.2 Quality and acceptability under pressure

Mental healthcare

In the early 1960s, mental healthcare was the first medical domain that met with fundamental criticism on an international basis. This domain had entered the modern health system, with a focus on cure and technology, relatively late. Traditionally, mentally ill persons were hidden from society in asylums, where they received care from nurses. As a consequence of medical successes in finding causes and treatment for the mentally disabled, however, this nursing regime was challenged by a redefinition of mental deficiency in the 1950s and 1960s. Mentally deficient individuals began to be perceived as "legitimate, treatable, and interesting to medicine" and even as "preeminently a subject for experts" (Tonkens, 1999). Rather than just providing care to mental patients, it was increasingly common to pursue practices aimed at testing them and "improving" their condition, if not curing them. New professionals entered the institutions, such as behavioral scientists. Policymakers in fact supported this "medicalization" of the institutions. In the Netherlands, for example, only institutions employing medical officers were granted an in-service education facility (Tonkens, 1999).

The redefinition of mental illness as a treatable disorder also had implications for "patients" and their relatives. For one thing, it prompted a gradual disappearance of shame and blame about retardation, degeneration, social backwardness and so on. Moreover, patients and their relatives increasingly evolved into important actors in the arena of mental healthcare. The same was true of behavioral scientists, who slowly started to "undermine the executive and steering position of the medical professionals" (Tonkens, 1999).

Together with this emphasis on "improving" patients' condition, there was mounting criticism of the new regime's cultures and practices, both from within the mental health domain and from outside of it. In 1961, for instance, the Hungarian psychiatrist Thomas Szasz wrote that the concept of "mental illness" was an inadequate metaphor, and that deviant behavior of psychiatric "patients" had a sociological basis rather than a medical one. He even compared modern society's eagerness to fight deviant behavior with the former Spanish Inquisition (Szasz, 1961; Mol and Van Lieshout, 1989). Canadian sociologist Erving Goffmann, who conducted participatory research in a mental institution in Washington, concluded that patients were "cured" in the sense that they were adjusted to their particular role within the psychiatric hospital (they were "hospitalized"), but they were not cured in a way that allowed them to live on their own in society again, outside the confines of the mental institution. In his view, psychiatric treatment was all but effective (Goffmann, 1961; Mol and Van Lieshout, 1989).

In 1967, British psychiatrist David Cooper introduced "anti-psychiatry" as a critique of the cure-oriented psychiatric regime. The ensuing anti-psychiatry movement fought against "authoritarian and patronizing power relationships in intramural psychiatry, against psycho-pharmaceuticals and electroshocks and against psychiatric hospitals as such" (Blok 2004). Cooper's book was published in Dutch in 1968. One year later, Ronald David Laing, Cooper's colleague and forerunner in anti-psychiatry, published *The Divided Self*, which became a bestseller. In the Netherlands, their sales figures were even outnumbered by a study entitled *Wie is van hout?* (Who is made of wood?, 1971), published by the Dutch critical psychiatrist Jan Foudraine (Blok, 2004). Aside from psychiatrists voicing criticism of dominant psychiatry, others have tried (and still try) to change the image and position of psychiatric patients in society. Since the late 1960s, for example, the Pandora Foundation has sought to re-educate the Dutch in this respect by relying on new marketing techniques and mass media. This organization initiated campaigns aimed at young people in particular, using slogans like: "Why 'mad'? Because he's different? So what!" and "Ever met a normal human being ... and did you like it?" It also organized excursions to psychiatric clinics and produced and distributed information films. Another Pandora project centered on making the formerly "hidden" psychiatric institutions literally more visible in society by designing and putting up public signposts – in collaboration with the official Dutch automobile association – in order to give directions to where these facilities were located. This was not just a service to visitors; it was also meant to increase the social recognition and acceptance of psychiatric patients.[2]

In the early 1970s, against the backdrop of mounting international pressure on modern mental healthcare, an experiment was conducted in the Netherlands that would become an icon of resistance against the dominant mental healthcare regime: the so-called "Dennendal case" (Tonkens, 1999). Essentially, it involved a dispute about "illness" and "health" and the position of the mentally handicapped in society and medicine. This case will be discussed in more detail below.

Dennendal: a Dutch niche experiment

In 1969, Carel Muller was appointed psychological director of Dennendal. His task was to modernize this institution for the mentally handicapped. At that point, Dennendal was a fairly old-fashioned facility. It employed only a few doctors and few patients were diagnosed; moreover, there was no medical director, the buildings were dilapidated, there was no research facility, and the focus was predominantly on nursing (Tonkens, 1999).

In the beginning, Muller lived up to expectations by replacing the prevalent nursing regime at Dennendal by a regime of experts, who aimed for a better understanding of the patients' condition by doing tests and experiments

(Tonkens, 1999). After a year or so, however, Muller began to move away from this expert regime, judging many tests and experiments to be more harmful to patients than good. In hiring new employees, Muller started to attach more importance to their personality and view of society than to specific expert qualities. Gradually, a new vision on patients and a new kind of regime emerged at Dennendal. Tonkens calls it the "self-development-regime," based on beliefs about individual development and relations between society and the individual that evolved after World War Two. This regime may be characterized as anti-expert, anti-authoritarian, informal as regards relations between patients and employees, and as having an entirely different perspective on the use of medication and means of coercion, such as solitary confinement. In essence, it involved a radically different perception of the mentally disabled. In the self-development regime, they were not seen as either ill or incapable of functioning in society, and therefore they should not be put away in clinics. It was even in the interest of society at large to intermingle with them.

At Dennendal, fixed visiting hours were abolished while ties with the patients' family were strengthened. These new ideas about (institutions for) the mentally disabled and their position and role in society was articulated in documents (De Rooy and Steers, 1971). But, so Muller reasoned, they should also be reflected in the architecture of the housing at Dennendal. He asked an architect and a landscaper to develop a new setting based on the notion that staff and patients live together in a community, characterized by small-scale integration, diversity, and a homely and cozy atmosphere.

Of course, the new ideas about how to deal with the mentally disabled and how to run an institution (in a less directive and more democratic manner, promoting self-development for employees, etc.) deeply influenced not only the patients, but also the employees and the organizational structure. The latter actually carried the seed for the downfall of the Dennendal experiment. Alongside the gradual replacement of the nursing regime (with small elements of an expert regime) by the self-development regime, the organizational structures linked to these regimes had to be dismantled and developed, respectively. As a result, responsibilities and decision-making changed, as did internal power relations. A shift in power from nursing to psychology and pedagogy took place. This in turn gave rise to forms of resistance and newly emerging problems, such as a lack of order and hygiene and patients' neglect. The self-development of employees, including their use of soft drugs, would often overshadow the patients' self-development, implying the disappearance of such conventional key features of nursing as self-sacrifice and a service-minded attitude.

To settle the disputes that had emerged, the Public Health Inspectorate was asked to examine the patients' situation at Dennendal. However, before the inspector reported his moderate findings, having observed no danger for patients nor any cases of medical neglect, *De Telegraaf*, a nationwide right-wing newspaper, published an article about abuses at Dennendal. Based on a story of a critical outsider, the newspaper created a picture of Dennendal as a disorganized free state ruled by long-haired hippies who were constantly on drugs. Within such libertine chaos it was no wonder that an epileptic mentally handicapped patient had drowned in the bath. Suddenly Dennendal was hot news, used by the establishment as a reprehensible example of what an alternative society would look like.

After investigations, Muller and others were suspended by the Board, but this suspension was withdrawn following widespread protest. Instead, the Board of Directors resigned. In their fight against the old regime, the reformers were supported by relatively new actors in the arena, such as nationwide organizations of psychologists and behavioral scientists, as well as by the parents' association of Dennendal.

This first victory of the reformers at Dennendal was followed by a dramatic defeat some years later, which put an end to the experiments. In January 1974, internal conflicts led to a schism. Some segments within Dennendal wanted to change the course, break away from the coordinating foundation and operate autonomously, under the direction of Carel Muller. The self-development regime, no longer the underdog, proved to come with hard-to-resolve problems and dilemmas. This new conflict was mainly about how to deal with them *within the regime* and was not a clash *between two regimes* (Tonkens, 1999). The strongly polarized conflict ended in a forced evacuation of the pavilions that were occupied by the "New-Dennendalians" on July 3 1974. Because Dennendal, as in 1971, was made into a symbol of a struggle between old-fashioned autocratic regents versus the anti-establishment, and because the eviction took place with heavy equipment (including a water cannon, a number of police assault vans and dozens of uniformed police officers), it received wide media coverage. The left-wing government led by Prime Minister Joop den Uyl, which had ordered the evacuation (or "deportation," as it was called by the "New Dennendalians") saw it as a defeat indeed. But it had no other choice, as Den Uyl admitted on the evening news.

Beyond Dennendal

The end of Dennendal was not the end of alternative mental healthcare. Although Dennendal was definitely a very famous and controversial case, it was suddenly not the only institution where experiments were carried out. Around 1970, for example, the men's ward of a psychiatric hospital in Deventer was transformed into a therapeutic community. Here, resistance against the "medical model" led to a central role for relation-, group- and family therapies, and hence for psychologists, nurses and group leaders, rather than psychiatrists. Among psychiatric institutions that in the 1970s embraced the ideas of Laing and Foudraine were those in Heiloo, Bennebroek and "De Hobbitstee" in Leiden (opened in 1978) (Blok, 2004). If there were many differences between these and other experimental alternatives in mental healthcare in the 1970s (Blok, 2004), the similarities were perhaps more strik-ing: a rejection of a medical pathologic approach toward psycho-social dis-orders; a rejection of hospitalization in psychiatric institutions; an emphasis on the control function of psychiatry in society, labeling people who showed maladjusted behavior as "ill" and locking them away in institutions; and an emphasis on positive elements of a psychosis (Trimbos, 1975).

A powerful symbol for critical psychiatry in its struggle against the dominant medical model was the use of electroconvulsive therapy (ECT). This treatment, by which electrical shocks are conducted through the head of a patient to trigger an epileptic response, was introduced in the late 1930s for schizophrenia in particular. It showed some remarkable results and became widespread in the 1940s and 1950s, when it was used to treat several mental disorders. It was introduced in the Netherlands in 1939 (Blok, 2004). The development and successful use of psychopharmacological drugs especially in the 1960s, however, would end the boom in ECT.

By the time the medical expert regime was under full attack, ECT had become marginal. This therapy nevertheless became a symbol of what was wrong in clinical psychiatry, not least because of the highly popular 1975 movie *One Flew over the Cuckoo's Nest* (based on Kesey, 1962). The film showed how ECT was used as a punishment for disobedient patients. The symbolic meaning of ECT as disputable even went beyond the domain of psychiatry. Manipulating the functioning of the human brain by means of technology could be misused by malicious people or regimes. It could be used – and was used (at least in the USA) – for example, to "cure" homosex-uality.[3] This labeling of homosexuality as an illness that could be cured was a slap in the face of gays who at the time found themselves in the middle of an emancipation process. To many, it proved that ECT was all but a harmless, objective technological tool, and although the therapy was marginalized in the early 1970s it was not totally abandoned. In 1979, 46 people in the Neth-erlands were treated with electroshocks. The Dutch National Anti-Shock Action (NASA), established in 1976, pursued a total ban of ECT. If it did not accomplish this goal, in 1984 the Dutch government issued strict formal guidelines for this treatment (Blok, 2004).

The anti-psychiatry movement shows how coalitions between critical professionals and outsiders were formed to point out abuses and to change existing practices of the dominant regime. Special interest groups like *Stichting Pandora*, the *Cliëntenbond in de Welzijnszorg* and *NASA* managed to attract larger numbers of people, and sometimes they radicalized and became a factor not to be underestimated. But while critical psychiatry was at its height in the second half of the 1970s, a resistance movement ("anti-anti-psychiatry") from within clinical psychiatry was on the rise as well: "As a result of the growing success of the biological psychiatry and the protest of parents of psychiatric patients, the dominance of the 'interpersonal' psychotherapeutic treatment diminished in the 1980s" (Blok, 2004). New technology opened up research of the brains of living people. It became possible to show differences in the state and functioning of the brains of both healthy and ill people. Neurobiological research made inroads into psychiatry (e.g. new professorships and research programs at universities) and this generated, together with new psycho-pharmaceuticals such as Prozac and Seroxat, a new optimism in the late 1980s and 1990s (Blok, 2004).

Pressure on the practices, routines and cultures of the dominant modern healthcare regime did not remain limited to mental healthcare, however. Issues associated with quality and acceptability began to be questioned in other domains as well, and female patients thereby took the lead.

Male specialists, female patients

After the 1960s, growing awareness of medical concerns and the rights of patients across the Western world led to the establishment of patient interest groups. These interest groups tried to overcome to a certain extent the unequal doctor–patient relationships (Titmuss, 1968: 146–147; Van der Maesen, 1987). Patients started to become more articulate, asking for more information about diagnoses, treatments, alternatives, etc. This change in mentality among the population toward medicine grew more prominent in the Netherlands as of the mid-1970s. As studies revealed, people responded more assertively to illness and symptoms of illness, and asked more from the medical system (Belleman, 1977; Van Doorn-De Leeuw, 1982). In this development, female patients served as trailblazers.

In 1970 a group of women in the USA became dissatisfied with the way they were treated by male doctors. They published a book entitled *Our Bodies, Our Selves*. This book, which was the outcome of a women health seminar organized in Boston in 1969, became very popular. A Dutch version edited by Anja Meulenbelt and published in 1975 was reprinted four times within six months. Women were urged to be critical and assertive, and not to take specialists' answers for granted (Snelders and Meijman, 2009). That women's resistance against practices of the gynecological specialized regime was successful is underscored by the following case.

Within the women's rights movement there was a lot of discontent about the huge number (*c.* 30,000) of surgical uterus extirpations in Dutch hospitals.[4] Some women organized themselves and made a blacklist of gynecologists who, in their opinion, decided in favor of surgical solutions too quickly. In 1981, these and other initiatives of women, such as discussion groups with gynecological cancers in the *Wilhelminaziekenhuis* in Amsterdam (AVRUEL group, established in 1978) and initiatives of women within Women in Menopause (VIDO, established in 1975), led to the foundation of Women Without Uterus (VZB, later VZG).[5] The initiatives received national media attention and in Parliament the Health Affairs Minister was asked about the high number of uterus extirpations (May 1981). Furthermore, the VZB cooperated with women's magazines, like *Libelle* and *Margriet*, to inform women about gynecological complaints; possible, regular and alternative treatments; sample questions for gynecologists; self-help groups and so on. Furthermore, the VZB served as partner in an episode of a TV series about a century of gynecology in the Netherlands. In 1987 the VZB joined the National Platform of Women's Self-Help Organizations.

Six years later, there was recognition and appreciation of the work of the foundation by the national government when it (then VZG) was asked to take part, together with gynecologists, in a national program to integrate expertise in gynecology. This resulted in VZG surgery hours at the Academic Hospital in Groningen, soon to be followed by other hospitals. In 2004 the VZG was renamed the Information Center Gynecology (ICG).

Aside from many different goals, such as informing and educating women, promoting and starting dialogues between women patients and gynecologists, and organizing self-help groups, the foundation also realized its initial aim: the number of surgical uterus extirpations dramatically decreased. This was the result of an increase in gynecological knowledge and techniques (hormonal treatments, hysteroscopical treatments), but also, to a large extent, of the struggle by women patients for their interests and rights.

Birth assistance is another example where the quality and acceptability of modern healthcare was at stake and where women played a leading role in questioning dominant practices. Along with the establishment in the twentieth century of a new medical regime, the childbirth process had gradually moved from the home environment to the hospital. This happened throughout the Western world and was completed in most countries by the early 1970s. For decades, the Netherlands basically followed this transition pattern (although at first it was late in doing so while it also proceeded at a slower pace). In the late 1970s, however, this process toward hospital childbirth suddenly stopped, probably as a result of the comparatively strong position gained by Dutch midwives in the course of the twentieth century. During the 1970s, Dutch midwives, general physicians and gynecologists struggled with competences and practices in providing childbirth assistance. This struggle had two remarkable outcomes: a diminishing role of general physicians in childbirth assistance, and sole supervision by midwives of many deliveries in hospitals and at home.

This "Dutch system" has been heavily debated up until the present day. Some specialists (mostly male) assume a correlation between a *relatively* high perinatal death rate in the Netherlands and the high number of home deliveries, and they advocate an increasing role of the hospital, specialists and technology in childbirth (Hoogendoorn, 1978). The Central Public Health Board (Centrale Raad voor de Volksgezondheid) had already advised in 1977 to end financial incentives to women wanting to deliver at home, by making hospital deliveries cost-neutral "even if a normal child birth is expected" (Hoogendoorn, 1978). Midwives (mostly female), on the other hand, emphasized the natural character of giving birth and concluded that, unless there are anticipated complications, there is no reason to go into hospital to deliver a child, nor for specialists to monitor and assist the process.

Today, the debate lingers on, as none of the parties has managed to convince the other side on such issues as the safety of the hospital versus the intimacy of the home, the role of medical specialists versus that of professional midwives, and a "desirable" natural (though painful) process versus an "undesirable" medical (but less painful) intervention (Van Erp, 2008). As Dutch midwives have suggested, an around-the-clock stand-by gynecologist in all (also small) hospitals will secure the necessary safety but keep childbirth out of the clinical environment of the hospital.

At the same time, several gynecologists have also pointed to the disadvantages of judging birth as an unnatural, medical act. Professor Lotgering agrees with WHO Director-General Gro Harlem Brundtland that "the epidemic in caeserian sections" in the Western world should be stopped (Lotgering, 2003). Others argue that Dutch gynecologists and midwives act in a too reserved fashion when accompanying deliveries. As some observed, there is too much fear to execute caesarian operations and a more pro-active attitude, especially in the last phase of pregnancies, should be pursued. One critic favors a shift in the Dutch "delivery culture," in order to reduce unnecessary deadly complications at childbirth.[6] Special maturity wards in hospitals and "birth-hotels," with specialists on hand if necessary, and with a friendly, non-technological aura may be seen as niche experiments trying to get the best of both worlds (Marland, 2001).

My two examples of contested modern healthcare thus far – the above-discussed gender aspect and the critique of the medicalized attitude toward the mentally disabled and the way society deals with them – underscore the increasing role of the articulate patient (and his or her family) within the medical domain. But these examples also show evidence of an emerging concern with the way in which "the body," "health," and "illness" are constructed through the rationality of the medical profession, rather than serving as "natural" givens.

Drugs and the pharmaceutical industry

Drugs are essential to modern medicine. Because drugs can be both curative and severely harmful, "trust" and "expectations" are key concepts when drugs are prescribed and promoted. When these concepts erode, two specified core values, quality and acceptability, are directly affected. Unknown or underestimated side-effects of particular medication may lead to pain and protests in society. Well-known examples are the sleep-inducing drug thalidomide (better known as Softenon), which malformed about 10,000 babies worldwide between 1957 and 1961, and the DES hormone, which was prescribed to pregnant women from 1947 to 1975 to prevent spontaneous abortions but increased chances of their daughters developing certain forms of cancer.

Criticism of the inaccuracy, carelessness and reprehensible strategies of the pharmaceutical industry is hardly a recent phenomenon (Robinson, 2001; Blech, 2003; Angell, 2004; Moynihan and Cassels, 2005). Drugs in general have a low price elasticity. In US congressional hearings in 1960 it was already argued that pharmaceutical companies indoctrinate physicians to pre-scribe high-priced trade market products, and exaggerate "their claims for the therapeutic value of certain drugs."[7] In the Netherlands, where the majority of medication is paid for via healthcare insurance premiums, the ties between doctors and the industry also raised concerns in around 1970. To provide doctors with impartial information about the dazzling developments in phar-maceuticals, since 1967 the Ministry of Health has published a "Drugsbulle-tin," inspired by the American *Medical Letter on Drugs and Therapeutics* (since 1959) and the British *Drug and Therapeutics Bulletin* (since 1962). This objective information was meant to compete for doctors' attention, with the increasing amount of (direct) advertising of pharmaceutical companies. In 1970 a Dutch PhD thesis showed (often hidden) "in-depth psychological seducers" in drug advertising aimed at doctors (Abraham, 1970). Medical professionals were misled and patients could be the victims of these tech-niques. It was emphasized, however, that there was no evidence that unrealis-tic advertising had harmed patients.[8] Inadequate and misleading information on the (side) effects of drugs or their high cost and reprehensible deals with doctors were made public and denounced at a time marked by social respon-sibilities for companies and first worries about the medical system's sky-rocketing costs (Van Meurs, 1976, 1978; Pollmann, 1976).[9]

The sector could not neglect this severe societal critique. In 1974 a "Council for Drugs Promotion" was installed by representatives of the phar-maceutical industry. This Council supervised, in retrospect, the "Code for the recommendation of drugs." It was one of the first initiatives of the Dutch Association of the Pharmaceutical Industry (Nefarma). In addition to this code, Nefarma put in place a "Central Board for medical representatives" in 1979 and a general "Behavioral code for Pharmacists" (1983). These self-regulating measures and image-building efforts were important for the sector in order to become a trustworthy partner in the negotiations arena characterized by rising government control during the late 1970s and 1980s (Ploumen, 1987).

Notwithstanding these measures, the pharmaceutical constellation was dis-puted throughout the period and its image perhaps even worsened. Illich judged the pharmaceutical companies as one of the actors that benefited most from the "medicalization" of life. For that reason, the sector had huge stakes in defending the existing "unhealthy" situation that fueled society's medicali-zation – and even in extending it. But doctors were also criticized for being too compliant.

Policy-makers continued to search for instruments to control the prescrip-tion and use of drugs in order to benefit public health – rather than raise the profits of the industry. The sector's expenditures for marketing have long been enormous (Illich, 1975). It is assumed that worldwide operating phar-maceuticals spend more money on marketing than on R&D (Van den Berg Jeths and Peters-Volleberg, 2002). In 2005, as Bouma has argued, Dutch pharmaceutical companies have spent 1 euro on marketing for every 60 eurocents they spent on R&D (Bouma, 2006). Today, policies are largely aimed at counterbalancing the "knowledge asymmetry" between doctors and the industry by providing independent knowledge to doctors, as well as at cutting the financial ties between doctors and industry (Mot and Windmeijer, 2002). The health insurance companies in particular are thought to play a prominent role in increasing the price elasticity of drugs. Taking this weapon from the hands of the pharmaceutical industry, "trust" can perhaps be restored and "expectations" made more realistic.

It is perhaps too easy, however, to paint a picture of an arrogant industry, merely aimed at quick profits and a natural enemy of healthcare policy-makers that can only be curbed by legislation. Triggered by a poor public image and pressure in particular from NGOs, some pharmaceutical companies have developed new business models. A front runner in this respect is Novo Nordisk. Already from the 1960s, this company has been very reflexive about its behavior. It started to take its stakeholders into account and over time broadened its business goals and integrated corporate responsibility into them. The company gradually adopted a proactive attitude in its worldwide fight against diabetes. It cooperates closely with NGOs and governments in several projects in many countries, not by fulfilling the role of a mere pill supplier, but by seeing itself as an actor in a complex global community, involved in "quality-of-life" issues, stakeholder dialog, prevention initiatives and political agenda-setting (Kingo, 2010).

Being an important actor in the medical regime, the pharmaceutical industry simply cannot ignore external pressure on that regime. Above all, a response like Novo Nordisk's, which is probably wise in terms of business strategy, is part of a much broader process of regime reconfiguration.

2.3 Accessibility and affordability under pressure

Restructuring and limiting healthcare

The crisis in modern healthcare, as noted by the WHO in 1978, has been largely related to economic determinants and the sector's productivity. While demand for healthcare was increasing, and the costs rose year by year, the health situation of the population in Western countries did not keep pace. Internationally, economic cost–benefit analysis in healthcare gained ground in the 1970s. Healthcare economics became a specialized discipline and research into, for example, productivity of healthcare technology and the hospital intensified and changed (Newhouse, 1970). The unit of analysis in health economics became ever smaller, while research methods and analytical techniques changed (Phelps, 2007).

In the Netherlands, the spiraling expenditures for the medical domain were identified as problematic in the mid-1960s. A 1966 governmental report signaled almost an uncontrolled growth of intramural medicine (Ministerie van Sociale Zaken en Volksgezondheid, 1966; Van Lieburg, 1995). From that time on, the growth of intramural healthcare and the costs involved prompted the government to take up a steering and controlling role. Legal and financial instruments were used to control the supply side of the system, as well as to (re)define and add or reduce medical operations. To concentrate top specialist medical facilities, the *Law on Hospital Facilities* was promulgated in 1971. It licensed the building of hospitals, as well as the purchase and use of expensive equipment.

In 1973, the new left-wing cabinet was determined to systematically restructure Dutch healthcare, among others by strengthening extramural healthcare to relieve intramural care. Although cost control was a central aim of its policy, it also addressed explicitly the quality and acceptability problems that healthcare faced by trying to overcome the demand–supply gap, focusing more on patients' needs and less on the possibilities of high-tech medical devices (Willems, 1995; Djellal and Gallouj, 2007). Here we see the unease about the position of the patient in the system and about the spiraling costs of the system come together. For the first time, patients were mentioned by the government as a defined category in the healthcare domain. Furthermore, this policy represented a shift from a confessional/liberal policy, marked by limited government interference and a strong role for social and professional players within the medical domain, toward government interference and planning, a more social-democratic approach in the 1970s (Ministerie van Volksgezondheid en Milieuhygiëne, 1974; Van der Maesen, 1987; Boot and Knapen, 2005). The revaluation of the demand side in healthcare was not abandoned when a right-wing government took over in the late 1970s (Ministerie van Volksgezondheid en Milieuhygiëne, 1980).

In spite of reorganization measures and a reallocation of means, the total expenditures for healthcare continued to grow in the 1970s from about 5.5 percent of GNP in the Netherlands to about 8 percent in 1980. In the late 1970s, the government tried to gain more insight into healthcare costs, and announced a cost-reducing policy (Ministerie van Volksgezondheid en Milieuhygiëne, 1977, 1979). By 1980, the economic situation and government finances had deteriorated and a general policy of austerity was introduced. A government document published in 1983 articulated a policy vision on how to manage an almost uncontrollable sector in economically difficult times. The document was called "Healthcare policy with limited means" and proposed general goals aimed at enhancing the autonomy and responsibility of the patient, as well as promoting a shift from cure to prevention, from clinical to polyclinical, and from specialist and intramural care toward the general practitioner. The role of advanced technologies, especially diagnostic techniques, such as laboratory determinations and imaging technologies, was viewed in a critical light. The policy document denounced the numbers in which diverse new and costly techniques were applied (Ministerie van Welzijn, Volksgezondheid en Cultuur, 1984). It explicitly mentioned the unwanted phenomenon of medicalization, arguing that "several societal problems are treated as if they were healthcare problems," and this caused a too broad application of healthcare functions (Ministerie van Welzijn, Volksge-zondheid en Cultuur, 1984).

With budget savings, concerns about the affordability and accessibility of modern healthcare started to conflict with concerns about its quality and acceptability. In 1983, the performance of ten medical interventions was pro-hibited without prior permission of the ministry, including dialysis, radiother-apy, neurosurgery, cardiac surgery, heart cathetcrizing, computer tomography and intensive care for neonates. Up until 1990, academic hospitals were excluded from these restrictions (Wladimiroff, 2002).

In 1983, the Public Healthcare Insurance Council (*Ziekenfondsraad*), which had a major task in coordinating and controlling the execution of the laws concerning public healthcare insurance, advised about limiting the package of healthcare supplies (Ziekenfondsraad, 1983). It emphasized that new technol-ogies should no longer automatically be added to the insurance system. In a subsequent policy recommendation, issued in 1986, a system of integrative evaluation of new technologies was introduced. Rapid advances were made in particular in heart transplantation, in vitro fertilization and liver transplan-tation, and this raised questions about limiting the care system. Some prelimi-nary cost-effectiveness analyses in IVF and heart transplantation, which had particular ramifications for policy-making, had already been made (Boer, 1999).

In the mid-1980s, the Dutch healthcare policy prioritized assessment of technologies and treatments, and their selection. A 1986 advisory report by the governments' highest advisory board, the Health Council, was called "Limits to healthcare." It proposed to the government annually to add, limit or adjust new and old technologies, based on scientific research aimed at the criteria "quality," "social effects" and "stimulation" (Wladimiroff, 2002). The first advice was given in 1989.

"Limits to healthcare" (1986), the government report "Nota 2000" (1986) and the report of the Commission Structure and Finance of Healthcare (also called the Dekker Commission; 1987) clearly marked a shift in Dutch health-care policy. Assuring the affordability and accessibility of the system had the highest priority. On the one hand, this meant an emphasis on disease pieven-tion and health promotion. The determinants of health served as a starting point of the national health policy: biological and hereditary factors, the phys-ical environment, the social environment and ways of life (Boot and Knapen, 2005). Scenario studies and health goals were part of this vision. Based on these factors, health policies in the narrow sense could be carried out – health policies aimed at determinants, for example, of cardiovascular diseases or dia-betes, including measures outside the health sector, in the workplace, in education and in construction. Policies in the broader sense – aimed at the overall health system, including health facilities and resources – were also to be based on these scenarios and aims.

On the other hand, the laws of the market were introduced into the healthcare domain. The government adopted many ideas from the Dekker

Commission in its own vision document "Change Ensured" and it made a plan to allow more market mechanisms into the system (Maarse, 2001; Boot and Knapen, 2005). At the time, however, a system of government-regulated free markets (Plan-Simons) proved too revolutionary to be politically accepted by the Christian Democratic/Socialist coalition, which was engaged in a dispute about the limitations of the welfare state.

It seemed impossible to sustain the welfare system at the same high level, but it was politically too sensitive to dismantle it overnight. A radical change in the health system, toward more "free market" but with a huge collective insurance system, met with many objections from both the left and the right, as well as from various stakeholders. "Change" as was proclaimed was therefore all but ensured. During the two socialist, liberal and liberal–democratic coalitions (1994–2002), which were marked by a strong economic revival, a more evolutionary approach of change was followed. By the end of this period, however, the debate about a fundamental change toward a regulated free market resurfaced.

Contesting limited healthcare

Limitations to healthcare met with resistance from regime players as well as from outsiders. At a conference of the Amsterdam Specialists Association in 1985, entitled "Who sells 'no' to a patient?" medical specialists expressed their frustration about the prevailing health system. A general manager of Philips led a plea for more technological innovations in healthcare, and a patient-lecturer asked the audience of specialists not to let him down. A more critical note from a general practitioner about the endless research and referral practices of specialists seemed less appreciated, since the professional group itself viewed it as their inherent qualities. In their education, medical specialists were in fact trained to study everything and exclude every risk. Furthermore, they assumed the willingness of the Dutch population to pay more for health, which was to be studied in a proposed survey (Achterhuis, 1988). Nation-wide, newspapers picked up the frustrations and critique voiced by specialists, offering them a platform for their grievances (Achterhuis, 1988).

In January 1990 a judge in Rotterdam took a decision that had far-reaching consequences for Dutch health policies in general. In particular, the governmental system of budgeting through which costs were kept under control was challenged by the judge's verdict. He stated that patients who have to wait too long for their heart operation according to their doctors may be treated abroad, while public and private health insurance had to pay for it. Two months earlier a judge in Den Bosch had passed a similar judgment when proceedings were instituted against a hospital that refused to perform percutaneous angioplasty on patients because it had reached the limits of its budget, while National Health Insurance refused to pay for additional treatments.

In both cases the judges decided in favor of the patients, stating that the law ordered hospitals a duty to provide for care and health insurance companies to make this financially possible. A budgeting system as a tool for policy-makers was subordinate to these patient rights. Nevertheless, in other cases judges decided that the National Health Insurance system was right in its decision not to pay for a bypass operation in London, because the patient could be operated on within a reasonable time span in the Netherlands. In addition, a decision by the insurer not to pay for a patient's stay in a non-recognized institution, because there was a long waiting list in such recognized institutions, was judged as right. All these examples took place between November 1989 and March 1990 (Leenen, 1991).

Several months later, the financing of scarce healthcare provisions once again attracted national media attention. The Social Affairs Deputy Minister prohibited the city of Nieuwegein from using its Fund for Social Assistance to financially help out a citizen who needed a lung transplant. Lung transplants (like heart transplants until the late 1980s) were not paid for by the regular health system. For that reason, local Social Assistance Funds had helped out people 47 times between 1983 and 1989. In 21 cases, money was paid for lung or heart transplants abroad. This was a figurative use of these funds and evaded the budgeting policy in healthcare. As long as there was no verdict of the Health Council on payment of lung transplants out of the Investigative Medicine Program, patients had to pay for these operations out of their own pockets. Because of the bitterness behind this situation, a number of local governments interfered. Now that they were legally forbidden to do so, some individual patients made collections, held lotteries and made appeals on TV shows to finance their transplants. The patient association of heart transplants (which also represented lung transplants) heckled this situation. The government, on the other hand, put the blame on the hospitals which had raised false expectations (Pols, 1990).

The problem of limitations in healthcare was studied by a Commission, called "Choices in Care," set up in the summer of 1990 (Roscam Abbing, 1991). The Commission, chaired by cardiologist professor A.J. Dunning, was ordered to broadly reflect on the problem of selection in healthcare. The more practical problem to solve was which healthcare provisions should be paid for collectively within a system with a limited free market. Dunning was inspired by the communitarian vision of American philosopher Daniel Callahan. This inspiration could be seen in a main conclusion of its report, "Take it and leave it." It was proposed that the package of collectively financed healthcare be mainly composed of the types of care that people need to participate in society.[10] Selection of healthcare provisions should be made based on criteria of necessity, efficiency, suitability and own responsibility. In the famous "funnel of Dunning," this process of selection was schematized. The Commission successfully stirred up the debate about responsibilities in healthcare. Discussions about the limitations of collective and individual responsibility for health and healthcare continue until the present day.

In addition to these discussions about choices and limitations of collectively financed healthcare, waiting lists and therefore the accessibility and, in its wake, the quality of the Dutch health system have been heavily discussed since the late 1980s. The existence of long waiting lists, especially in times of economic growth (since about 1994), was regarded unacceptable. In addition, the decreasing quality of healthcare due to savings in the care domain was contested. The appearance of Jolanda Venema on national television in 1988, naked and tied to the wall of her room in a mental institution, elicited many protests. This was all but an image of a modern health system. Healthcare was stripped to the bone as opposition parties argued.

In the late 1990s, the economization in healthcare, especially within the nursing domain, and the introduction of the (regulated) market dynamics in the domain became a focus of critique. Professional institutions in welfare work and healthcare were pushed to reinforce economic rationality in their work. "Taylorizing" homecare services, by dividing up the work into small sections ("stopwatch care"), as well as introducing economies of scale and the merging of organizations and institutions seem to prevail over important non-economic values in healthcare, such as "the human standard," as one critic put it. Furthermore, introducing market mechanisms and the supervising role of the government shifted responsibilities and required new forms of account-ability, often leading to increased bureaucracy. Today, healthcare professionals spend much of their time on the input of data – time that should be spent on patient care. Moreover, the distrust among financers, suppliers, government, institutions, clients, professionals and intermediaries appears to have risen.[11]

Last but not least, excessive bureaucracy is also reported as a problem for a substantial group of users of the so-called Personally Assigned Budget (PAB) in healthcare. This financing tool was introduced in 1995 to enhance freedom of choice for healthcare consumers. Up to a certain limit, users may purchase care from care suppliers and even from family or friends. In terms of the number of users and evaluations of the first group of users, the PAB was a success. But not everything in the PAB garden was lovely. Next to the bureaucracy, due to strong governmental regulation in indications, and budget assignment, control and sanctioning, which hindered 20 percent of PAB users, there were other problems. Many care suppliers were monopolists in a certain region and very few small suppliers were available. Furthermore, the Association of Consumers concluded in 2002 that users had too little information about suppliers to make rational choices. To help PAB users in their choices and with the bureaucratic procedures, a network of intermediate actors arose (WRR, 2004). Aside from the bona fide ones among them, others tried to make profits out of patients' ignorance and use weak spots in the system to commit fraud on a large scale, as a national newspaper reported (Bruinsma, 2009).

2.4 Unlimited healthcare: more is not enough, better is not good enough

Since about 1970 the health system has been contested in many countries throughout the Western world. The main targets of the criticism put forward are rooted in the regime. Table 2.1 shows this relationship, based on the Dutch examples provided in sections 2.2 and 2.3.

The Dutch case reveals that the dominant healthcare regime has been in a constant reconfiguration process trying to meet the criticism and pressure from the landscape. In recent years the regime has been directed at "individually aimed quality" (Van der Grinten and Kasdorp, 1999). Here we see the rational–reductionist paradigm in medicine, with its focus on illness and the doctor, meet the human–integrative paradigm, focusing on health and the patient (Bensing, 2000). Often in experimental settings, such as patient-centered hospitals, "birth hotels," transmural care, "health coaches" linked to health insurance companies, and tele-medicine, solutions were sought to meet the specified core values of healthcare.

These and other niche experiments in healthcare are an effect of pressure on the regime. The paradox of a very healthy population with many diseases and complaints reveals itself here (Schnabel, 1995). The aging of the population and the quality of life of the very old puts new demands on healthcare: "almost half of medical expenditure now [1999] is being incurred in the last 60 days of a patient's life" (Le Fanu, 1999, 2000). The affordability and accessibility of the system asks for solidarity; a debated principle in a secularized, individualized, and *"de-pillarized"* society, which stresses own responsibility. Furthermore, due to scientific and social developments, the quality and acceptability of the regime have been questioned, giving the current healthcare debate width and dynamics previously unseen.

Scientific developments in genetics force us to rethink "illness" and the boundaries of modern medicine. Furthermore, recent disputes about national vaccination programs in the Netherlands show that resistance against collective prevention programs is no longer limited to religious minorities. Top-down measures and self-responsibility are judged differently today than 40 years ago. Although the articulate consumer patient has existed for centuries (Snelders and Meijman, 2009), increased information and education has "proto-professionalized" him or her, asking more from doctors and from the health system in general. Articulate patients defend their rights for "the best of the best and much of that" (De Swaan, 1982; Achterhuis, 1988). If the development of the articulate patient over past decades did not so much lead to a changed balance of power between patients and doctors (an initial aim),

Table 2.1 Relationship between the main targets of the criticism and regime features

Targets of criticism	Related to regime features
Depersonalization; not patient-centered but deficiency-focused	Specialization/evidence
Costs → limited healthcare; dehumanization	Technology/hospital
Medicalization: "constructivism" through the rationality of the medical profession	Cure

it did cause a spiraling growth of the entire system (Krol, 1985). Today's healthcare regime has to reckon with patients' opinions, often developed at discussion forums on the internet, in trying to achieve goals when fighting determinants of diseases (genetic or social) and influencing lifestyle.

Furthermore, medical boundaries are challenged by a culture of enhancement. Starting with commercial cosmetic surgery in the 1980s, today medical human enhancement has gone way beyond the top sportsman taking drugs to improve performance. In the third quarter of the twentieth century, the so-called "worried well" were pulled into the medical domain (Le Fanu, 2000). In the last quarter of that century the "unhappy well" also knocked at the doors of medicine. Living up to particular norms of beauty and strength is perhaps a feature of all eras and cultures, but new insights and technologies now and in the near future enable modern medicine to enhance bodies and the "unhappy" not to take "abnormalities" for granted. Where for centuries the medical constellation was focused on finding, curing or preventing illness, it is now also involved in making "better" (wo)men, next to making ill (wo)men better.

Can technological and organizational innovations keep up with rising and changing demands and expectations? Will expenditures raise questions about choice, selection and priorities that a democratic and civilized society, based on solidarity, can answer in a satisfory way? Undoubtedly the healthcare regime will continue to be contested in the years ahead. Only in retrospect we will be able to say whether or not the 2010s or 2020s proved to mark a new turning point.

Notes

1 Video, *A Day in the Life of Sheffield Royal Hospital*. Available at www.dailymotion. com/video/x88770_sheffield-royal-hospital_creation.
2 Available at www.stichtingpandora.nl.
3 In 1972 American magazine *Horizon* published (without irony) an article about therapists using conditioning techniques "try[ing] to cure a homosexual by giving him electric shocks when pictures of men appear and the 'reward' of no shocks for pictures of sexy women." Available at http://santitafarella.wordpress.com/2008/08/15/would-james-dobson-approve-electroshock-therapy-for-homosexuals/.
4 Available at www.icgynaecologie.nl/geschiedenis.php.
5 This part is mainly based on VZG (1996), *15 jaar VZB = VZG, 1981–1996* (Utrecht 1996) and the website of the icg available at www.icgynaecologie.nl.
6 "Denk niet dat de natuur het voor je oplost," *De Volkskrant*, February 21, 2009.
7 Cited in: "Prescription for change. A survey of pharmaceuticals" in *The Economist*, June 18, 2005, 4; for a recent study in the Netherlands see Mot and Windmeijer (2002).
8 Arts wijst op gevaren van geneesmiddelen-reclame "Met ons produkt bent u een goede dokter," *Leeuwarder Courant*, November 6, 1970.
9 Some examples: "Zegen met keerzij" in *Leeuwarder Courant*, November 15, 1971; "Huisartsen schrijven te vaak dure recepten" in *Leeuwarder Courant*, July 24, 1972; "Publiek betaalt veel te veel voor pinstillers" in *Leeuwarder Courant*, October 23, 1973; R. van Meurs, "De fraude met geneesmiddelen gaat nog steeds door" in

Vrij Nederland, December 6, 1975; R. van Meurs, "Bonussen, kortingen, cheques, belastingvoordeel en bootreisjes: wie schrijft de meeste antibiotica voor?" in *Vrij Nederland*, April 8, 1978.
10 Advies Dunning kan Simons vertragen, *NRC*, November 15, 1991.
11 Available at http://canonsociaalwerk.nl/1987commDekker/1987commDekker. html.

3 Key features of modern health systems

Nature and historical evolution

Roel van Raak and Fjalar J. de Haan

3.1 Introduction

This book centers on the persistent problems in present-day healthcare and the transition to a more sustainable healthcare in the future. As the previous historical chapter highlighted, such a transition poses quite a number of challenges. The Dutch health system has been contested since the 1970s, without a clear resolution being in sight. This chapter takes the reader further back in time, to the preceding one-and-ahalf centuries (1820–1970), when the last major transition in the Dutch health system took place.

To assert that the last transition took place a century ago may come across as a downplaying of the fierce debates, the many innovations in medicine, and the financial reforms of recent decades. Although we are aware of this, we argue that the foundations and paradigms of the health system have not changed fundamentally over the past decades, especially in comparison with the period covered by this chapter.

We will elaborate this claim systematically here, but first we illustrate our point through a series of thought experiments. In each experiment a young, ill person is transported back 50 years, as if in a time machine. In our first experiment, we transport him back in time from the present to the 1960s. To address his illness he has to depend on the health system of that era. He would probably need to adapt, but still manage to find his way through this system. First, he would consult a general practitioner (GP). His GP would have many of today's major pharmaceuticals at his disposal, and like today he would refer his patient to a specialist if the patient's condition was beyond his abilities. Our time traveler would know where to find such a specialist: in the hospital. Such a hospital would look much like today's hospital: a busy space dominated by specialists assisted by nurses and full of high-tech equipment. The hospital would prefer to treat him as an outpatient in one of the specialist policlinics, while the costs would typically be covered by compulsory insurance.

Next, we teleport our young, sick person from the 1960s to the 1910s. He would still recognize the general outline of the medical world, but would be unpleasantly surprised by the limited options and accessibility. His GP would simply be "the doctor." Only if the patient was a complicated or interesting case might he be advised to seek a specialist's opinion. The doctor he was stuck with had a much smaller therapeutic arsenal at his disposal. He could disinfect and tranquilize, but rarely tackle the root of a health problem. If the patient's condition worsened, he might be transferred to a hospital, where he would most likely be admitted as an inpatient. He would be familiar with hospitals as clean places, where patients can rest and be nursed. But he would scarcely see a specialist and basically need to get better on his own. He would be covered by insurance only if he belonged to the minority of people having such insurance.

As a final step in our thought experiment, we teleport this same patient from the 1910s back to the 1860s, and he would be at a complete loss. At the time, a doctor was just one among many practitioners trying to earn a living by soliciting to help the ill. He might recommend baths or herbs, or simply be satisfied by having diagnosed the problem. He would not touch the patient, as he considered that to be the task of a surgeon. This surgeon, on the other hand, would barely have any theoretical knowledge. In fact, surgery was an ordeal that often ended in a deadly infection. The ill person would do best to completely avoid the hospital, because being in such an institution, virtually without medical staff, basically meant that one was only one step removed from death. Our time traveler would have found that health insurance was hardly known. At the time, the rich simply paid for the doctor, while the poor had to beg their quartermaster or church to pay for them. This thought experiment suggests that Dutch healthcare has been continuously changing over two centuries, but at times more fundamentally and at a higher pace. Between 1860 and 1910 there were dramatic changes that reverberated up until the 1960s – a transition occurred. After the 1960s, the system stabilized to such a degree that we negatively refer to its stability as "persistency."

The above accounts serve rather as descriptions of this transition than as explanations of it. Our analysis in this chapter is aimed not only at increasing our understanding of the historical transition in Dutch healthcare by moving from describing to explaining, but also at presenting the methodology used. Given that we study the past to better understand the present regime, including its persistency and possible alternatives, we develop our argument based on the following research questions: (1) how did the present system come about?; (2) can we trace the roots of its current persistency and contestation in its past?; and (3) could other transition paths have been possible historically, and if so, why did these alternatives founder?

Several factors complicate our effort, in particular the time span considered (nearly two centuries), the vastness of the health system (in its more recent stages amounting to as much as 10 to 15 percent of the Dutch economy; see OECD, 2007), and its intrinsic complexity, consisting as it does of myriad different services in various institutional settings (Boot and Knapen, 2005). Although thorough research has been done on the history of Dutch healthcare (e.g. Houwaart (1991) on the hygienist movement and Geels (2006) on sewage systems), an encompassing study of the developments leading to the current Dutch healthcare system as a whole seems to be lacking. This may be for good reasons: such an overarching study runs the risk of paying for broadness with shallowness. At the same time, many have voiced the idea that Dutch healthcare seems to, or at least should, go through a major transition (LOC, 2009; Neuteboom et al., 2009; VWS, 2006), which gives rise to the question of whether such transitions have occurred in the past. To formulate tentative answers to this question, a method is required that systematically describes long-term and large-scale transition processes in order to reconstruct the paths of change. As outlined in the following section, the method adopted here uses the Multi-Pattern Approach (De Haan, 2010; De Haan and Rotmans, 2011). Next, in Section 3.3 we systematically describe the history of the various constellations in Dutch healthcare, and reconstruct the transition paths in which they were involved. The analysis in Section 3.4 provides a synthesis of these various paths. The research questions will be answered through critical reflection on these analytical results in Section 3.5.

3.2 Methodology

Like the WHO's (2000) definition of a health system, we start from what we call societal systems: a system geared to meeting societal needs. The health system, in our case, has the function to "promote, restore or maintain health"; that is, it meets society's health needs. *How* a societal system meets such a need is called its functioning. As social theorist Niklas Luhmann (1984) pointed out, societal systems have a tendency to differentiate when dealing with increasing complexity. This suggests that a complex societal system such as the Dutch health system is composed of several subsystems, which we refer to as *constellations*, each of which is concerned with a specific aspect of the health system's overall functioning. This allows us to unravel "the complex network of activities" constituted by the "different forms of prevention, cure and care" (WHO, 2000). Constellations deal with different types of patients or cases, and different constellations entail different infrastructures and paradigms for addressing these differences. Obviously, Dutch healthcare itself may be considered a constellation within a larger societal system, such as global healthcare or the Dutch public sector.[1]

Constellations should not be viewed mechanically, as mere cogwheels in a "healthcare machine." The function of any constellation is subject to internal and external debate. This also implies that constellations are known to those associated with it, rather than serving as abstract analytic entities. Furthermore, we allow these constellations to interact with and adapt to each other, as well as to the system's environment. They can be in competition or complementary, or both. A constellation's share in fulfilling a particular social need may vary over time; if it is possible for small *niches* to gain *power*, large *regimes* may become marginalized. Constellations can merge or split. We will label constellations based on keywords such as "doctor" or "financing"; to avoid confusion we demarcate constellations in this text by using guillemets (e.g. «doctor»).

Moreover, we consider the system – and thus its parts – to be open. Interactions occur not only between the parts within the system, but also between the parts of the system and the environment. The function of each part, and consequently the function of the whole, is the result of both internal dynamics and interactions with its environment (De Haan, 2006). This environment is conceptualized as *the landscape* (Rip and Kemp, 1998), which comprises all other relevant societal systems of greater scale than the scale of the system under study (see De Haan (2010) and De Haan and Rotmans (2011) for this kind of interpretation). Because large societal systems, such as our political system, our economic system and our knowledge system, slowly – and sometimes abruptly – evolve over time, the landscape is hardly a static entity; instead, it is a dynamic force on the developments within the societal system under study.

The interactions between the constellations and the system environment shape the system as a whole. As such, a constellation is an ontological notion, yet one that provides an epistemological advantage. The complexity of the system under study requires a methodology for mapping the processes of change without having an overview in advance at the system level. If we know which constellations are relevant we can establish a systems overview bottom up. Although this does not eliminate demarcation issues, it is less controversial to identify potentially relevant constellations than in the traditional approach, which conceptualizes transitions in terms of the old and new regime. Our approach to explain transitions from constellation dynamics comprises four steps:

1 Demarcating the societal system, especially in function and time, and broadly based on particular research interests.
2 Describing the constellations over the course of the demarcated period, in order to understand *what* changes.
3 Describing *how* the constellations change, which entails decomposing the histories of the constellations in terms of typical *patterns*.
4 Reconstructing the overall transition in terms of the changes in the constellations and aggregating these constellation-level dynamics to system-level dynamics.

Below, we further elaborate these steps by applying them to the case at hand. For a schematic depiction of the whole process, see Figure 3.1.

Step 1: demarcation

Initial demarcation should be done on the basis of initial observations and common sense, such that the scope of study may reasonably be expected to be sufficient to address the central research questions of this chapter.

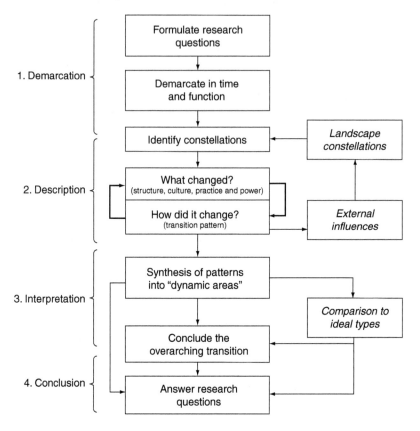

Figure 3.1 Schematic depiction of the methodology

Conceiving of common sense as "the collection of prejudices acquired by the age of eighteen,"[2] such demarcations in function, space and time need to be transparent – and thus open for discussion – and need to be revised along with the findings in the next steps. The constellation concept can help in explicating what is and what is not being investigated (see step 2).

Iterations will lead to the exclusion of elements that turn out to be irrelevant, but not necessarily to the inclusion of relevant elements initially excluded. The demarcation should therefore be broader than the expected extent of the transition dynamics. This is especially relevant for transitions, which are characterized by long predevelopment and stabilization phases that may not be immediately visible.

We chose to limit ourselves to healthcare within the Netherlands. In the nineteenth century, Dutch society faced a shift of power from the local to the national level in the emerging nation-state (see e.g. Van Sas, 2005). International influences have been addressed as "landscape" influences. Healthcare is a distinct sector, but it overlaps with many other sectors in society, varying from sanitary engineering and social security to politics and nutrition. These sectors are described as part of the landscape. With regard to the temporal demarcation, the most profound changes in Dutch society apparently took place between 1865 and 1965. As a broad, preliminary demarcation of our study, then, we chose to begin in 1800 with the "French period" (the French military and political presence in the Netherlands) and to end in the 1990s, when new preoccupations had arisen, as described in the previous chapter.

Step 2: identifying and describing constellations

Given the system boundaries, we identified a set of constellations to be studied, which may be revised upon further study. The choice for a limited number of constellations should be made such that:

- Each constellation can be treated as a single unit of analysis. For example, in our case, our initial constellation of «doctor» had to be split into «specialist» and «general practitioner», as these come with different paradigms, structures and routines.
- Constellations are defined on a similar level of abstraction, and in such a way that secondary literature is available. For example, we discarded the idea of using «care», «cure» and «prevention» constellations, because no literature was available at such as level.
- Constellations that significantly influenced the development of others are included; for this reason we included the «financing» constellation.
- Constellations of research interest are included. For example, as this book pays attention to integrative care and initiatives from civil society, we take «Cross Work» and «public health» constellations into account.

These considerations led us to identify and select the following constellations in the Dutch health system:

- The constellations concerning medical practitioners:
  - *The «surgeon»* (until 1865): constellation around using traditional skills to physical-mechanically intervene in patients' bodies. The «surgeon» represents the "old" skills-based approach to healthcare. The «surgeon» constellation was one of the two elements constituting the «physician» constellation, which has been a dominant factor in the transition.
  - *The (academic) «doctor»* (until 1865): constellation around using academic knowledge to interpret symptoms of patients in practice. The «doctor» is the other constituting factor of the «physician» constellation. In the Netherlands, the doctor constellation was crucial for incorporating the landscape trend of increasing the societal relevance of academics and science into the health system.

- *The «physician»*[3] (1865–1930): transient constellation around the near-universal practice of medicine and counseling. Dominant around 1900, this constellation was pivotal in uniting very different approaches to healthcare.
- *The «specialist»* (from 1900): constellation around providing specialized medicine for severe illnesses and/or specific treatments. As the name suggests, the «specialist» was a reflection of – and a driving force toward – a more specialized, technical health system.
- *The «general practitioner»* (from 1900): constellation concerned with gatekeeping and medical practice of non-specific and mild illnesses. It is the direct successor of the «physician» constellation, although much less dominant. Still, as gatekeeper and practitioner closest to patients we included it in this analysis.

- *The «hospitals and nursing»*[4] (entire period): constellation around the nursing of and providing for the ill (and the weak in general) that would later transform into a supporting role for curative therapies of «specialist» healthcare. We included this constellation because of the emblematic current role of the «hospital» in healthcare and the pivotal role played by the «hospital» in transforming the universal «physician» into highly specialized professions.
- *«Financing»* (from 1900): constellation around distributing the healthcare costs for individuals among a larger group, as a means of risk spreading and solidarity. Originally, most developments in healthcare were driven by direct payments from the middle and upper classes. Late in the transition, however, financing arrangements became crucial to funding «specialist» healthcare, which even the rich could not afford.
- *«Cross Work»* (from 1900): constellation around providing a broad spectrum of healthcare at the district level with a proactive involvement of the district's citizens.
- *«Public health»* services (from 1920): constellation around the practice of healthcare in a public and collective way, rather than privately and individually, typically through direct government involvement.
- *«Mental healthcare»* (entire period): constellation around care and treatment for those with a psychological condition, behavioral illness or mental disorder. We included this constellation because of its significant power. In addition, it allows for an analysis of conformation to the somatic regime.

It is at least as important to account for the constellations that in the end were not included. (1) We excluded many paramedical approaches, such as «midwifery», «physiotherapy» and «dieticians», because they did not appear to have played a significant role in the coming about of the current or transitional regimes. They also seem of slightly less interest for solving the current persistent problems than other constellations.[5] (2) We excluded «homeopathy». Homeopathy does not appear to have had a major material or cultural magnitude within or impact upon the health system. (3) We excluded «civil engineering». Undoubtedly water and sanitation infrastructure has contributed tremendously to improving people's health. However, our framework starts from what appeared to have been the institutional, socially constructed boundaries of the health system, not from the objective determinants of health. Engineering works may be said to have been part of engineering and public works rather than the health system (for a history, see TIN19). Accordingly, we placed them outside of the health system, even though we will address their cross-fertilization with healthcare. (4) We excluded the modern «well-being» sector. There is a blurry distinction between health-related well-being and general well-being. We addressed this partially by describing the influence of «poor relief»[6] (and the split of its successor of the «well-being» sector). (5) We did not consider «regulation» to be a separate constellation: regulations may be considered as part of specific constellations (e.g. insurance directives and disciplinary rule for physicians); however, especially in the second half of the nineteenth century, the forming of an effective regulatory apparatus was pivotal in the coming about of the first regime while it also served as a basis of many preventive measures. (6) We did not include «pharmacists». Although the pharmaceutical options and the pharmaceutical industry transformed dramatically as part of the international landscape, pharmacy (both as a profession and a form of retail) has remained remarkably stable in its structure, culture, practice and power.

Having identified the constellations, we need a method to describe them systematically. We describe these constellations by their "structures," "cultures" and "practices" (Rotmans and Loorbach, 2006; Loorbach, 2007; Van Raak, 2010; see also the introductory chapter of this volume). These three aspects shape each other: structure and culture support (or constrain) behavior of actors in practice. As a result of the exercise of agency in these practices, however, structures and cultural elements also change. Figure 3.2 depicts the continuous interactions within this triplet. Structure and culture are grouped together as the structuring elements (in the sense of Giddens, 1984). They both enable and constrain the practices in which actors are engaged. This take on structure and culture, as enabling practices are similar to the view of the WHO (2000) on "organizations, institutions and resources … producing actions" within health systems.

The constellation as a whole facilitates particular societal functioning. Although the actors' agency is central in shaping the constellation, individual actors are not explicitly taken into account here. Unless specified otherwise, a term such as «physicians» refers to the constellation, not to individual physicians. Still, actors are crucial of course, for instance, in determining whether two constellations interact in a symbiotic or competitive pattern. This exclusion of actors from the definition of the system is also in line with the definition formulated by the WHO (2000).

The constellation may be distinguished from the wider societal system in that it fulfills some (perceived) societal need in a certain way, by providing

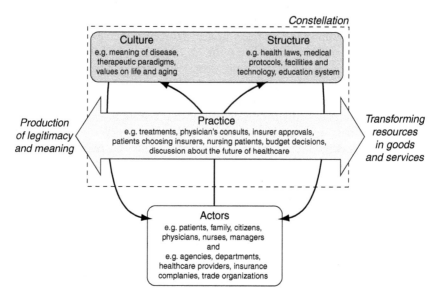

Figure 3.2 Schematic depiction of the structure–culture–practice triplet for describing constellations

certain goods and services. But societal needs have cultural dimensions as well and therefore one should look beyond the material goods and services provided. The values, legitimacy and perceptions at issue are continuously reproduced and adapted by the actors involved. This holds true for healthcare in particular. Explicitly or implicitly, the health system – through its constituent constellations – does not simply provide services; it also engages in giving meaning to these goods and services.

Patterns of transitional change in conditions

Every answer to the question of "what changed" needs to be accompanied by an answer to the question of how it changed. In other words, a description of a changed constellation needs to be complemented by a description of the *pattern* that changed it. The Multi-Pattern Approach is a method for such description and explanation. It was put forward by De Haan and Rotmans (2011) as part of the larger Pillar Theory presented in De Haan (2010). In this approach three patterns are distinguished: "empowerment," "reconstellation" and "adaptation" (see Box 3.1). Each one of these patterns describes a typical way in which a constellation can undergo transitional change: the top-down reconstellation; the gaining of power by a constellation through empowerment, and the adaptation pattern in which a constellation transforms itself by incorporating elements "alien" to its current structure, culture and practice.

Box 3.1 Patterns of transitional change

EMPOWERMENT: *Bottom-up constellation change*
A new constellation emerges, or an existing one gains power, either on itself or through interacting or merging with other constellations within the societal system.

   Examples: A niche around a novel medical approach finds its way into the medical mainstream or the merging of medical professions. Although not part of the theory of De Haan, we also needed a term for a constellation dwindling away, which we will call *depowerment*.

RECONSTELLATION: *Top-down constellation change*
A new constellation emerges, or an existing one gains power by interacting with constellations outside the societal system.

   Examples: A macro-economic downturn favors a constellation that employs inexpensive staff or the postwar individualization that favors individual approaches over community initiatives.

ADAPTATION: *Internally induced constellation change*
A constellation alters its functioning either through interacting or merging with other constellations within or from outside the societal system.

   Example: The «Cross Work» approach that adapts from the fighting and prevention of epidemics, to community care, and later to individual homecare.

The approach makes use of the conceptual language of transition studies. Yet its familiar concepts, such as regimes and niches, are reframed in the context of a more rigorous theory. This allows for more systematic case analysis, as well as the description of transitions where technology is not such a prominent factor – such as in healthcare. The patterns themselves are *deduced* from the theoretical frame, which is in turn construed from the transitions studies state-of-the-art (for a thorough overview, consult Grin et al., 2010) and informed by various recent empirical insights.

Some comments on the process of classifying patterns of change are relevant here:

- Different patterns of change can occur within the same constellation at the same time. In the application to our case, some change patterns in some constellations in time overlap (partly) with a subsequent change pattern. This complicates a simple periodization of the histories of constellations. We have addressed this by grouping multiple change patterns in a single period of change where two patterns mostly overlapped or, in other instances, by allowing the time periods of description to partially overlap.
- Interactions between constellations have directionality: if constellation A gains power at the expense of constellation B, we will classify this as

constellation A being empowered (by its own strength or under landscape pressures). One could say that constellation B is "depowered."

- In most cases classification is quite straightforward, but in complex interactions discerning patterns of change can be more complicated; we will give some examples of this.
- In many typical accounts, niches are empowered or thrust into power by reconstellation, and the regime constellation subsequently adapts. However, this sequence of patterns does not occur by definition, and our case study shows different combinations.
- Instead of first describing an event or development and then classifying it, for practical reasons one may also use the pattern terms directly for brevity (e.g. "constellation A is empowered").

Step 3: interpretation (analysis), and Step 4: conclusion

When the results of the previous step are plotted against one timeline, a detailed, systematic overview emerges. As many separate patterns are identified, however, this overview needs to be simplified into a few overall developments. This step also allows one to construct the transition as a whole, at last, by addressing the following questions: (1) During which period did major change occur and which pattern (or patterns) dominated? (2) Which structural, cultural and practical changes occurred in many constellations and how did the total power of the constellations change? And (3) In which constellations does this new structure, practice and culture manifest the strongest? With the answers to these questions and the previous results, it becomes possible to answer the research questions (step 4).

3.3 Histories of constellations

This section describes the constellations and the landscape and corresponds to step 2 of our methodology. This includes classifying events and developments into patterns of transitional change.

The medical practitioners

The medical practitioners'[7] constellations are distinct constellations, but they are related through splits and mergers, as displayed in Figure 3.3.

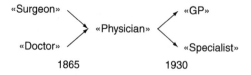

Figure 3.3 The merger and split of the medical practitioner constellations

The «surgeon» constellation

The abolishment of the guild system of surgeons during the French period (see below in this section) led to a vacuum that would be filled only slowly over the next decades. This process of change was obviously driven from the landscape level (the European geopolitical turmoil), and we therefore classify it as a "reconstellation" pattern. Surgeons were licensed locally, and later regionally, but there was no organized training. Without training (standards), licensing was ineffective. This reluctantly convinced government to establish state "clinical schools." This is a typical example of adaptation, whereby the regime adopts new elements. By 1840 the «surgeon» constellation represented an important healthcare approach, if unorganized, lacking theoretical education as well as methods for controlling infections following surgery. Table 3.1 provides an overview of the history of this constellation, by characterizing it in terms of structure, culture, practice and power at moments of relative stability (1800, 1818, 1840, 1864) in four, slightly overlapping periods of change.

The academic «doctor» and «physician»

Around 1800, falling ill was still attributed to divine will, although scientific explanations were gaining ground. Until 1840, however, these scientific interpretations tended to be quite nostalgic or Romantic. Disease was considered to be the result of the move from the countryside to urban life – an irreversible process. After 1840, modern scientific paradigms became more important. This development on the landscape level boosted the «doctor» paradigm, indicating that disease was caused by specific sources (e.g. bad odors) and could therefore be mitigated by intervention. Because it again involves a landscape influence that increases the power of a constellation, we label it a reconstellation pattern. In the regulation of the medical professions, the «doctor» gained superiority over the «surgeon» (even though this power shift was only slight it still classifies as an empowerment of doctors) and it was seldom enforced. The improved economy created a modest income surplus for the middle classes. Over the following decades, government-organized care and poor relief by charities would also reimburse doctors and surgeons. The status of the «doctor» constellation thus began to improve and acquire a legally exclusive position.

In the emergence of the modern Dutch state, 1848 was a landmark year: the monarchy was "constitutionalized" and power shifted to Parliament and government. This progressive-liberal climate was also reflected within Parliament and in the first modern, liberal government. Enforcement of medical licenses became a real option, and this in turn created specific options for empowerment patterns.

Consequently, the market competition between the «doctor» and the «surgeon» spilled into the political arena and resulted in a long turf war. At

Table 3.1 History of the surgeon constellation

	Structure	Culture	Practice	Power
1800	Embedded in guild structure, masters and apprentices, located near each other	Practical skills transferred from master to apprentice Surgery as craft	Bone setting, wound treatment, crude surgery (stone removal, amputation)	Mainly dealing with injury Surgery is last resort option Exclusive rights —— (niche regime)
1800–1820	Reconstellation:			
1818	Very little structure, ineffective local regulatory committees	Unchanged	Unchanged	Mainly dealing with injury Surgery is last resort option No exclusivity —— (weakened niche regime)
1808–1830	Reconstellation (and empowerment):			
1840	Education in clinical schools, some regulation by provincial committees	Surgeon as professional	Unchanged	Mainly dealing with injury Surgery is last resort option Regained exclusivity but inferior to doctor —— (weakened niche regime)
1840–1864	Adaptation:			
1864	Unchanged	Part of medical community	Bone setting, wound treatment, simple surgery	Mainly dealing with injury Surgery is last resort option but more survivable Regained exclusivity and professionalism but inferior to doctor —— (weakened niche regime)

the same time an opposite movement presented itself: in 1849 the Dutch Medical Association (NMG – "Nederlands Medisch Genootschap") was founded, a modern professional organization representing both surgeons and doctors. As such, the NMG was quite different from the old guild structure. Whereas the guilds themselves were in charge of regulation and training, based on the privileges granted to them by government, the NMG put pressure on the government to ensure adequate medical regulation and education. Rather than advocating training on the job, as in the apprenticeships of the old guild system, the NMG favored formal education and qualification through degrees.

In the period between 1850 and 1865, the constellations were framed as complementary instead of competing. This *rapprochement* continued up to the point where the constellations merged within a single profession: that of "physician."[8] Such a merger, marked by a shift of power within the system to a (new) constellation, is a clear case of an empowerment pattern. In 1865 a series of medical laws established the boundary between medicine and quackery. Dentists, pharmacists, physicians and midwives came out of this process as the "winners," while all others active in medical professions (including, for instance, owners of drugstores) lost out on institutional recognition and were potentially going to be labeled quack doctors.[9] For more than a century, the incumbent medical professions held legal exclusivity over novel medical professions, such as nurses or physiotherapists, who received full legal recognition by the end of the twentieth century.

From 1860 to 1920, favorable landscape conditions furthered the rise of the «physician», not only as a result of their gaining power from outside of the health system and the ongoing modernization (thus a reconstellation pattern). The use of inventions such as antiseptics and anesthetics greatly improved surgery and reduced infections. The constellation also gained power over other constellations. In fact, such other constellations were actively dismissed as forms of "quackery." we classify such change as an empowerment pattern because the constellation strengthens its position at the expense of others.

From 1880 onward, a more social-progressive climate strengthened the «physician», extending their role to the general hygiene of society (a reconstellation pattern). The physician would also become involved in public sanitary works, food safety, occupational safety, hygiene in public places (notably hospitals), assessing the fitness of potential civil servants, and verifying the illness of those who sought admittance to hospitals. In particular the *Rijksinspectie* (national medical regulatory agency) was a powerful mechanism. At the height of its power, the «physician» approach was dominant in every corner of the health system. Some aspects should be classified as empowerment, such as the rise of health insurance funds for doctors.[10]

The most powerful instruments of physicians remained hygiene and diagnostics. Hygiene led to better survival chances in cases of surgery, but most health was gained in non-medical sectors where hygiene was applied (such as sanitation and food safety). The diagnostic strength was contrasted with the barely increased therapeutic possibilities. Physicians would stress their role as a friend and counselor to the family of a sick person, and they mainly adopted a reassuring and mitigating stance.

The «specialist» and «general practitioner» («GP»)

From 1900 onward, the unity within the «physician» constellation began to erode The emancipation of *specialized doctors* at the expense of *general doctors* again led to a decades-long turf war, culminating in two separate constellations with a shared academic degree, but distinct structure, culture and practice (for a good account of the emergence and consolidation of the specialist profession, see Lieburg et al., 1997).

Although the «specialist» constellation would not become a significant constellation until the 1920s, its roots go back to the "unity of profession" regulation of 1865. This gave rise to a large, homogeneous group of physicians, as it began by grandfathering licenses for all previously licensed surgeons and doctors. Initially, this was not a problem, as the physicians won ground over the unqualified "quacks" and the physician constellation expanded. Eventually, however, there was again a surplus of medical professionals. This led some physicians, toward the end of the nineteenth century, to stress that they were "specialist." Often this meant that they specialized in treatments involving a specific instrument (such as the eye mirror).

These specialists were not the most esteemed physicians and mostly did not have a lucrative private practice with a middle-class clientele. Instead, they ran policlinics (Greek for "city clinics") for ad hoc clients from the lower classes. Aside from this class difference, the use of increasingly larger, hard-to-move devices confined the specialists to their clinics. Until about 1900 to 1910, the transition patterns were mainly driven by stress within the physician constellation, with specialists simply seeking to secure their livelihood. After that, the «specialist» constellation slowly became a force on its own (an empowerment pattern), putting the dominant «physician» constellation under pressure.

The change in dynamics had a number of causes. First, the clients of city clinics could easily be used as research and teaching material, whereas for a private doctor it would be out of the question to take a student with him on house calls (see e.g. Mooij, 1999). Slowly, specialists would become teaching authorities and the physicians of choice for new, interesting or complicated cases. A subsequent change involved the move of specialists from private practice to the hospital. Treating patients in hospital was hardly new for physicians, but it used to be confined to admitted patients. However, the advances in hygiene, the presence of a qualified nursing staff, and the high investment costs of X-ray and other machines drove the specialists into the hospital. It gave rise to a quid pro quo deal with hospitals, in which specialists treated admitted patients as teaching material, and the hospitals provided support staff (and technology) for the specialists' work in their policlinics. In the 1920s private policlinics were virtually extinct and the «hospital» constellation became more centered around the «specialist» constellation. If at one point the nurses (especially nuns) contracted a specialist, now a nurse would work under the supervision of the specialist. From the point of view of the interaction between hospital and specialist, we would label this an adaptation. However, in relation to the nursing profession, the «specialist» constellation empowered itself at the expense of the nursing profession. From the point of view of «nursing», their transformation from independent caretakers to assistants (in Dutch legal terms "extended arm of the physician")[11] could be seen as an adaptation to the emerging regime.

The symbiotic relationship of the «specialist» constellation with the «hospital» constellation is in sharp contrast with the long institutional turf war of the «specialist» with the «general practitioner», reminiscent of the struggle between the «surgeon» and the «doctor» half a century earlier. Although for some time general doctors had felt threatened by the rise of specialists, serious rivalry started only with the prospect of national legislation on healthcare financing in the early 1910s (which in the end was never enacted). The specialists founded their own group in order to have their interests better represented. Over the decades, the general doctors and specialist doctors would not only battle over issues pertaining to financing, but also education, professional registration and similar matters. With the rise of (voluntary) collective forms of health insurance for low-income groups (so-called "*ziekenfondsen*" or, literally, "sick funds"),[12] the financing of healthcare shifted from individual to collective arrangements in the first half of the twentieth century. These funds operated with a fixed reimbursement per patient (not per treatment) for physicians and pharmacists. In this way the income and expenses of the financing system were predictable and balanced, and physicians had a negative incentive to perform unnecessary treatments.

The specialists however did not fit into this system. Many alternatives were proposed and some were tried, ranging from fixed reimbursement for specialists to imbursement per patient. The battle ended in the 1930s with a stalemate: recognition of specialist care as a separate category and per treatment reimbursement for specialists, but only on referral by the general physician (Schouwstra, 1995). This introduced a new inconsistency, however, because it made it possible for general physicians to control the growth of the specialist constellation by limiting referrals. Each individual general physician, however, had a strong incentive to refer as quickly as possible. Treating a patient himself would increase his workload, not his income.

During World War Two, the German occupier ended the decades-long debate on a national healthcare financing arrangement by formalizing the status quo in legislation. All of a sudden, both the membership of a collective health coverage fund and a compulsory reimbursement regime were fixed. From the 1950s onward, the «specialist» constellation grew intensely. In the early 1960s, for the first time more specialists than general practitioners were

registered. At its peak in the mid-1990s, there were three times more specialists than general practitioners. Ironically, especially the explosion of expensive
«specialist care» necessitated collective «financing» for virtually everyone.
Because in this case two constellations mutually reinforce each other, we refer
to it as an empowerment pattern.

The «specialist» constellation was aided in outcompeting the «GP» constellation through advances in the «hospital» constellation. By the 1920s, modern
hospitals and operating theaters bore no resemblance to the nineteenth-
century "houses of death" anymore; at the time, people were even willing to
pay for separate insurance to be able to afford hospital care. After surgery's
modernization, the invention of antibiotics and similar drugs suddenly led to
near miraculous recovery of severely ill patients. In the following decades,
specialist care would continue to amaze the general public by new and at
times stunning showcases of the advances of the medical profession, such as
organ transplantation. The odds changed in favor of medical specialists, who
with their scientific knowledge and widely publicized technical abilities
increasingly outshone, and became the preferred choice over, the traditional
reassuring-friend-of-the-family type of physician – a development also stimulated by ongoing individualization.

The number of specialists in the Netherlands would continue to increase
until the 1990s. The «specialist» power peaked perhaps slightly earlier.
Growing individualization and a more critical attitude in society at large
undermined the notion of the specialist as an authority figure, That this led to
some loss of status is suggested by the appearance of patients' requests for
second opinions and popular media attention to medical mistakes and the
exorbitant costs of specialist healthcare.

The «general practitioner» was a residue of the physician constellation after
the specialist constellation diverged and entered into a symbiotic relation with
the «hospital». The limits of what general practitioners could achieve began to
show during the interwar period (Bremer, 2006). Although the «general practitioner» constellation would still show steady growth, it was outflanked by
that of the specialists. The stress following from the now infeasible ideal of
the universal physician led to a "if you can't beat them, join them" type of
behavior vis-à-vis specialization. In the second half of the twentieth century,
GPs sought recognition as a separate medical specialization. In the 1930s,
one-third of all GPs were members of the Dutch Association of General
Practitioners within the NMG. This emancipation as a specialty was concluded in 1973 with a separate registration as medical specialty. From this
point on, general practitioners were no longer "physicians without specialization," but so-called "basic physicians," a term denoting their eligibility to
enter the trajectory of further medical specialization or further medical training toward becoming a general practitioner. This is a typical case of a pattern
of adaptation to the regime.

The «hospital» and «nursing» constellation

The period between 1800 and 1850 (or even from as early as 1650) is often considered the dark age of hospitals. During the French period – in a typical reconstellation pattern – hospitals run by the clergy were repressed. This stimulated the gradual decline of the importance of religious institutions in public life over a longer period of time. The hospitals that remained became fully part of the care effort aimed at the poor. At the same time, the boundaries between hospitals, madhouses, poorhouses and jails were often unclear. From 1850 to 1950, however, the «hospital» would undergo a spectacular transformation, turning into an icon of modern healthcare (Houwaart, 1996).

In 1848, the new Dutch constitution granted equal rights to Catholic citizens, causing organized Catholic life to resurface. At the same time the *Protestants Réveil* (Protestant Awakening) took place, adding a more compassionate component to Protestantism's rational worldview.

During the same era, around 1850, the general attitude toward poverty in Dutch society shifted from regarding it as a natural phenomenon, to be addressed by pity and alms, to an avoidable condition of bad morale. Therefore, the poor were to be alleviated from their dire conditions by force, by limiting their access to poor relief resources. Unconditional support, such as in hospitals, was prohibited by the Poor Law of 1853, except for the care of the sick. Suddenly, Dutch hospitals, by reconstellation, became much more specific places, exclusively devoted to the sick. The Poor Law also gave rise to the active involvement of state-funded physicians, as admission to hospitals needed to be monitored. In time, the hospital would adapt toward a singularly medical function.

As a medical profession, nursing did not exist prior to 1850. The "nurses" who comprised the lay staff in hospitals were barely trained. Initially, the only ones trained in nursing were nuns associated with medical orders. The *Protestants Reveil*, however, created a different kind of nurse. In neighboring Germany, for example, deaconess hospitals took on female volunteers from the upper middle classes. In this context, Theodor Fliedler set up an advanced training program which trained Florence Nightingale and many others (Dane, 1980).

Unlike in Germany, the Dutch «hospital» constellation did not swiftly incorporate the modern nurse, possibly because physicians saw her as a challenge to their medical monopoly (and, more practically, middle-class women needed their own private accommodation). Many Dutch nurses, then, would enter the progressive niche of «Cross Work», locally based organizations interested in setting up networks of "district nurses," a new professional who would make house visits to provide care to those who signed up for it. In an adaptation pattern, hospitals slowly improved their standard of care, incorporating nurses trained by «Cross Work» organizations (Binnenkade, 1973). Combined with new hygienic insights, hospitals changed from exceptionally filthy to exceptionally clean environments. The function of the «hospital» constellation thus shifted from offering material refuge to providing a clean and caring environment for the sick.

Although the combination of «hospitals» and «specialists» served as an icon of the curative ideal, as discussed above, hospitals also hosted chronic patients who had no prospect of being cured whatsoever. After World War Two, these patients were perceived to occupy hospital beds that could better be used for "treatable" patients. For the original function of hospitals, the new constellation of «nursing homes» (or more broadly a system denoted as "care") emerged. This constellation saw further expansion after 1965, when such homes began to be funded by collective insurance rather than by municipal budgets. This pattern clearly reflects the empowering of nursing homes as a new niche, even if it was inspired, paradoxically, by the intent to reduce the resources invested in nursing. Still, it is difficult to say which of the two resulting constellations gained most power in the long run. The new function of hospitals speeded up the growth of the curative «hospital» constellation (until the budget curbs of the 1980s), as well as to its "glossy" image (no more chronic or senile patients). On the one hand, care facilities and nursing homes have outgrown hospitals in number of beds. The reduced significance of extended family in providing care and counsel greatly increased the need for professional care. As this is broad societal change fueling the growth of a niche, we identify it as a reconstellation pattern. On the other hand, because nursing comes with a much lower cost per bed, hospitals began increasingly to rely on these professionals

In the late nineteenth century, it was progressive for a woman not yet married to take on a volunteer job and be trained within a hospital. But by the 1950s and 1960s the social landscape had changed, and this implied that several aspects of nursing had become outdated, such as the lack of theoretical training, the low wage, the "calling" (as opposed to "profession") paradigm and the subordinate role to the male physician (Zwols, 1985). As of the 1970s, nurses evolved into professionals with normal pay and advanced training in the higher education system. Such developments that force change upon a societal sector or that fuel the growth of some particular niche may be seen as a reconstellation pattern.

«Financing»

Around 1800 one had to pay one's healthcare costs directly to the health provider. Even though typical costs were low, many lacked discretionary income and needed to apply to local Poor Relief organizations. Some guilds had a limited system of "sick funds" to spread costs. But during the French period, guilds and organized labor were prohibited. This prohibition briefly included the sick funds. Industrial decline between 1820 and 1840 impeded their re-emergence. From 1840 to 1880 many different initiatives similar to the old forms of coverage surfaced. These varied from funds organized by commercial insurers, the predecessors of welfare work and mutual funds. As curative therapy was rarely an option, many of these forms of insurance were largely concerned with funeral costs and compensation for lost wages.

The developments until 1890 were marked by the emergence of several niches, which however failed to grow due to an unfavorable landscape. In the period between 1880 and1920, large-scale manufacturing changed this landscape by creating large groups of (organized) workers. Moreover, fewer and fewer people could pay for long hospital stays, the use of expensive devices and advanced surgery. As noted above, cost-spreading arrangements and advanced medicine reinforced each other's development.

For some time, civic, voluntary initiatives were the only ones active in this domain, because debates on government regulation stalemated between conservatives, liberals, and a strong lobby from both workers' unions and physician organizations. Plans took longer to develop than a single term of government, and thus they were always vulnerable to political shifts in the country's fragmented political landscape. A lack of government interference did not hamper growth, and neither did the continuous rivalry between the different approaches toward health insurance and the turf war between physicians and particular insurance funds over the profitable middle and upper classes. But these developments did introduce stress and inconsistencies when the sick funds were institutionalized in the 1930s and 1940s (some of which have already been discussed in the context of the «specialist» constellation).

At first, income support was institutionalized. Many health insurance funds already separated income support from medical expenses, as these required a more specialized reimbursement system. In 1930, income support was separately legislated, being seen as less complicated and less controversial.

From 1940 to 1945, the German occupier froze the conflicts over reimbursement of medical care (a typical reconstellation pattern). Participation in sick funds became mandatory for all workers up to a certain wage. Although most of those involved had voluntary coverage already, this was still an irreversible breakthrough in institutionalization.

Up until World War Two, healthcare for the poor was still part of care for the poor in general. The underlying paradigm was still the "tough love" approach of the mid-nineteenth century. Based on this approach, the reaction to the mass unemployment of the 1930s crisis was to set up large-scale employment projects, such as manually digging new waterways. This confronted many skilled workers and clerks with strenuous physical labor, antagonizing a generation against the traditional approach of dealing with care for the poor. Subsequently, in the 1950s, the paradigm shifted from the view of unemployment as a matter of individual morale to its framing as a macroeconomic phenomenon. For the next several decades, income support was a right of the modern welfare state. The traditional form of poor relief was transformed into government-run social security. This paradigm shift from alms to right would spill over into healthcare financing.

Over the following decades all low-income groups would become compulsory members of sick funds. The private insurance market was regulated to conform its reimbursement policy to the sick funds, leaving only additional insurance for special treatments (e.g. alternative medicine) as a true insurance market. This harmonization of the financing arrangements for curative care was finalized in the early 2000s by a universal and compulsory "basic health-care insurance plan" for all.

The financing of long-term care (such as nursing homes) was transformed from a municipal budget matter into a national "collective insurance,"[13] pro-viding a resource base for an empowerment pattern. Other forms of care – such as home nursing or mental healthcare – were also transformed from local collective provisions to a national individual right.

Efforts were made after 1973 to curb expenses. The postwar economic boom had ended and the steadily shrinking welfare state could no longer afford to support the rapidly growing health system. The number of hospital beds was reduced and "budget ceilings" were introduced. Over the following decades the system was "tinkered" with, which – at best – reduced the growth rate of expenses temporarily (see Figure 3.4).

«Cross Work»

«Cross Work» is a specifically Dutch phenomenon that was in operation from approximately 1875 to 1980. It consisted of so-called cross organizations, civic healthcare initiatives that started out as organizations to prepare for and prevent epidemics. They developed into comprehensive neighborhood-oriented healthcare organizations and finally evolved into present-day home-care providers (Knoop and Schuiringa, 1998).

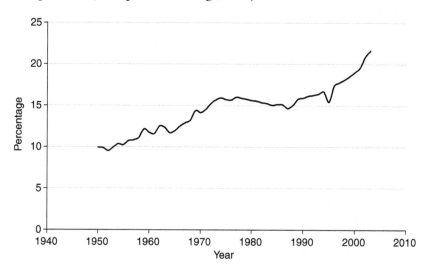

Figure 3.4 Dutch collective spending on healthcare as percentage of total collective spending

Data source: CPB.

Cross organizations were a response to a growing dissatisfaction with the lack of effort of municipalities in implementing adequate healthcare and epidemic prevention. The «Cross Work» constellation follows a typical empowerment pattern. The first cross organization was founded in 1875 as a volunteer organization by a health inspector who turned his attention to civil society with other members of the higher classes, envisioning a "peacetime Red Cross."

The original cross organizations primarily prepared for an epidemic that in the end never came, which in fact was perhaps partly the fruit of their preventive, hygienic program. In response, «Cross Work» underwent an adaptation pattern by widening its organizational scope to general healthcare. It grew into a broader movement and became a source of local pride, especially in rural communities – where municipal health services were absent. As such, this organization serves as a perfect example of an adaptation allowing for an empowerment pattern. Its buildings, originally used for storing materials to be used during epidemics, now also stocked materials used in long-term care such as crutches.

The upscaling of cross organizations fostered a further empowerment pattern. In the 1920s' liberal-confessional political climate, they managed to outcompete the municipal health services of the «Public Health» constellation. Importantly, cross organizations were ideologically neutral, and this was unusual in Dutch society at the time, marked as it was by strictly segregated religious and political "pillars" that each had their own social and cultural organizations (see also "landscape developments"). Initial Protestant and Catholic protests against government support for such neutral organizations ceased after the founding and funding of separate Protestant and Catholic cross organizations.

This period also introduced inconsistencies, however. «Cross Work» was marked by a bottom-up paradigm, but de facto it partly evolved into a top-down implementer of public health tasks. Moreover, cross organizations were no longer neutral, but each belonged to an ideological faction or social pillar. Originally this was a strength, since it allowed them to embed their effort in a larger societal structure. But in the 1960s, when Dutch society quickly grew more individualized, the social pillars lost much of their relevance. Another byproduct of individualization was a drop in volunteer work. People regarded their membership of a cross organization rather as a subscription on homecare, not as support of integral community care. All these factors weakened the cross organizations, forcing them to accept more government funding. In the 1970s, budget cuts forced scale increases, leading to a vicious circle as it further alienated these organizations from their original locally based community structure. In the 1980s the cross organizations were integrated into the care (financing) as providers of homecare.

«Public health»

During most of the nineteenth century, government became increasingly involved in funding poor relief organizations that provided healthcare but refrained from other involvement. During the French period an ambitious plan for a state-run health system was devised, but was never implemented. Decades later, a new governmental plan to employ more "state physicians" was struck down in the liberal climate of the 1850s.

Social matters were a municipal responsibility in the new "decentralized and unitary state." National involvement was limited to the licensing of medical professionals, keeping statistics and advising municipalities. The latter had little affinity with healthcare. In contrast to other constellations, the landscape was unfavorable from 1850 to 1900, leaving no room for reconstellation patterns. From 1890 onward, the role of government grew; large cities in particular increasingly bore the costs for poor relief, including healthcare. To manage costs, they wanted to verify the necessity of specific expenses by employing government physicians, who started rudimentary quality regulation of the institutions they inspected or monitored.

A new generation of physicians, the so-called hygienists' movement, pressed for a more proactive agenda. These hygienists argued that in the new political era, liberalism should include extensive provisions for a health infrastructure and health services by the government. Moreover, health regulations pertaining to food, working conditions and other aspects were introduced. This needed to be verified by more government physicians and biologists.

Starting in the late nineteenth century, the Netherlands changed from an early industrial society (with dispersed industrial production) to a full-blown industrial society (with concentrated production in large factories in industrial districts). This brought crowding, poor living conditions and industrial accidents, which in turn required pest and disease control, emergency aid, school physicians, etc. These types of activities were difficult to provide for by commercial and charitable parties, especially as some would require intrusion of the private sphere (Querido, 1965).

Initially, there was little coordination between the various medical tasks of the municipalities. From the 1920s, large cities started to merge their medical services into integrated public services. These aimed to provide healthcare directly, especially to the poor. The growth of municipal services under urbanization is a reconstellation pattern, and their integration – to strengthen their position – an empowerment pattern.

Still, the new constellation only filled the void left by other constellations in the largest cities for clients who could not afford private practice physicians, as well as for problems that required government enforcement (Kerkhoff, 1994). Throughout the period under study, proposals were launched to expand this marginal role to a more comprehensive public health service in at least five attempts.

After the attempts by the French in the early 1800s and the conservative attempt in the mid-1850s, a third attempt was made in 1920 under a center-left government that proposed compulsory public health services for all municipalities, but the proposal failed to gain enough support. The fourth attempt was made in the 1940s and 1950s. During the war, the Dutch government in exile had witnessed the start of the National Health Service (NHS) in the UK. On its return in 1945, its enthusiasm was met with the skepticism of a segregated society. A law was eventually passed in 1965, but it reconfirmed the primacy of private parties, while public health services and councils were reduced to marginally coordinating and stimulating it.

After 1960, the «public health» constellation lost its central function as healthcare provider to the poor, as this function was transferred to sick funds. Many of the subsequently unemployed municipal doctors became the first "organizational or company doctors," contributing to a new «occupational health» constellation. This may be seen as an empowerment pattern (with «public health» on the losing side), followed by an empowerment pattern into a new niche.

In 1974, the political climate again shifted to the left and the financing constellation approached the limits of its growth. A window of opportunity opened to reintroduce a national health system and a law was passed in 1982. During the same year the law was retraced as the window of opportunity was closed by a political shift to the right and the start of an economic crisis. During the 1980s, new activities such as venereal disease education, preventive disease screening and disaster management were undertaken. In the end, in 1990, 70 years after the first proposal, it was mandatory for all municipalities to run a (joint) public health service.

«Mental health»

Initially, mental health*care* was restricted to locking up the insane in madhouses or prisons if they were a burden to society. The French Revolution introduced the paradigm that an insane person was mentally ill and ought to be treated as a patient. This led to a series of legislation that organized «mental healthcare» around the asylum (Schut, 1970). The practice remained institutionalization, but culturally the insane gained recognition as patients.

In the second half of the nineteenth century the somatic approach from «hospitals» became prevalent in mental institutions (Vijselaar, 1982) in a typical adaptation pattern. The mentally ill were treated like patients with a physical illness: in beds. From the beginning of the twentieth century, the more traditional, conversational relationship with the mental patient re-emerged under the influence of Freud and Breuer, a process sometimes referred to as *re-psychologization* (Dankers and van der Linden, 1996)

From the 1920s, «mental healthcare» went through patterns of adaptation and empowerment, leading to a *medicalization* of mental healthcare. New mental illnesses were diagnosed (notably schizophrenia) and medication led to a depopulation of the asylums. The joint rise of clinical psychology and social psychology led to a process of deinstitutionalization. From the 1950s the WHO started to recognize mental disorders as diseases. After World War Two, societal welfare became important, leading to the establishment of several (public) institutions for mental healthcare, such as the RIAGGs,[14] and various arrangements under collective financing for long-term care in 1980.

Landscape developments

From the histories of the individual constellations, we can infer the landscape developments that influenced the dynamics of the Dutch health system by reconstellations, but also by influencing shifts of power within the system and forcing constellations to adapt.

- *Medicine and philosophy of science:* The French period accelerated the Enlightenment in the Netherlands and gave primacy to academic explanations. Academic explanations of the early nineteenth century were holistic and Romantic, and were thus less suited for specific interventions. Half-way through the century, the modern, reductionist, scientific method gained ground. From 1850 to 1900, a general theory on the origin of infectious diseases was established and antiseptics and anesthetics were invented. Between 1900 and 1960 these were complemented by therapeutic pharmaceuticals and diagnostic equipment. After 1960 medicine would continue to become ever more sophisticated. At the end of the period under study, medicine was at the forefront of scientific standards and rigor.
- *Religion and society:* Initially, the Netherlands was dominated by a Protestant ethics with a hard-hearted tendency. From 1850 onward this rational Protestantism was complemented by a more compassionate Protestantism that aimed to elevate the weaker (the *Réveil*, or Awakening). At the same time, the repression of Catholicism ended, which allowed organized Catholic care. As a result of the emancipation of Catholics and the rise of Socialism, from 1900 to 1950 Dutch society became denominationally segregated or "pillarized." This segregation abruptly fell into decline from the late 1960s and early 1970s, when individualization became the predominant cultural paradigm.
- *State and politics:* In the nineteenth century, Dutch political life was marked by a struggle between monarchy and democracy. Initially, the monarchy dominated, but a wave of revolution (attempts) in Europe around 1850 gave momentum toward a constitutional monarchy. In the resulting political system, no single ideology dominated. Until 1900, power shifted back and forth between conservatives and liberals, and from 1900 to 1990 the confessional parties (Catholic, Protestant, Dutch-Reformed) entered into different government coalitions, often with liberals. Aggregated over the decades, this favored combinations of publicly funded civil organizations (which aligned with confessional parties) and private insurance and practice (which aligned with liberal ideology). The Dutch state itself slowly built an apparatus of civil servants and legal authority capable of intervening in previously local matters, such as healthcare.

- *Economy:* In the early nineteenth century, the Netherlands was impoverished after a century of wars and internal strife. The medieval system of guilds as basis for quality regulation, education and market protection gave way to a more liberal market. Although this happened throughout Europe and medieval structures such as the guilds and clergy had already grown weaker, the abolishment of such structures occurred in the Netherlands over a very short period after French domination. Alternative structures according to ideals of the Enlightenment and the French Revolution never materialized. This created a void in areas such as regulation and education, which stagnated much of the transition in healthcare. It would take until 1840/1850 for the economy to pick up steam again. In the late nineteenth century, industrialization introduced large-scale manufacturing, leading to safety- and crowding-related health issues. The first half of the twentieth century was characterized by economic ups and downs (such as the two wars and the Great Depression), followed by a postwar economic boom. Arguably this boom allowed for comprehensive, compulsory, national arrangements instead of the previous fragmented, voluntary, municipal budget financing arrangements.
- *Social security/poor relief:* The nineteenth-century care for the poor played an important role in financing medical practitioners, while hospitals were initially more part of poor relief than any other societal constellation. Poor relief underwent two transitions itself: from alms to "tough care to social security as right." In the first transition, specifically the 1854 Poor Law, hospitals were redefined as places exclusively for the sick (Van der Heyden et al., 1994). Enforcement of this rule was put into the hands of the predecessors of municipal health services. The "aid as right" paradigm strongly influenced the heavy government regulation on curative healthcare insurance. The new financing structures of social security – national collective insurance – became a model for chronic care financing.

3.4 Interpretation

In the previous sections we gave a detailed account of the histories of the individual constellations. Although it is clear that virtually all constellations have changed and that these processes of change are interrelated, the interactions are complicated. Constellations interact and experience autonomous change, leading to an overall pattern and direction, but not without significant amounts of "noise." This makes any inference of the overall dynamics somewhat dependent on interpretation. In our interpretation we move from patterns to dynamic areas (step 3 of the methodology) and from dynamic areas to overall conclusions (see below).

To render our interpretation more transparent, in Table 3.2 we indicate for each constellation the patterns described in the previous section over time. We propose to aggregate those patterns into the following areas, as listed in the lower half of Table 3.2.

Table 3.2 Overview of patterns in each constellation over time (upper half) and aggregation into areas of dynamics (lower half)

	1800–1820	1820–1840	1840–1860	1860–1880	1880–1900	1900–1920	1920–1940	1940–1960	1960–1975	1975–1990
Mental healthcare	Reconstellation				Adaptation	Adaptation	Adaptation	Adaptation	Adaptation	Reconstellation
Hospitals and nursing				Reconstellation	Reconstellation	Adapt and empower	Adapt and empower	Adapt and empower		
Specialist (no hospital)										De-powerment
Surgeon	Reconstellation	Reconstellation								
Physician/GP			Empowerment	Empower reconstellation	Reconstellation	De-powerment	Reconstellation			Empowerment
Doctor		Reconstellation								
Financing	Reconstellation		Reconstellation		Reconstellation	Reconstellation	Adaptation	Reconstellation and empowerment	Empowerment	Reconstellation
Cross Work			Empowerment and reconstellation			Empowerment	Empower and adapt		Reconstellation and de-powerment	
Public health				Empowerment	Reconstellation	Reconstellation	De-powerment	De-powerment	De-powerment	Reconstellation

	1800–1820	1820–1840	1840–1860	1860–1880	1880–1900	1900–1920	1920–1940	1940–1960	1960–1975	1975–1990
Mental healthcare										
Hospitals and nursing										
Specialist (no hospital)						Adaptation to regime	First regime (empowerment)			New era
Surgeon	Breakdown by Reconstellation	Void					Original regime as "niche within the regime"			
Physician/GP										
Doctor							Final regime (empowerment)			
Financing				First transitional regime						
Cross Work				Reconstellation and empowerment		De-powering of alternatives				
Public health										

Breakdown of the system by reconstellation, resulting in a void
(1800–1840)

From 1795 to 1815, the French presence in the Netherlands led to a strong reconstellation. Various old societal structures, such as guilds and socially active religious orders, went into decline or disappeared altogether. Often, these structures received a "final blow" in this era, as many had already been weakened by modernization.

The French attempts to rebuild the system were overambitious and not implemented after the French left the Netherlands, causing a decades-long void. This void was not caused by a lack of new alternatives or potential in the health system, but by adverse landscape conditions. The country was impoverished and the state weak. Because of the prevalence of a religious-Romantic attitude toward illness and a hard-heartedness toward the weak, there was no fruitful soil for any of the new approaches to healthcare to gain momentum.

Growth of many alternatives under reconstellation (1840–1875/1940)

During the period from 1840 to 1850, the Netherlands entered a new era. The attitude among Protestants changed from resignation to a more positive and uplifting stance, while Catholic institutions were reinstated and Catholics as a social group became visible again in public life. The economy resurged, creating income surpluses. A liberal political climate replaced the absolute monarch with an early form of democracy. The state grew stronger, but left most policy areas to the local and regional governments. The combination of new religious and liberal attitudes limited intramural care to the disabled and sick (instead of to the poor), thus medicalizing the «hospital».

From around 1880 until 1920, there was a second wave of reconstellation patterns, driven not only by innovations in medicine, but also by a changing Dutch society. In the early nineteenth century the Netherlands was quite urbanized, yet on a small, pre-industrial scale. After around 1900, large-scale industrialization and urbanization took place, and the social structure grew more strongly segregated. This made it possible for initiatives such as «Cross Work» to become funded by public means, without them becoming public themselves.

Taken together, these developments created tremendous potential for growth of the health system. Many constellations were initiated or gained power. Overall, the constellations reinforced each other, as exemplified by the hospitals' adaptation of the "nurse" as a trained professional from «Cross Work».

Empowerment of the «physician» (as simple regime) as a result of the merger of «surgeon» and «doctor» from 1840 to 1900/1940

Within the process of the growth and reinforcement of the different alternatives, one constellation gained an early lead over the others and would become the dominant approach to healthcare. Especially around 1900, the culture, structure and practice of the general physician were the focal point of the health system. Aside from being a medical authority, they also acted as "friend of the family" to the middle and upper classes, while apart from practicing medicine they advised and promoted health in many other domains.

The main constituent, the old "doctor" constellation, combined a strong past with a potent image of the future. With the fall of the guild system and the decline of religious rule over secular life, the academic system was one of the few remaining respected institutions in which medical occupations could be embedded. At the same time, the sciences gained in academic and societal prestige, making the physician's approach a promise for the future. The merger with surgeons provided practical, surgical skills to the constellation. The merger transformed the competiveness between the surgical and academic approach into a combined approach of highly educated and skilled medical professionals.

Empowerment of the physician, hospital, specialist and healthcare financing (into a compound regime) from 1930 to 1970

This hegemony of the «physician» constellation did not last, however. The focal point of healthcare shifted to the combination of individually practicing «specialists» and the larger scale «hospital». In a long process of co-evolution, the «hospital» (and its nurses) became subservient to the specialists' practice.

The original « physician» constellation lived on in that of the «general practitioner». On the one hand, the GP was the very opposite of specialist medicine. After all, GPs had lasting relationships with their clients and practiced individual care at a neighborhood level. On the other hand, GPs were pivotal in the specialist system as the central referring actor. This even held for the GPs' role as confidant, where patients would be referred to psychotherapists.

Financing arrangements originally tried to provide the lower classes with the same level of services already available to the middle classes. In the twentieth century, the financing arrangements grew to the extent that any constellation needed some form of cost spreading, also for the middle classes. These arrangements began to shape healthcare. The emancipation of specialists took place through changes in the financial regulation sick funds. Healthcare financing became an industry in its own right, fueled by the growing need for coverage of new and costly medical possibilities. In the second half of the twentieth century, the sick funds changed from voluntary risk pooling to a public instrument of solidarity and even a basic right. The separation of chronic care from the normal budget removed many limits on growth within the early «financing system», in particular with respect to specialist healthcare.

Conforming to the regime by adaptation, split-off and merger («mental healthcare», «hospital», «Cross Work») between 1860 and 1990

The constellations that were not part of the new compound regime went into an adaptation pattern and so conformed to the regime. The «hospital» incorporated the specialists and even split off its traditional nursing task to a new constellation (that of nursing and caring).

The «mental healthcare» constellation modeled itself in part after the somatic hospital and physician. In the nineteenth century, «mental health» adopted the practice of putting people in beds from hospitals. Twentieth-century psychotherapy was partly a turn away from medical paradigms, but the ambulatory type of practicing was taken from developments in somatic care. The twentieth-century ambulatory care centers (RIAGG) resembled hospitals in the way they were organized. Highly individual psychotherapy was often practiced from large semi-public institutions. This is remarkable, as the reasons for somatic therapy to embed itself in large-scale institutions – such as hygiene, large devices and nurses – have no equivalent in psychotherapy.

What today remains of the original «Cross Work» constellation has also adopted the paradigm of delivering specific care to the individual, as a replacement for a collective, neighborhood approach.

Depowerment of «Cross Work», «public health» in the period 1925/1950 to 1970/1980

The difference between relevant developments in the years between 1865 and 1900 and those during the period between 1910 and 1990 is that empowerment patterns occurred between the constellations, instead of between constellations and the environment of the system. This may be seen in Table 3.2 in the occurrence of more empowerment patterns and much less reconstellation. This means that power was not gained from the environment, but shifted within the system. Although the health system as a whole expanded, the dynamics started to resemble that of a "zero sum game," with some constellations gaining at the expense of others. Examples are the specialists (and the specialist hospital), who gained power at the expense of nursing, public health and the "general doctor," but also «Cross Work», for example, which gained power at the expense of «public health».

Slight depowerment of compound regime in the 1970s and 1980s

The compound regime has continued to grow in absolute, economic terms up until the present. We can however observe a weakening of the power of the regime relative to other constellations and in cultural aspects. «Hospitals» have faced a renewed preference for extramural (home) care and have faced reductions (in beds) and budget ceilings since the 1980s. Second opinions and attention to medical mistakes and excessive incomes of specialists have gained media attention. Financing arrangements have been questioned since the 1970s. Largely symbolic deductibles and exclusions were introduced.

Changes in structure, culture, practice and power

After having aggregated the "how" question, we can do the same for the "what" question by finding which trends may be identified within the diversity of structure, culture, practice and power changes within constellations. These findings are summarized in Table 3.3.

We find that the structure of the primary process has remained unchanged, whereas the financing and regulation have been subject to upscaling. We further note a tendency toward specialization. The know-how has shifted from traditional sources, by holistic means, to scientific sources. This is accompanied by a shift in attention to very specific causes. Interestingly, care (nursing, alleviating pain), the most important paradigm at the start, shifted to prevention (sanitation, hygiene) in combination with the "caring" physician, but with the rise of the specialist and therapeutic hospitals there was eventually a shift to "curing." Practices have changed from typical routines focused on permanent institutionalization to routines that try to efficiently route patients into, through and out of the health system.

Over time, the boundaries of the system shifted considerably. First, in the late nineteenth century healthcare expanded to infrastructure, nutrition, etc. and diffused the hygienist approach in these sectors, but ultimately these fields themselves would not become part of what is considered healthcare. Second, healthcare was originally mainly reserved for serious illness, to be later expanded to tackle minor ailments as well (for example, slight depression, light allergies). Third, in the context of mental health the world of healthcare was expanded to include large new domains, pertaining to issues associated with the "soul," "happiness" and "public order."

3.5 Conclusion

We can now finally move on to step 4 of the methodology and reflect on our research questions as formulated in the introduction to this chapter.

How did the current system come about?

The current regime, characterized as it is by a focus on curing, came about in two dynamic phases between 1820 and 1970, after the vulnerable old regime was basically destroyed by French influences and the Dutch nation's ensuing impoverishment. Note that we thus found the actual transition in fact

Table 3.3 Overall changes in structure, culture and practice

	From	Via	To
Structure:			
Organization of primary process	Individual practices and larger institutions		Individual practices and larger institutions
Specialization	Some specialization	Some specialization	Highly specialized
Organization of financing and regulation	Individual voluntarily	Collective individually and municipal budgets	National and compulsory
Culture:			
Knowledge and know-how	Philosophy and craft	Holistic, romantic science	Reductionist, scientific method (evidence-based)
Cause of disease	Divine will	Environment	Specific causes
Paradigm	Care	Prevention/care	Cure
Practice:			
Process of treatment	Complaint → diagnosis → institutionalization *and* Complaint → diagnosis (→ treatment)	Complaint → entry check → diagnosis → institutionalization (→ release) *and* Complaint → entry check → diagnosis → treatment	Complaint → initial diagnosis and referral → specialist diagnosis → specialist treatment (DBC)
Power *(within society)*	Limited for minor ailments and last resort	System for prevention and cure of somatic disease and serious mental illness	Iconic, authoritative and resource-rich for *treatment* of virtually all diseases and unhappiness

occurring between 1820 and 1970, within the research period between 1800 and 1990.

First, in the decades after 1820 many different alternatives reinforced each other and competed with each other to fill the void. From this period, the physician – as a merger of the classical surgeon and academic doctor – emerged as a simple regime. The focus shifted to prevention. This particular professional approach gained dominance because it was a strong combination of the practical surgeon and theoretical doctor, in a society with a belief in science, which was confirmed by a series of medical innovations. However, this factor in combination with the abundance of physicians also led to the rise of the specialist.

Subsequently, as powers shifted and dynamics internalized, a compound regime of the specialist, the hospital and the compulsory financing arrangements emerged with a firm focus on curative therapies. Specific financial arrangements enabled the spectacular growth of specialist healthcare. Other approaches, such as «Cross Work» and public health, were marginalized, also because of an individualizing society, or had to adopt elements from the approach of this specialist-hospital-financing combination. Healthcare became more sharply demarcated and much broader than it once was, including approaches for minor ailments and mental health.

Can we find roots of the current persistency and contestation of the regime in its past?

With regard to contestation, we found in our study that the regime is not a monolithic entity; rather, it is a combination of different constellations that strengthen and lock each other in. This compound nature of this regime brings ambiguity. This regime is a compromise between centralization and individualization. The financing is collective and centralized,[15] while the practice (and culture) of healthcare is highly individualized (the specialist treating the patient). This is expressed by some awkward combinations; for example, many specialists work as small private commercial firms within large not-for-profit private foundations (hospitals) that provide a public service, delegated, financed and "inspected" by the government.

This stress was built in by the 1930s' reimbursement of specialists, which removed the traditional checks-and-balances that made the system fundable from modest contributions from workers. As a result, healthcare entered a spiral of more expensive treatments and a growing financing constellation. For this reason, it is hardly surprising that after the postwar economic boom this stress resurfaced.

Furthermore, this regime is a "child of its time." The major changes occurred at a time when society was dealing with infectious diseases, against a backdrop of an impoverished lower class and an urbanizing and industrializing society. The authoritative role of the physician and hierarchically organized institutions were molded to the late nineteenth- and early twentieth-century organizational and cultural ideals.

Finally, from the 1970s onward, the contestation could also be the result of the cultural expectations versus actual increases in health (see Figure 3.5). Barring fundamental breakthroughs in, for example, genetics, the maximum lifespan of a human being is a little over 100 years. Thus the present potential for lengthening life expectancy seems only to be an additional ten to 20 years (*c.* 20 percent), instead of the 40 years gained between 1860 and 1960 (*c.* 100 percent). And for these ten to 20 years it is highly questionable if it can be fully obtained by a curatively focused healthcare (see also Le Fanu (1999 and 2000) for this argument). Of course lifespan is not a comprehensive health indicator, but the potential gain in healthy years may not be that different. Nevertheless, society continues to increase its investments, especially in curative care, leading to a diminishing return effect that puts pressure on the system.

This particular case may have some wider implications for transition studies. We found indications in line with the literature that other constellations tend to conform to the regime, potentially limiting diversity and innovation and thus a factor in the persistency of the status quo. However, this may or may not be an undesired factor. For example, the "somatic approach" in the mental healthcare of the second half of the nineteenth

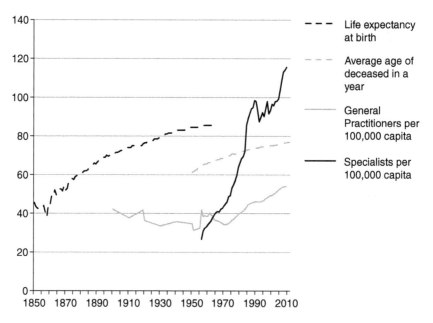

Figure 3.5 Medical professionals versus available longevity indicators

Source: CBS Statline.

Note
For increasing longevity, the average age of those deceased in a year trails the actual life expectancy at birth (approximately by the average age/life expectancy). In reality, longevity will probably be determined by healthcare over an individual's entire life span.

century, characterized by putting people in beds and "treating" them by water boarding and lobotomies, may be seen as the negative side of regime conformation. But the twentieth-century conformation of the same constellation to the regime turned out to be quite positive. Pharmaceuticals affecting neurological processes were very helpful in controlling psychological problems, even though it could be argued that they are currently overused. The mimicking of the somatic hospitals' approach through ambulatory or short-stay treatments also liberated many from lifelong institutionalization.

Moreover, the correlation between a regime and the failure of alternatives to succeed does not imply causation. The landscape can easily be the underlying third factor. For example, the «Cross Work» constellation diminished as a result of a changed society, not because of the specialist-hospital-insurance regime. Arguably, «Cross Work» conforming to this regime as "homecare" saved it from being obliterated altogether.

Why and where did the alternatives founder?

This last point relates to the third question. We can reframe this question as: Why did the «Cross Work» and «public health» constellations specifically decline and, ultimately, become marginalized?

The history of «Cross Work» has been closely interwoven with landscape developments. It was the *Protestants Réveil* and appreciation of civic initiative that led to its inception and growth. It successfully adopted a new approach when its original aim, namely fighting epidemics, was no longer necessary. It survived societal tensions over segregation (*pillarization*) by itself becoming segmented into different ideologies. Its position within the health system was strong: it redefined nursing in hospitals through its education programs and it acquired "public functions" such as vaccination at the expense of the «public health» constellation. «Cross Work» thus had considerable power within the health system and was not a plaything of "the regime." Its strong decline, however, is much more closely related to changing circumstances in the wake of World War Two. Dutch society individualized and people were less willing to work for free or for low pay. People started to interpret «Cross Work» as a subscription service instead of as a community-based initiative. «Cross Work» adapted toward more central public financing, but this would introduce stress within its decentralized, diversified organization.

A similar story may be told for the "direct public health" approach. It has been a "logical next step" for over one-and-a-half centuries, owing to either the public nature of health or the heavy government involvement in health-care financing. However, being a logical next step was never sufficient. During most of the nineteenth century public health initiatives failed, because of a mismatch with a very limited role for the (central) government in society. Public health services started to develop during the first half of the twentieth century, but did not align with the segregation of society. After World War Two, this segregation was still too strong to allow the NHS example of the

UK to be taken over. The 1970s' progressive left climate did not last long enough for cost and fragmentation concerns to be addressed by «public health».

The histories of direct «public health» and «Cross Work» demonstrate the decisive influence financial arrangements can have – arrangements which are sometimes changed by politics, but mostly frozen in time, because changing the status quo seems to require much more force than maintaining the status quo. This points to the necessity of relatively long, stable political climates to achieve change.

It should also be noted, finally, that the absence of a strong constellation within a societal system does not equal the absence of societal impact. Looking only within the boundaries of what is generally considered to be part of healthcare, prevention seems a weakly represented part. However, from the histories of the constellations we learned that many preventive successes could take place because these ideas diffused out of the health system into other societal systems. It is a non-trivial judgment whether it is better to develop a strong approach within a single societal system or to diffuse particular ideas or practices broadly across into other societal systems.

3.6 Discussion

The framework and its application to this case study demonstrates the potential for using methods from transition studies to research developments in healthcare. It allows understanding of both the bottom-up processes of change (such as those identified by e.g. Schrijvers, 2008) and top-down influences (such as many accounts of the history of medicine). The use of constellations allows the unraveling of the diversity and complexity noted by the WHO (2000) in its perspective on health systems.

As main advantages of our specific approach within transition studies for retrospective case studies, we already mentioned that (1) what the transition entails does not need to be a priori decided, nor does it need to be technological in nature; and (2) system demarcation and inferring overall dynamics can be done in a systematic, transparent way.

In other words, our approach *systematically* opens up the layer underlying societal transitions. If our approach does not cover even lower level dynamics, we touched upon some of these small-scale dynamics in the constellation descriptions. Sometimes these small-scale dynamics have been compellingly and rigorously studied already, such as the uniting of doctors and surgeons in the mid-nineteenth century (see Houwaart, 1991) and the emancipation of specialists through the reimbursement war during the period 1920 to 1940 (see Lieburg et al., 1997).

In other instances, this kind of high-level case study might identify areas of interest for lower level case studies such as in our case: (1) the "decision" by the general physicians' community to paradoxically turn their profession into "a specialization," instead of maintaining the idea of the universal physician;

(2) the introduction of nurses into the «hospital constellation» from the Cross Work organizations, as a typical example of innovation arising in niches; (3) the failure of a more encompassing public health service during the period from 1970 to 1980s and, more in general, the forming of an early awareness that the current regime may not be sustainable; and (4) the choices and deliberations within the Cross Work organizations to accept government funding, even if seemingly against their core value of communal autonomy. The identification of key moments to be studied in detail may very well be another application of the framework presented in this chapter.

Finally, we would like to comment on the implications for policy-making for transitions on societal systems in general. Hitherto societal transitions were usually described by tracing the incumbent regime back in time to one (or more) small niches or innovations. The resulting innovation journey describes how, against the backdrop of the landscape, a niche changes or becomes the regime. Instead of such a long and winding road view, our framework offers more of a "spaghetti" view on developments. Many different alternatives interact with each other and the mainstream, resulting in the emergence of a new regime. Although the winding road may be appropriate for an entrepreneur or pressure group focusing on a single alternative, the helicopter view of complex interacting alternatives may be more suitable for governmental policy-makers, trade associations or broad societal movements. It puts the focus on the strategic stimulation of many alternatives and their interactions over fostering one "winner," who may be impossible to identify in advance.

Notes

1 Constellations and societal systems may be seen as the larger (or more general) and smaller (or more specific) elements of a scalable, nested concept.
2 Attributed to Einstein.
3 Dutch: "arts." Note that for such specific Dutch terms for medical practitioners, there is often no direct equivalent in English. In such instances we will use the closest term available in English.
4 Nursing could also be interpreted as an independent component, first coupled to the Cross Work constellation, later to the hospital constellation, and again later also to the "nursing and care" sector of course.
5 These constellations may provide useful insight as they seem to have been subject to some typical turf wars with the regime constellation(s) over the boundary of what is medical and what is not medical. In particular, midwifery would be interesting, because the Netherlands is quite unique in its high degree of home deliveries and system of maternal care.
6 Dutch: "armenzorg." Note that although the label of the constellation is translated as "poor relief," this does not necessarily imply a "relief" attitude toward the poor.
7 The meaning of English equivalents for Dutch names of particular professions may differ slightly from that in English or American contexts. In particular, "surgeon" (Dutch: "chirurgijn") should be understood as the guild-based profession, not the modern medical profession (Dutch: "chirurg").
8 Although physician (Dutch: "arts") was not a new notion, before the 1860s it occurred sporadically (WNT, 1998).

9 One should be careful in extending this conclusion about labeling to other forms of alternative medicine. In the nineteenth century, many such forms that are now clearly in the domain of pseudoscience were not immediately disqualified for research and teaching. In fact, unconventional therapies, by today's standards, such as "scaring" patients out of mental illness by near-drowning, were taken quite seriously.

10 Dutch: "Artsenfondsen."

11 In Dutch: "verlengde arm van de arts," a legal construction in which physicians mandated tasks to "their" nurses. These tasks were then performed by the nurses as if by the physician. This practice ended in 1993 when nursing became an independent profession again.

12 "Ziekenfondsen" are a Dutch healthcare financing arrangement, originally started as very small-scale solidarity funds among apprentices (and sometimes among masters) to pay for costs related to sickness and death, later more resembling a typical insurance (and after the 2006 changes to the healthcare insurance Act (*zorgverzekeringswet*), all sick funds became insurance schemes).

13 Dutch: "Volksverzekering," or, literally, people's insurance. More specifically it involved the AWBZ ("Algemene Wet Bijzondere Ziektekosten"), or, literally, General Act on Extraordinary Expenditures in Case of Illness).

14 *Regionale Instelling voor Ambulante Geestelijke Gezondheidszorg* – literally: Regional Facility for Ambulatory Mental Healthcare.

15 Of course, the curative sick funds and insurers have never been nationalized or centralized. However, they are so heavily regulated and institutionally embedded that de facto the system comes close to a national health insurance.

Part II

Innovative practices at the niche level

4 Unraveling persistent problems through analyzing innovative practices in healthcare

Tjerk Jan Schuitmaker and
Erica ter Haar-van Twillert

4.1 Introduction

Over the past decades there has been increasing criticism in the Netherlands of the accessibility, acceptability and quality of healthcare. At the same time, the Dutch health system has become ever more costly, and the growing number of chronically ill patients has contributed to the fear of unsustainability in terms of affordability (De Nationale Denktank, 2006; RIVM, 2010). Because it seems difficult to solve these long-standing problems, either by policy interventions, care measures undertaken by health professionals or new small-scale care initiatives, these problems have been labeled "persistent problems" (see e.g. Dirven et al., 2002; Rotmans, 2005). Persistent problems are believed to be structural, inherent to the current health system, and therefore seen as system deficits. Accordingly, they are presented as both the reason for and the legitimization of the need for a system innovation or transition (see e.g. Grin et al., 2010).

More specifically, persistent problems are problems in which the system reproduces itself (Schuitmaker, 2010, 2012, 2013): a system actively creates barriers for innovations that are incompatible with the existing regime within that system. A better understanding of the systemic reproduction of problems helps innovative practices to survive or have a broader impact. Furthermore, an instrument for analyzing how enduring problems in daily practice are linked up with underlying systemic features may help policy-makers to redesign interventions geared to overcoming these long-standing problems.

This chapter is proposing such an instrument. The point of departure is that the unraveling of flaws of current systems should be based on an analysis of the opportunities and especially the problems encountered in new or innovative practices that try to overcome enduring problems. The iterative method we propose consists of (1) a historically informed system analysis: features that may be seen as the strongholds of the current system but that are said to have negative side-effects are identified. (2) The systemic reproduction of these negative side-effects can be unraveled by analyzing how new or innovative practices give shape to their agency in relation to their direct environment. This chapter explores this method by applying it to two new care practices: one dealing with patients with medically unexplained physical symptoms (MUPS), and one developing psychotherapy through the internet.

In the first section we present our theoretical and methodological considerations, leading to a five-step method for systematically unraveling system deficits – conceptualized as persistent problems. In the second section we discuss the stories of, and reasoning behind, the new care practices and how systemic problems manifest themselves. Finally, in the concluding section we briefly reflect on the merits of the method applied.

4.2 Unraveling persistent problems

The idea that large social systems (like the health system) come with enduring problems that are difficult to solve is hardly new. The concepts of the "wicked problem" (Rittel and Webber, 1973) and the "ill-structured problem" (Hisschemöller and Hoppe, 1995) were developed to describe and analyze such processes. Building on these concepts, the concept of the "persistent problem" was introduced in transition management and system-innovation literature. Loorbach (2007) talks about a specific type of "unstructured" problem; problems for which there is no agreement on values, facts and relevancy of facts, and that are firmly rooted in our institutions and structures. Bos and Grin (2008) perceived persistent problems, first, as problems that are obstacles for sustainability, and second, as problems that will not be solved by the market alone, or whose partial solutions will probably have negative side-effects, if solved in isolation.

However, persistent problems identified following these conceptualizations are diverse in nature, ranging from tangible problems, such as the cost of hybrid cars, to more fundamental problems, such as a systemic technological bias in possibilities for problem-solving. A further operationalized definition separates enduring problems – which may be seen as concrete, tangible – from the features and pathways that lead to their systemic reproduction, i.e. from that which makes them persistent (Schuitmaker, 2012, 2013). Here, persistent problems comprise the features underlying an enduring problem, as well as the pathways and mechanisms through which their (re-)production is effected. These pathways and mechanisms exist because agents act out regulations, financial structures, institutional structures (Schuitmaker, 2013), discourses (Arts and Van Tatenhove, 2004), etc.

Rotmans (2005) and Dirven et al. (2002) defined persistent problems as being complex, uncertain, difficult to manage and difficult to grasp. Rotmans and Dirven explicitly position the complexity of persistent problems in the actions of different actors or "stakeholders in several systems, institutions and domains." This notion of actor involvement is elaborated by Grin and Van Staveren (2007). While working on the governance of system innovations they identified "perverse couplings": connections between positive effects of progress in a production system and negative side-effects. The essence of this concept is that this coupling does not reside autonomously in some external systemic environment, but is actively effected by actors who think and act through institutionally and culturally paved pathways.

Actors, or agents, thus act out systemic properties, which (have) come into being because of actions of agents. A system, including all its material elements (buildings, people, money and so on), came into being as the result of earlier actions of agents. In turn, this system heavily influences the actions of the agents in the system. This notion is known as the "duality of structure" (Giddens, 1984). According to this theorem, the structural properties of social systems are both the medium and outcome of the practices they recursively organize.

Important here is that Giddens makes a distinction between structures and systems. A system is what you can see and touch, like the health system and all its actors, buildings, money and written laws. A structure on the other hand is only instantiated when people make use of this set of rules and resources (Giddens, 1984). In acting, agents draw upon features of the system in which they function (Stones, 2005) because they consciously or unconsciously decided it is in their best interests for whatever reason – and because of these actions the structure of the system exists. For instance, a medical protocol only structures a part of the health system if medical practitioners actually adhere to it. Because some do so, it creates the context in which other agents recognize the importance of this protocol and take it into account when planning their own actions.

The conduct of agents is heavily influenced by this structure via the process of "reflexive monitoring": actors not only monitor continuously the flow of their activities and expect others to do the same for their own; they also routinely monitor the social and physical context in which they move. This concept is developed by Giddens in the stratification model, in which actors reflect on their actions, their – sometimes unintended – consequences, and adjust their forthcoming actions accordingly (Giddens, 1984).

The underlying structure of a system, effected through the actions of agents, is usually formalized in rules and institutions, which agents follow, neglect or make use of, and reflect upon. Within these institutions "arrangements" exist, which may be seen as the temporary stabilization of the structure and agency around an issue or problem (Arts and Van Tatenhove, 2004). In the health domain, an arrangement can exist around a patient or a group of patients, or pertain to the health sector as a whole. Structuring features may also be seen as forming part of a dominant culture, structure or practice, and thus as part of the *regime* (Loorbach, 2007; Rotmans, 2005), or as an element of the "deep structure" or grammar of socio-technical systems: the "socio-technical regime" (Geels, 2004; Rip and Kemp, 1998).

When agents act, they make use of the resources of the system in which they function. What is considered a resource for one agent may be considered a constraint for another (following Giddens (1984): structure is both constraining and enabling). Resources, as any systemic feature, are inherently contested: agents make use of resources and in the process try to foreground the value of their resources, while potentially discrediting the value of resources of opposing agents. Resources are "symbolic capital" (Bourdieu, 1990): their value is not objective, but based in the subjective perception of agents. More powerful agents are able to impose the notions of a particular capital's value upon other agents, who recognize its value because of the power the agents possess (Bourdieu, 1990). Thus, Bourdieu points to a circular and self-fortifying process in which symbolic capital is always defined by the system in which it is valued. Accordingly, a recurrent problem for new practices is legitimizing their product in the context of the regime that they (try to) function in or change.

Bourdieu explicitly points out the unintentional part of this process. That is, actors actively and intentionally draw upon capital, but are not aware that it may be seen as symbolic. Systems can thus emerge and retain elements whose generation no one intended. As such, human history is created by intentional activities, but is not an intended project (Giddens, 1984). A system, then, has no conscious goal or opinion. It just is. And it is because every piece of it is enacted by agents.

With the theory of the (re-)production of systems laid out, we now turn to the aim of this chapter: the development of a method for systematical analysis of the persistence of enduring problems in a system. This analysis implies both the unraveling of the structural properties of specific regimes through which resistance to change is effected, and an (abridged) description of which system deficits exist – thereby generating the legitimization of transitions or system innovations. This is done by iteratively combining a historically informed system analysis with an analysis guided by the perspective of a new or innovative practice or care arrangement.

Part one: historically informed system analysis

To be able to understand and unravel how enduring problems are embedded, the historical context and the process of co-evolution that led to the current structure need to be examined (Bos and Grin, 2008; Grin, 2004; Grin and Van Staveren, 2007). Specific attention is paid to those features that are part of the *success* of the system, such as generally improved health conditions. These features are likely to be internalized by the agents involved through education and upbringing, thereby structuring their actions. When agents' actions effect structural properties, the communal actions of many agents have a strong structuring effect on a system via the influence this has on the behavior of other agents.

The positive effects of progress in a production system and the negative side-effects seem connected through perverse couplings (Grin and Van Staveren, 2007). According to Beck (1997), current techno-social systems and institutions have yielded significant progress and improvement of the human condition over the last couple of centuries, but, along with these benefits, risks and side-effects have been produced as well. These issues, logically, cannot be dealt with based on current paradigms that dominate the system, because the regular solution-producing pathways are also the producers of the problem (Grin, 2004). Institutions, as described by Hall and Thelen (2006), are solidified power structures, well equipped to solve problems. The tools, or "resources" (rules, laws, financial structures, guidelines), used by these agents to solve those problems are also symbolic capital; besides being helpful in solving a set of problems, these tools are bound to positions and power of agents. These agents will (unconsciously) foreground the value of those resources, even when the tools have become counterproductive in some cases.

Within these institutions, arrangements are the hinge between strongly structuring system factors, and the concrete or day-to-day problems agents try to solve. When trying to deviate from preferred solution pathways, innovative agents are constrained by other agents who (1) are themselves part of arrangements, which (2) are in turn structured by the underlying success factors. This would mean that exactly the success factors of a system may be seen, first, as features that produce problems, since some identified enduring problems that appear difficult to solve may be understood as negative side-effects of these success factors; and second, as the underlying reason why these enduring problems are *re*produced, and hence become persistent. These systemic features cause a bias because some solution pathways are preferred and acted out by agents, even though they systematically fail to lead to a satisfactory solution.

A persistent problem may be seen as a systemically reproduced negative side-effect of a success factor of the system-in-focus. To identify system deficits and unravel their pathways of (re-)production, one thus has to start with a historically informed system analysis focused on features that may be seen as the strongholds of the current system, which are said to have negative side-effects (see Figure 4.1).

Part two: actor-guided system analysis

The process of social reproduction explains the persistence of enduring problems, but holds no clues as to how to identify or unravel inherently social persistent problems themselves. In order to unravel the production and reproduction of negative side-effects, we propose to select, based on the earlier historically informed system analysis, a practice that implicitly or explicitly deals with identified negative side-effects: a new care arrangement that, while trying to device solutions, challenges regular paradigms. Such an arrangement would inevitably clash with the current regime, since its approach would require a revision of regular solution pathways. A problem without active intervention might be enduring, but only becomes *persistent* when those performing the intervention are facing serious inertia or resistance. Hence, a persistent problem only becomes *visible* if people are working on it – an approach very much in line with Kurt Lewin's remark that trying to change something is the best way to true understanding (Broerse et al., 2010b).

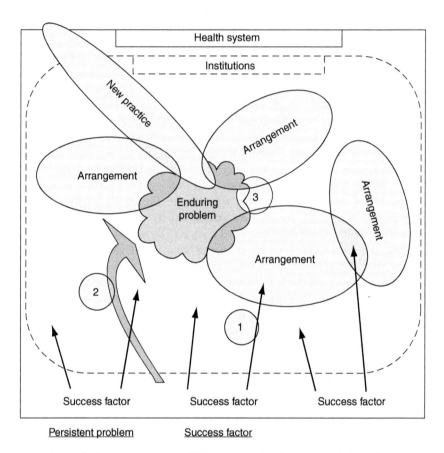

Persistent problem	Success factor

Systemically reproduced negative side-effect of a success factor (as described by practice and literature)

1) Structures system/arrangements in system

2) May have negative side-effect: enduring problem

3) Causes a bias in solution pathways: (re)production of enduring problems

Figure 4.1 Identifying persistent problems

The identification of persistent problems in a given system needs to be an *iterative* process to overcome two related problems: by relying on a historically informed literature review the researcher runs the risk of imposing (theoretical) views upon the practice, thereby rendering the analysis powerless. This problem may be countered by focusing on what systemic features are made relevant by the practice in focus. An isolated focus on one particular practice runs the risk that this researched practice is nothing more than an instance of itself. If no systemic background information is included, there is no reason to assume that findings are transferable to other practices or settings. The practice, in iteration with problems described in the literature, can point toward relevant enduring problems – which may be systemically reproduced, and thus become persistent. The researcher thus needs to have a dual-perspective in investigating the practice: analyzing the practice in focus shows what the problems are, after which the researcher may identify the problem behind the problem, based on the iteration with the historically informed system analysis (see Figures 4.1 and 4.2).

Our actor-guided system analysis draws upon the formulation by Stones (2005) of how to reconstruct a system through the eyes of an agent. Stones' "strong structuration" builds a bridge between ontology and empirical evidence, translating Giddens' structuration theory to the practical level of particular social processes and events in particular times and places.

To unravel the interaction between structure and agency, Stones first breaks down the notion of the duality of structure into four analytically separate components and defines for each the role it plays in the cycle of structuration: (1) external structure, the forming conditions for actions; (2) internal structure within the agent, itself analytically separated into the "general-dispositional" type of internal structure, which encompasses the unconscious, by bringing up internalized ways of seeing the world, and the "conjuncturally-specific," referring to the agent's more specific knowledge of particular settings and contexts; (3) active agency, which includes a range of aspects involved when agents draw upon internal structures in producing practical action; and (4) the outcomes of action as external and internal structures and as events (Stones, 2005). He draws up this quadripartite model of structuration to identify a central starting point for empirical analysis. If agency and structure are constantly interacting and changing, the question is where to start investigating this inherently fluid construct. For Stones this would always be the internal structures of an agent-in-focus, situated in a position practice (Stones, 2005). Such a practice may also be seen as an arrangement around a certain (healthcare) problem.

It is particularly helpful to investigate the *projective part of the agency*, since this combines the internal structures of agents with an analysis of the system in which these agents function. Projectivity encompasses the imaginative generation by actors of possible future trajectories of action, in which received structures of thought and action may be creatively reconfigured in relation to actors' hopes, fears and desires for the future (Emirbayer and Johnson, 2008; Emirbayer and Mische, 1998). Looking at the projectivity of a change agent thus leads to identifying systemically embedded problems, comprising both the insight of an agent into systemic problems – which is why the agent feels that a new practice is needed – as well as insight into the mechanisms and pathways by which these systemic problems are reproduced – formulated in ideas about how to circumvent problems concerning the construction of the practice within its systemic context (see Figure 4.2).

Building on the conceptual framework laid out above, we combine the work of Stones with the notion of "interpretive frames" (Grin and Van de Graaf, 1996). To guide the empirical work, and the analytical part, we

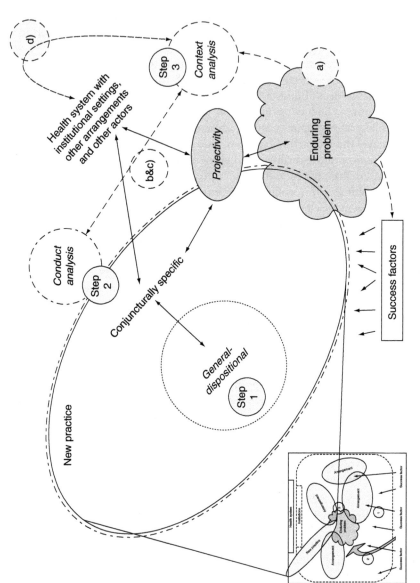

Figure 4.2 Unraveling persistent problems

formulate five questions (see below). The formal reasoning behind these questions, and the legitimization and theoretical grounding of our method, is based on four recurrent steps, as defined by Stones (2005). Starting from the internal structures of the agent in focus, these steps are based on the methodological bracketing of the analysis of the practice-in-focus into an agent's "conduct analysis" and an agent's "context analysis." Our method draws upon these steps, as well as specifying them.

According to Stones (2005), an agent's *conduct analysis* refers to unraveling and structuring the internal structures of the agent: her reflexive monitoring, her ordering of concerns, her motives, the way she carries out the work of action and interaction within an unfolding sequence. An agent's *context analysis* refers to unraveling the social nexus of interdependencies, rights and obligations, asymmetries of power and social conditions and consequences of action from the perspective of the agent-in-focus.

Within arrangements, agents function according to their own internal structures. These may be separated into a "general-dispositional" part and a "conjuncturally specific" part. The first part may be seen as corporeal schemas and memory traces, and are best understood as existing in a taken-for-granted and unnoticed state. Conjuncturally specific internal structures consist of knowledge of the interpretive schemes, power capacities and normative expectations and principles of (other) agents within the arrangement. Because of the reflexive monitoring of agents, the arrangement structures these internal structures, whereas the internal structures of the separate agents shape the arrangement-in-focus, because of the subsequent actions of the agents. The conduct and context of agents can be identified in arrangements.

Step 1 Conduct analysis: general-dispositional frames of meaning

The first step is identifying the general-dispositional frames of meaning of an agent-in-focus. This can be done through interviewing the agents who initiated the practice by making use of *interpretive frames*: a quadruple set of problem definitions, preferred solutions, and empirical and normative background theories, linked to each other by the question *why?* The first layer contains the solution preferred by the actor, or what the actor perceives as a (possible) solution to the identified problem. Next, the problem definition of the actor (i.e. the problem put forward) constitutes the second layer. The third layer contains the assessment of the problem by the actor (i.e. the reasoning why the solution put forward is preferred for the identified problem). This layer thus contains all knowledge of the actor, including knowledge of the (institutional) context in which he works. Finally, fundamental preferences and normative ideas constitute the fourth layer (Grin and Van de Graaf, 1996). A new practice is a new arrangement around a certain problem. The path to the general-dispositional frames of meaning of an agent thus begins in talking about what solution for what problem has been devised. The fourth layer then represents these taken-for-granted, unconscious notions.

Step 2 Conduct analysis: conjuncturally specific internal structures

The next step – still within the agent's conduct analysis – is to work from an identified general-dispositional frame and go on to focusing on the *conjuncturally* specific internal structures of the agent-in-focus. The goal is thus to identify how the agent *perceives* her immediate external structural terrain from the perspective of her own project, whether in terms of helplessness or empowerment, or a complex combination of the two. This part of the analysis may be done by structuring the information found in the third layer of the interpretive frames into clusters of important issues (e.g. diagnostic problems or endless referrals of patients).

Step 3 Context analysis

In the third step, one can identify, as a researcher, relevant external structural clusters, including the overall frames of the agents within these clusters. This pertains to the wider context of the arrangement, and leads to the structural properties that constrain or enable the practice-in-focus. These structural properties manifest themselves in the support or impediments encountered by the practice, such as policy themes, legislative rules, material structures, the actions of other agents, or the structural properties on which *those* other agents base their actions. This *context* analysis thus requires interviews with relevant actors within and outside the arrangement, participant observation, literature research and so on, but it should always be guided by the information from the first two steps. Furthermore, we argue, this third step must be guided and constrained by the above-mentioned historically informed system analysis. This is how the link between the underlying success factors, their negative side-effects and systemic reproduction may be constructed. These three steps constitute the actor-guided system-analytical part as such.

Step 4 Feedback of analysis into arrangement

The final step is to investigate the possibilities for action, and for structural modification allowed by external structures, as well as the constraints and influences imposed upon the agent-in-focus by these external structures. In doing so, the knowledge gained is iteratively used, fulfilling the recurrent element of the steps as specified by Stones. This means that the fourth step may be used to aid the practice-in-focus, or other new or innovative practices, to survive or have a broader impact. The first three steps provide insight into the success and failure of the practice-in-focus, as well as the underlying reasons. First, this makes it possible to help practices circumvent identified obstacles. This may be done by providing the practice-in-focus with the analysis: improving the knowledgeability (see Giddens, 1984) of the agent will empower the agent to better capitalize on the available resources. Identified obstacles, then, may well be external in terms of institutional arrangements, or interfering actions of other actors, but they may also be internal in the sense that the practice-in-focus itself reproduces impeding structural elements. Second, the knowledge gained may be used by policy-makers to create room for practices or new care arrangements that potentially contribute to a system innovation.

A method for unraveling persistent problems

The preceding discussion has yielded five guiding questions as a method for analyzing system deficits (see Figure 4.2).

Part one: historically informed system analysis

1   In historically embedded debates about enduring problems, which under-lying features of the system have been described as both success factors and factors that lead to problems, in terms of healthcare's affordability, accessibility, acceptability or quality?

Part two: actor-guided system analysis

2   How does the new care practice-in-focus organize itself; which solutions fit what (care) problem? (*interpretive frames layers one and two, projective part of agency*).
3   Premise and expectations underlying the practice; how does the current (health) system function? (*interpretive frames layers three and four, conduct analysis, projective part of agency*).
4   What kind of support or impediment does the practice experience: fin-ancial, managerial, organizational, non-cooperative colleagues or patients, etc.? (*context analysis, projective part of agency*).
5   What is the link, if there is one, between the success factors described to have negative side-effects (question 1), the way the practice tries to over-come this (questions 2 and 3) and the way the practice is supported or impeded (question 4)?

These five questions comprise the framework of the following section, where our method is applied to two cases in healthcare: patients with medically unexplained physical symptoms (MUPS) and the development of psycho-therapy through the internet.

4.3 Unraveling persistent problems in healthcare

In this section we apply the method developed in the previous section in an explorative way. As part of a historically informed system analysis we describe a few strongholds of the current health system that have negative side-effects, in the sense that they cause a bias in solution pathways. An actor-guided system analysis is followed by an integrated analysis. We follow the guiding questions above, but discuss questions 2 and 3 together in one section, as is true of questions 4 and 5.

Neither one of the practices discussed here has the deliberate intention to initiate a system innovation or transition. They are geared toward improvement of accessibility, acceptability and quality of care, and by doing so challenge systemically embedded notions. The first practice tries to overcome the mind–body dichotomy, the second the traditional doctor–patient relationship. The comparison between these two practices is interesting: the first operates from within the heart of the medical system, based on the problem that the current system fails to adequately treat a group of patients, trying to shield its practice from its surroundings; whereas the second is an outsider trying to get its innovative care method adopted by the incumbent regime. Both practices run into systemic resistance while doing so. As a background for analyzing both cases, we start with answering question 1: a historically embedded system analysis.

Historically informed system analysis

As explored in Section 4.2, a system emerges over time, based on the results of countless actions of actors. In the case of most modern Western health systems – the Dutch health system is no exception – the current system may attract many critiques, but does what it was meant to do. As a result of the ever-increasing medical knowledge, acting as the base on which new care techniques and practices are built, healthcare has made enormous progress over the past two centuries. In combination with the emergence of Western state-based care systems, a smooth and well-operating health system emerged, which was able to prolong people's life expectancy considerably and stamp out many deadly diseases (Grin, 2004). The features highlighted below – based on iteratively analyzing practices and literature – are said to have contributed greatly to this progress, but have also been singled out as factors that cause problems.

Foucault (2003) has described how the modern discourse of medicine developed in the late eighteenth and early nineteenth century. Until then, diseases were classified in terms of symptoms, and combating symptoms was at the center of medical action. Around that time the medical gaze turned inward, revealing the inner workings of human bodies, and, as a result, diseases became classified in terms of bodily abnormalities. The central focus of diagnosing diseases thus changed from symptoms to physically discernible deviations. This development marked the start of impressive medical achievements, based on the meticulous descriptions of the inner workings of bodies, and the resulting standardized interventions based on this knowledge. The history of modern medicine shows that the medical profession benefited greatly from the uniformity generated by recruitment, selection and performance standards. Standards have been explicitly used to rid medicine of quacks, impostors and alternative forms of healing, and to put the human body under the jurisdiction of physicians, nurses and other officially sanctioned medical groups (Timmermans and Berg, 2003).

The first question logically following from this is whether "standardization" and classification will change the human body into something it is not: a standard machine. Not only do people differ in how their social context or diet influences their health; also physiologically the human species comprises six billion varieties. Standardization of healthcare thus leads to a uniform treatment of a disease based on a statistical analysis, proving that a significant number of people profited significantly from a treatment in a *clinical* setting. Thus by definition this treatment is not suitable for *all* patients. Furthermore, if standards are formed based on what products pharmaceutical companies develop, the question is whether people profit in a *therapeutic* setting, and if the standard-generating supply side does create a demand or the other way around (Medawar and Hardon, 2004).

Furthermore, as Achterhuis (1983), building on the work of, for instance, Illich (1976), has demonstrated, the improvement of the quality and quantity of care leads to an interrelated growth in care dependency. Personal health has become extremely important, while suffering is not accepted. Care is demanded by all, instead of asked for by the sick. Healthcare has become the more or less exclusive field of government, insurance companies and medical specialists, instead of something that people do for themselves or for each other – leaving the responsibility for good health in the hands of care professionals.

According to De Swaan (1996), this is partly the result of the diffusion of the medical professional way of thinking of healthcare professionals to laypeople, a process he framed with the term "protoprofessionalization." According to De Swaan, already during the early development of the modern health system, and especially since World War Two, medical discourse has found its way outside the professional world. Through popular publications by medical experts, conversations with patients on what they were told, hygienic living rules and so on, laypeople adopted the professionals' way of talking about and dealing with their health. This process greatly contributed to improving general health. Such protoprofessionalization probably makes it easier for laypeople to gain access to professional care. This is not only because laypeople know how to express their problems as problems that health professionals should be able to deal with, but also because professionals tend to be willing to grant these care requests because they feel competent in dealing with these problems. As a result, it is likely that the demand for professional healthcare will rise, because problems people will have anyway are likely to be explained in medical terms and are thus directed at the medical system (De Swaan, 1996).

It is said that laypeople, although they have internalized the medical stance, are nowadays less capable of utilizing their own potential to become and stay healthy; they externalize the responsibility for and the coordination of their care to professionals. These professionals, on the other hand, because of institutional arrangements, are not always capable of taking up this role.

In the construction of an effective and professional health system, *specialization* has led to enormous progress. In the decades after the war, the Dutch government seemed mainly interested in realizing adequate health services. In the period between 1955 and 1970, this led to an impressive increase in hospitals and the emergence of specialized departments, in concurrence with differentiation and professionalization (Hendrix et al., 1991). This specialization also had a major negative side-effect: clients were eligible to receive the care health professionals had to offer. If the caregiver could not offer a solution, the patient was referred. Compartmentalization was the result. Moreover, specialized health professionals seem little inclined to participate in multidisciplinary care teams, precisely because their specialty is not easy to integrate with other specialties.

The medical rationality present in the above-described features was further formalized by a relatively recent development: the progress of "evidence-based medicine" (EBM). Since the introduction of this term by the Evidence-Based Medicine Working Group (Guyatt et al., 1992), it has become increasingly popular. EBM is the practice of medicine based on the best scientific data available as a solid foundation of the problem-solving approach. In other words, it is a conceptual framework that professionals and students in the healthcare sciences use for gathering information, processing it, and attempting to utilize what is most important, relevant and useful (Brown et al., 2005). According to the ideas of EBM, clinical practice guidelines should be based on scientific evidence, preferably a meta-analysis of randomized clinical trials offering probability estimates of each outcome.

Although the original description stated that this information should be integrated with the personal clinical expertise of the practitioner (Guyatt et al., 1992), proponents of EBM nowadays are wary of reasoning from basic principles or experience; they distrust claims based on expertise or pathophysiological models. They prefer to remain agnostic as to why something should or should not work; instead, they measure objectively whether or not it works in real-life settings (Timmermans and Berg, 2003).

EBM has become a powerful discourse with a strong structuring effect; many actors draw upon this feature to inform and legitimize their actions. This includes not only healthcare professionals: insurance companies tend to reimburse only EBM-validated treatments, and policy-makers rely on EBM as guardian against inefficient deployment of healthcare provisions. EBM has thus become more than a tool to promote sensible and cost-effective care; it has become *symbolic capital*, bound to institutional positions, and is therefore used as a resource for other purposes than for what it was originally developed.

The question is whether this paradigm always dictates appropriate treatment. For instance, the regular paradigm of evidence-based medicine appears to have difficulties with two-way causality. Furthermore, the evidence is only rarely available to cover all the decision moments as laid down in medical guidelines (Timmermans and Berg, 2003). What is more, the evidence itself may have a bias because it is based on research done on an artificially composed treatment group (Hardon and Van Haastrecht, 2005). EBM, meant as a tool to support clinical decisions, has become a guiding principle supported by other parties than just medical professionals, dictating particular interventions also when other solutions may be more helpful.

We now turn to our method's second part. For the purpose of this chapter this exploration does not deliver a full-scale system analysis (if such a thing is possible), but it highlights what this approach can reveal in terms of system deficits and their reproduction, which in itself can help draw out opportunities open to the practice-in-focus. As said, this part of the method is actor-guided, and therefore departs from the reasoning of the practice itself, positioned in its new care arrangement.

Case 1 Clinic for unexplained diseases

It is estimated that approximately half a million people in the Netherlands suffer from physical pains and impairments for which medical doctors have no explanation (Brandt, 2005a; Vermeulen, 2008). For patients with these "vague complaints," a diagnosis is often difficult to make, because no underlying pathology can be identified. After a long diagnostic process, the illness may be classified as, for instance, "chronic fatigue syndrome" or "fibromyalgia," but these diseases are themselves contested. One of the more commonly used classifications is Medically Unexplained Physical Symptoms (MUPS), and an estimated 2.5 percent of all patients going to a general practitioner (GP) fall into this category (Verhaak et al., 2006). However, specialists in (academic) hospitals are also often confronted with this group of patients (Dirkzwager and Verhaak, 2007). This section analyzes a clinic that aims to treat this complex group of patients.

The (conduct of the) practice: solutions for which care problem based on what notions

The point of departure for the clinic for unexplained diseases was the question of why some people with relatively minor physical complaints turned into chronically ill patients after 18 months of going through the health system. The main problem they were trying to tackle was basically frustrated doctors as well as patients. Their multi-layered solution, which is described below, is grounded in two lines of reasoning: one based on the organization of the current health system, and one based on neurobiological knowledge – as explicated by the initiators of the practice, and substantiated by other literature. The information in this section departs from interviews with the initiators of the practice, and is supplemented with observations of consults.

According to the initiators, patients come to a general practitioner (GP) with difficult-to-diagnose physical complaints. GPs, as a start, frequently order blood tests when they see patients presenting unexplained complaints. GPs tend to focus on physical complaints, ignoring other signals, like when a patient complains about insomnia (see also Kappen and Van Dulmen, 2008). The risk of false positive test results is fairly high. These result in unnecessary further testing, unfavorable effects such as patient anxiety, high costs, somatization and morbidity. A policy of watchful waiting is expected to lower both the number of patients to be tested and the risk of false-positive test results, without missing serious pathology. However, many general practitioners experience barriers when trying to postpone blood testing by watchful waiting (see also Van Bokhoven et al., 2006). When further tests provide no conclusive answer, the patient is referred to a specialist, even when the GP suspects that the specialist will not find anything either.

The reasons for referral are two-fold, according to the initiators. The GP would not want to overlook a potential serious illness, as this could diminish the patient's confidence in the GP (see also Kappen and Van Dulmen, 2008; Van Bokhoven et al., 2009). Furthermore, the patient him- or herself often puts pressure on the GP for further testing. This is based, first, on the patient's fear that some serious illness is hiding, and second, on the idea that a *physical* explanation for the pain must exist, and therefore a *medical-physical* reason – in contrast to a psychological one. However, when the specialist does not find tangible evidence for physical abnormalities, he or she refers the patient back to the GP, or to another specialist. As a result, the patient, after many inconclusive diagnostic tests, feels something *must* be wrong, and becomes even more stressed and anxious.

At some point in this trajectory the patient may be referred to a psychologist – a referral which patients often refuse because he or she is experiencing *physical* pain. Patients whom we interviewed confirmed this, stressing the physical nature of their pain. Even when the patient visits a psychologist, he or she may be referred back because the psychologist feels insecure about treating patients with physical pain which may point to a life-threatening illness.

These dynamics accumulate in an uncured, stressed, rejected and chronically ill patient, and medical practitioners who feel either helpless or inclined to reject "whiney" patients. Meanwhile, societal costs are high, based on used diagnostic equipment, consulted doctors, and the patient's inability to work.

A neurobiological mechanism called long-term potentiation explains how patients with vague complaints, after an initial physical trigger, become trapped in vicious circles of monitoring their symptoms and pain. Combined with the stress about what they feel, patients become hypersensitive about their symptoms, which causes them to increase, which further restricts their activities and leads to frustration and demoralization. This in turn gives rise to new and/or more symptoms, concerns and physical changes – so much so that what started it is no longer what keeps it going. The trigger of this (neurological) distress is no longer detectable.

Although the illness is not the fault of the patient, he or she has a vital role and responsibility in combating it: physiology and behavior are inseparable.

The health system, however, is not equipped to organize adequate care, because its organization starts from a specialized division between body and mind. Therefore, the clinic for unexplained diseases embarks on its cure-trajectory, first by taking an extensive anamnesis. Where a regular consult takes 15 minutes, this anamnesis could take up to an hour. The treatment then comprises five important elements, which we derived from observations of consults: recognition of complaints, reassurance, the notion that improvement is possible, but not without the personal effort of the patient, and coaching. It is first made clear that the physical pains and problems experienced are real and not imaginary, even though no physiological evidence is visible. Since patients feel they have lost control, the immediate goal is to reinstate the patient as the person in control (see also Brandt, 2005b; Knepper, 2007). This means in practice that the diagnostic trajectory is stopped: there are no more referrals, no new medical examinations. Furthermore, the basis of trust is established based on medical authority, which is used to reassure the patient: the neurologist explains the above-described explanation of long-term potentiation to convince the patient that there is no underlying life-threatening pathology. The logic behind this is that, as long as the patient stays focused on his physical impairments they will not go away; de-sensitization is needed. When this point is established, the patient is coached on learning to deal with the pain, and subsequently on reactivating him- or herself. According to the clinic, two or three sessions usually suffice.

The (context of the) practice: support and impediments, and systemic reproduction of problems

In the abridged version of the reasoning of the practice-in-focus above, several systemic features appear to manifest themselves in the way they are (re-)produced by the actions of agents. For the purpose of this chapter, we now discuss some of the support and impediments observed, and link this to the way the practice tries to overcome identified problems and the systemic features identified earlier (question 5).

First of all, compartmentalization and standardization show a perverse coupling here. A prerequisite for standardization of practices is classification: a diagnosis is indispensable for prescribing further action. In the case of medically unexplained physical symptoms, no univocal classification based on medical standards exists – the classification "unexplained" itself is contested (Van Dieren, 2007). No other action than further testing or referral appears possible.

In addition, the clinic for unexplained diseases can only exist, first, because of its setting in an academic hospital, and second, because of the academic and contractual position of the head of the department. Both appeared to be needed to create room for innovation and experiment. However, this position at the heart of medical science dictated two things. First, the immediate surrounding required that the treatment was tested in a medically approved manner, because – residing in the conjuncturally specific internal structures – the initiator knew his treatment needed to be approved in a manner deemed valuable by his colleagues; otherwise the academic hospital would never support the clinic. And second, the head of the department, because of his medical upbringing (stored in his general-dispositional internal structures), is just as inclined to validate its new approach to treatment in the conventional way: by making use of randomized controlled trials (RCTs) as part of the EBM approach. For that reason a medical trial was started, which immediately ran into tough methodological problems. Although EBM leaves room to incorporate context and complexity, RCTs, which are considered the most reliable form of EBM, are mostly used. And in carrying out RCTs an important element of the dynamic and social component of disease is considered to be irrelevant for measuring effectiveness. Overall, in RCTs a bias exists in research design favoring simple causal connections and immediate solutions.

In the case of patients with MUPS, this leads to two major difficulties. First, the interaction between body and mind has not been theorized and conceptualized extensively, making it difficult to design intervention studies. Second, patients basically suffer from bad *quality of life*, which is extremely difficult to measure before and after the intervention, implying that – ironically – the main concern of patients is not incorporated into the research methodology. EBM is thus part of the projective part of the agency of the head of the clinic, structuring his current behavior into reproducing the underlying problem.

Finally, protoprofessionalization plays an interesting dual role. The patient is inclined to turn to the medical system for help for his or her problems. In doing so, he or she focuses almost solely on a medical diagnosis. This is meant to deliver objective proof of the reason for the physical impairments, thereby providing peace of mind. It also places the blame outside the patient's self. But by blaming an external factor the solution is also externalized, whereas the patient is the one who has to change behavior to improve. Furthermore, it is not the patient alone who propagates this externalization: friends and family consistently suggest different approaches and possible diseases. Recurrent themes in interviews and casual talks with patients and family were "other treatment options," "trying an experimental treatment" and "I read on the internet...." Partly because family and friends want to be helpful, partly because they feel a patient is not *allowed* to give up searching in the medical discourse. The dual role of protoprofessionalization shows itself via the internal structures of the head of the neurology department: he himself draws upon this resource by using his medical authority to win the trust of people. He is thus aware of the value of his knowledge on purely physical medical issues, and he uses this (symbolic) capital to actually turn his patients away from a physiological focus.

Case 2 Interapy

Interapy is an innovative practice which developed psychotherapy through the internet. It combines new technological possibilities with traditional psychotherapeutic treatment. Several advantages of this approach are recognized: high accessibility (treatment is available when and where patients find it feasible), the patient has more control over treatment, the program and time-span is manageable, and tools for self-management are included. Although interapy is not set up to improve healthcare in a broader sense, the advantages of this new treatment, interestingly, in fact collide with current healthcare arrangements. Far-reaching impact is worked against by, for instance, expectations of health professionals and patients, financial, planning and other rules, and compartmentalization of the health system.

The (conduct of the) practice: solutions for which care problem and based on what notions

Interapy provides a treatment developed by the Departments of Clinical Psychology and Social Science Informatics at the University of Amsterdam. The idea of interapy treatment arose from an informal meeting between a professor of clinical psychology and an internet expert. The treatment follows a protocol in which clients make an assignment and therapists react to the contribution of the client, leading to instructions for the next step. The client communicates with his or her therapist via a secure website. All information exchanged will be preserved, so the client can reread the whole process. At its launch, it was one of the first psychological treatments accessible via the internet.

The main characteristics of interapy are: high accessibility, client's own responsibility for the treatment, a transparent program, and development of personalized instruments for self-management. With these features, interapy offers opportunities for early intervention and prevention, preventing the patient's drop-out from social and working life, as well as relapse. On average there are two contact moments in a week, which is why the duration of the total treatment is shorter than in face-to-face therapy. Furthermore, interapy treatment increases the accessibility of healthcare not only through quick access, but also by offering the opportunity for taking part in treatment the moment it suits the patient, instead of within the working hours of the care provider. As a result, the patient is more in control of his or her treatment, which in turn stimulates the capacity to regain one's own health, as well as to keep fit. "I had the feeling I did it myself, which made me proud and gave me hope for the future" (client's story, presentation workshop for professionals, 2007). This implies that the traditional role for professionals changes, altering the power balance between professional and patient.

From 2001 onward, interapy has become an independent treatment organization. Up until 2008, the organization developed treatments for short-term psychological care for people with posttraumatic stress syndrome (PTSS), mourning complaints, job–related stress, depression and panic complaints, and provided help to adolescents after sexual harassment. Interapy provides only evidence-based treatments. It first offered treatments for diseases with a high incidence, such as PTSS, burn-out and depression, to assure there was a large target group.

At the start of interapy, this practice was not acknowledged as an Exceptional Medical Expenses Act (AWBZ; *Algemene Wet Bijzondere Ziektekosten*) institute. This means that interapy treatment could not be reimbursed according to public reimbursement rules. With the AWBZ permit acquired in 2004, interapy could function as a traditional mental health institute. During the course of the case study the law changed; secondary psychological help was transferred from the Exceptional Medical Expenses Act to the Health Insurance Act (ZVW; *Zorgverzekeringswet*), where primary psychological help was already in place. Since January 2008, all acknowledged psychological help – as well as interapy – falls under the Health Insurance Act, and interapy treatment became part of the basic reimbursement rules. The interapy organization was purchased in 2008 by six mental healthcare institutes, and as such it has become institutionalized in the traditional arrangement.

Rather than having been explicitly set up to solve problems in healthcare, interapy aims to improve care for a specific group of patients. The new practice departed from the problem definition of these patients, which implied that a new institutional arrangement was needed to create patient-centered care, whereas interapy strived to become part of existing arrangements. Although the features of interapy could improve the quality and accessibility of care, the development of interapy has been a "bumpy ride." A manager of interapy said in an interview in 2007 that its development went well content-wise, but that it has been difficult financially.

The (context of the) practice: support and impediments, and systemic reproduction of problems

Owing to the patient-centered characteristics of interapy, struggles with traditional structures were anticipated. Furthermore, because interapy originated from traditional arrangements, reproduction of the system by interapy has been visible as well. For most psychologists and psychotherapists today, the healing part of the therapy is grounded in the unique relationship between professional and client, which is automatically linked to actual face-to-face contact. This professional value is deeply embedded in the general-dispositional structures of mental health professionals. Interapy's development is influenced by this in two ways. The first became visible during the request for an AWBZ license. Although the admissions committee communicated that it judged interapy to be ineligible for an AWBZ license based on the criteria of complex psychiatric help, and that its new mode of offering therapy had nothing to do with it, professional values about treatment via the internet seem to have played a role. "If problems can be dealt with over the internet, it cannot be that serious" (interview, committee member, CVZ, 2007). Interapy fought back, however, by providing evidence of their results with treating patients with severe psychiatric problems. After almost a year the license was granted, even though the professionals on the admissions committee remained unconvinced.

The second way this professional value influenced the development of interapy shows itself in the (contested) use of interapy treatment in large mental healthcare institutes. Many of the professionals seemed barely motivated to use the interapy treatment, because they had no faith in a healing relationship without seeing the patient. If the interests of interapy are to be advanced, the connection between a trustful relationship and actual face-to-face contact will have to be decoupled.

Our context analysis of interapy also reveals formal institutional resistance during the process of interapy treatment being integrated into regular care arrangements. When professionals *are* motivated, external structures – of the arrangement in which they function – constitute an obstacle, such as planning rules and referral problems. The flexibility in time and place functions well in the interapy organization, but planning problems occur in traditional healthcare institutes when clients did not deliver their contribution at the desired moment. Planning and registration rules in the traditional arrangements and habits in how work should be performed – located in the general-dispositional internal structures of the professionals in those arrangements – are not equipped to deal with clients who themselves control the time schedule.

In the majority of mental healthcare institutes, interapy treatment in the end remained a marginal element of the treatment program, and some stopped the new treatment altogether. At the same time, several institutes tried to use interapy treatment in more profound ways, as part of a larger effort to deploy new technologies to reach clients.

It is interesting that some clients demonstrate the same misgivings as professionals. In one mental health institute, the introduction of interapy treatment initially went smoothly. The positive outcomes of effect research of interapy were convincing to professionals, but although the practitioners promoted interapy, which in this case had the added value of beginning the therapy almost instantly, circumventing the existing waiting lists, most clients turned down the offer. They had the feeling that they were being refused regular treatment, and being offered an unfavorable alternative. In particular, those clients who registered themselves at a mental health institute explicitly expected face-to-face therapy.

Where clients followed interapy treatment, most reported positively, and some saw benefits compared to face-to-face therapy. Those clients seemed to experience more independency, and more responsibility for their own treatment, in comparison to the traditional therapy to which they were exposed. Although the interapy treatment is programmed, the client is in control of the planning process, not only in terms of doing the planning (within limits), but also through the rule that the therapist is supposed to react within 48 hours to the client's contribution. Furthermore, clients felt less ashamed and less influenced by the appearance of the professional. They were also more motivated to start interapy treatment because of the more customized, personal context – as reflected in the flexibility offered or the role of their writing skills – and the motivation of the professionals involved.

Specialization, leading to an increase in health services as well as professional values, and protoprofessionalization, which transfers responsibility and potential for one's own health to the medical specialist, have formed arrangements for treatment that favor control by the professional. In the above examples, professionals as well as clients reproduce these structures, which have impeded the development of interapy. Furthermore, interapy requires a clear diagnosis for treatment to begin. The traditional mechanism of having the GP classify a person as either a burn-out patient or a person suffering from stress directly interfered with the goal of high accessibility of the treatment.

Finally, the development of interapy centers on providing *evidence-based* psychotherapy treatment only. The professionals involved are structured by their own professional values – valuing treatment over guidance or advice – as well as by their acknowledgment of the importance of those professional values within the regular care arrangement: officially sanctioned treatments for more severe psychiatric problems come with opportunities of reimbursement by the public reimbursement rules. A health service worker of a company who uses interapy treatment in occupational health stated that interapy could have been more successful if the focus had been on prevention in learning courses, instead of on (EBM) treatment. Managers are willing to pay if workers are treated in a way that they can continue working, or in a way that they return more quickly to the work process.

4.4 Evaluation

The aim of this chapter was to develop an instrument for analyzing system deficits – conceptualized as persistent problems. We argued that this can be done by unraveling systemic production and reproduction of enduring problems by iteratively combining a historically informed system analysis with empirical research into the problem definition of new practices, in concurrence with the opportunities and, especially, the problems they encounter. We applied our method to two differently situated practices to explore and illustrate what this method can reveal. By showing systemic reproduction, it is possible to unravel structural properties of regimes through which resistance to change is effected.

This application showed that several success factors of the Dutch health system – and arguably most Western health systems – such as standardization, protoprofessionalization, specialization and evidence-based medicine can have negative side-effects that are systemically (re-)produced through the influence they have on the actions of agents.

Based on the two cases described above, there are two interesting, additional observations to be made. First, EBM and the medical rationality structure the behavior of many agents in the two arrangements described, including the actions of the change agents themselves. EBM may, for instance, be found both in the general-dispositional and the conjuncturally specific part of the internal structures of the head of the clinic for unexplained diseases. The first is because he had been working as a neurologist in an academic hospital: he internalizes, and thus takes for granted, the notion that all medicine should be evidence-based. The second is because he also feels that if his new practice wants to be successful, he has to validate his treatment with a RCT, because he knows that other professionals and insurance companies expect him to work accordingly.

For the initiators of interapy, the value of EBM treatment is also recognized, because they need this validation to become eligible for adoption by the conventional mental care regime – in terms of reimbursement and referrals – and to be accepted by patients as a "real" treatment. EBM thus structures the behavior of this practice through its conjuncturally specific internal structures, as part of strategic behavior. This line of approach worked well, but also led to a bias in the perception of opportunities open to the practice, because a possible market of work-related prevention courses remained unexplored. The same systemic feature thus manifests itself in both practices, even though the first practice is operating from within the heart of the medical system, whereas the second is an outsider trying to get its innovative care method adopted by the traditional regime.

The second interesting observation derived from this is: if one wants to circumvent the problems posed by this reproduction, it may be an option to take the following two-step approach: reproduce this knowledge as much as possible by convincing patients that the treatment offered is EBM-validated, while developing new methods for doing EBM that, other than traditional EBM, can actually prove the validity of the care intervention by recognizing the multiple causation and patient agency involved in pathologies, rather than assuming a linear relation between an intervention and health outcome. Based on the fourth step, as described by Stones, this could inform a new practice, or new policies aimed at tackling enduring problems concerning the affordability, accessibility, acceptability and quality of healthcare.

5 System innovation

Workplace health development

Lenneke Vaandrager, Ingrid Bakker,
Maria Koelen, Paul Baart and
Tamara Raaijmakers

5.1 Introduction

Workplace health[1] reflects fundamental needs of employees who require both a safe and health-promoting work environment. Within such an environment, a high quality of working life provides opportunities for personal growth and learning, and enables employees to balance working and non-working life. In industrial nations, a long tradition of attention to workplace health exists. Although the standard view is that work-related health problems and risks should be prevented, the potential of satisfying work for life fulfillment (Graetz, 1993) and thus a positive contribution to health and well-being is virtually neglected. As we will argue, much potential in this respect is still untapped, and this is due to a number of underlying factors inherent in the incumbent system of work and health. In this chapter we discuss these factors and propose specific suggestions for system innovation pertaining to workplace health development.

The aim of this chapter is to describe an innovative perspective on workplace health development processes and to discuss three cases in which attempts were made to implement these processes. The latter analysis will also reveal how the incumbent regime influences these practices, thus providing an indication of changes in the regime. We start with historically contextualizing workplace health development processes, after which we discuss the current definition and determinants of workplace health. This provides a basis for considering a pathogenic and salutogenic orientation of workplace health. Examples from case studies involving three Dutch companies which have tried to implement an innovative approach to health promotion in the workplace serve to illustrate the opportunities and barriers for system innovation in this field. We conclude by discussing strategies for the transition needed in this area.

Historical overview

Changing perspective on health

In the nineteenth and (early) twentieth century, the European labor movement, supported by progressive liberals such as Helene Mercier and Aletta Jacobs (Bosch, 2002), actively pursued legislation aimed at protecting the rights of working people. Health and safety in the workplace was one of the issues of concern. From the late nineteenth century up until the present, countless new laws and regulations that protect and promote health at work have been enacted or introduced (Jones and Basser, 1999). For example, in 1919 the International Labor Organization (ILO) was asked by the International Labor Conference held in Washington to "draw up a list of the principal processes to be considered unhealthy." This prompted the ILO to conduct a careful investigation of working conditions and working environments; of the substances used at work and their hazards; of possible sources of disease and injury; and of methods of treatment and prevention and existing protective legislation (www.ilocis.org). As this example underscores, in the early twentieth century it was mainly occupational safety that urged governance of workplace health, setting in motion a (still ongoing) series of societal efforts to protect employees against work-related injury and disability. Over the years, occupational safety laws and regulations evolved into high-quality standards that in turn gave rise to and were facilitated by an array of institutions and executive organizations such as the ILO.

In addition, new developments in medical science during subsequent decades resulted in an acceleration of specialist medical care for workplace health. In large companies, doctors increasingly provided medical care for workers and their families. It may be argued that the various domains of working life in general were increasingly brought under medical control (Baart et al., 2003).

Largely unintentionally, yet crucially, the effort aimed at addressing employee health began to coincide more or less with applying the biomedical model of health, whereby health is generated through the elimination of the specific risks of contracting a disease and where the medical profession has enormous power in defining what does and what does not constitute a disease. Obviously, much was gained from the many technological advances of medicine. At the same time, however, it became increasingly clear that this biomedical model was also reductionist, in the sense of neglecting the more sociological notion that health and disease have a variety of social roots. Especially since the end of the 1990s, this safety and biomedical perspective on workplace health has been critically scrutinized from this angle (ENWHP, 1997).

When it comes to understanding this recent change against the backdrop of three crucial landscape trends – aging, growing pressure from the global economy on labor costs and taxes, and the rise of the neoliberal paradigm – it is possible to identify several major factors:

- the transition from infectious diseases to the predominance of chronic diseases, which are products of the modern age itself (see the Introduction to this volume);
- the dramatic rise in numbers of disability benefit recipients;
- the fact that people who did not participate in the labor market were in fact unhealthier due to the importance of work for social and mental health.

These developments have stimulated a more holistic view on workplace health development, seeking to integrate services of medicine, human resource management, well-being and safety policies for the development of health and well-being (Baranski et al., 2003; Houtman, 1997; Kompier and Cooper, 1999).

In fact, this emerging discomfort is quite understandable from the perspective of what transition theory would analyze as the co-evolution of problems, knowledge and discourses. Curative and safety measures were never meant to solve the problem of falling ill or getting injured. Yet, around 1990, due to the emergence of non-communicable diseases, the increase in the number of people with disabilities, and the rise of a neoliberal climate of concern about welfare state spending (Helderman et al., 2005), preventive measures were re-appreciated. As a result, views and approaches gradually started to change in occupational health services, as well as in disciplines like medical science, psychology and business management (Cooper et al., 2009). The perspective on workplace health changed from an entirely *negative* orientation with a focus on "ill-health"[2] and dysfunctions toward a more *positive* orientation aimed at health, well-being and optimal functioning. Work was no longer seen solely as a potential threat to health, but also as a resource for self-enhancement (Shain and Kramer, 2004). But ideas about improving employees' health and well-being were largely translated into a focus on the individual (lifestyle behavior change), while wider organizational and societal factors that also determine health and well-being were often ignored (Chu et al., 1997). Even worse, existing identities and divisions of labor made those actors who were needed to deal with these challenges reluctant to take proper action. For instance, the Ministry of Labor and the Ministry of Health referred to each other for taking action on health and work issues. Another example concerns the problems of establishing collaborative practices in between different fields: human resource management, safety and health, also referred to as integrated health management (Zwetsloot et al., 2003; Zwetsloot and Pot, 2004). Up until the 1990s, when the above-mentioned problems fueled an interest in a more integral perspective, each of these domains had become strongly specialized as part of "early modernization" processes, or tailored knowledge-based social and economic processes (Beck, 1997). As such, the above-described situation can be labeled the "incumbent regime" (Geels and Schot, 2007) of workplace health management.

New stimuli for change in workplace health actions

At present, increasing awareness of the complexity and perseverance of problems related to workplace health serve as a new stimulus for change. Current health problems are related, for example, to sedentary work (the automation of work and decreasing share of physical labor have been leading to a lack of exercise, which negatively affects cognition and physical health), high levels of stress (a partial cause of some of the more prevalent chronic and other non-communicable diseases), growing sick leave and unintended side-effects of the welfare state (reduced mobility) and an increased share of disability pensions (WHO, 2002c).

By the early twenty-first century, the need for profound change has come to be emphasized by government, healthcare workers and companies alike (Raaijmakers et al., 2009). This sense of urgency is felt because of the challenges stemming from new work arrangements, skills needed to succeed in careers, and an aging population. Significantly, there is an increasing appreciation of work itself as health-promoting, even for those who traditionally may have been considered unsuitable for employment, such as people with physical and mental disabilities.

Defining workplace health

To clearly understand the underlying factors in the system of work and health, it is important to first clarify how the notion of health has been historically conceptualized. This question is much less trivial than one might expect. "Health," like "happiness," is difficult to define because it is a very general and open-textured concept (Callahan, 1973), and views regarding what has to be understood by health differ across and within disciplines (Koelen and van den Ban, 2004). In 1946, the World Health Organization (WHO) defined health as "the complete state of mental, physical and social well-being, and not merely the absence of disease or infirmity" (WHO, 1946). In this definition, health was perceived to be broader than the absence of disease, while it also recognized the importance of the social environment (including affectionate relationships and group membership). Health was placed in a broad context referring to the interaction between the body and the mind. Well-being in this definition includes such aspects as happiness and prosperity (Koelen and Van den Ban, 2004).

This definition, which was formulated when the WHO was set up in 1946, must of course be seen in its proper historical context, in the wake of two world wars and a major economic crisis. At the time, further modernization of society was seen as key to economic recovery. More specifically, the belief was that the improvement of world health would make an important contribution to world peace. After recognizing the fundamental right of all individuals to health, the WHO Constitution's Preamble (WHO, 1989: 1) states:

[T]he health of all people is fundamental to peace and security and is dependent on the fullest cooperation by individuals and states .... Unequal development in different countries in the promotion of health and control of disease, especially communicable disease, is a common danger.

For at least three decades, the 1946 definition was used rather generally. It was hardly debated; the main issue of debate concerned the problem created by the word "complete." This has been criticized as being too utopian and unachievable (Callahan, 1973). Furthermore, since physical and mental functioning and participation in society can differ over time and place, the WHO presented a new definition in 1986, suggesting that "health is a resource for everyday life, not the object of living," in order to stress that health is not a state, but a process on a continuum with a dynamic nature. It was also added that health "is a positive concept emphasizing social and personal resources, as well as physical capacities" (WHO, 1986). This broader and more process-oriented definition fitted better with the development of the welfare state.

Since that time, various authors have written about the definition of health, for example, regarding the nature and process through which families play an active part in their own health (Novilla et al., 2006), or by conceiving of health as a process enabling people to develop healthiness through their assets and thus having the opportunity to lead a good life (Eriksson and Lindström, 2008). Following these debates, health may be defined as an important prerequisite for being able to work, rather than as a state of being.

This redefinition of health has also inspired the definition of health in the context of work, as the ability of the workforce to participate and be productive in a sustainable and meaningful way (Vaandrager and Koelen, 2013). Workplace health is of course not a matter of chance. It depends on everyday technical, social and personal resources, as well as on mental, social and physical capacities of employees to use these resources (Antonovsky, 1993; Beddington et al., 2008; Hanson, 2007; Huber et al., 2011). In terms of the more positive and dynamic understanding of health, satisfying and meaningful work in itself has the potential to create health. Taking both aspects together, which implies an even broader definition of workplace health, we may speak of circular causation, with several interconnected causes and effects. Work has effects on self-esteem and social recognition. Employment provides time structure, social contact, collective effort and purpose, social identity and regular activity. On the other hand, health is a prerequisite for being able to work. Re-employment has been shown to be one of the most effective ways of promoting the (mental) health of the unemployed (ILO, 2000).

The salutogenic and pathogenic orientation for health

This contemporary definition of workplace health presumes a strong, multi-directional interaction between environmental, social and individual determinants. The individual determinants include the characteristics of the individual such as age or gender and personal behavior or lifestyle. The physical environment encompasses the architecture and infrastructure of buildings, information technology, the nature of working equipment, and beverage and food services. The social environment consists of business models, management structures, leadership skills, availability of health(care) services, opportunities for personal development, skills training, and company culture and ambience.

The biomedical and more holistic orientations for health may also be labeled pathogenic and salutogenic perspectives. From the pathogenic perspective the concept of ill-health is a dichotomy. Ill-health is a state in which clinical and/or experienced health is disordered and, as a consequence, normal functioning may be disrupted. For the pathogenic perspective, risk factors (why people become ill) serve as the starting point of thinking about workplace health. Essentially, this perspective assumes a biomedical orientation. In contrast, the salutogenic perspective understands the concept of health or well-being as an ongoing process of (re)producing health through self-regulation in a given socio-ecological environment, such as the workplace. When assuming a salutogenic perspective, the resources for health are the main focus.

For the workplace, health resources include healthy lifestyles, enhancing management structures, and sufficient opportunities and warranting room for personal development. Risk factors (the pathogenic perspective) include environmental hazards, illness and high working demands (see Table 5.1).

Salutogenesis and pathogenesis play a simultaneous and complementary role and they interact in real life. Employees (re)produce their health continuously in time, making use of the available resources. An individual can simultaneously experience positive aspects of health (e.g. a nice flow in work) and negative aspects (e.g. a physical disability like asthma). Furthermore, individuals will differ from each other: risk factors such as high stress levels may be harmful for one employee, whereas someone else will experience job pressure (e.g. deadlines or challenging special projects) as fulfilling and stimulating. To most people, on the other hand, resources like team spirit or fellowship at work will help minimize the impact of risk factors, be of

Table 5.1 The salutogenic and pathogenic orientation

	Resources	Risk factors	
Salutogenesis	• Healthy lifestyle • Management structures • Opportunities for personal development • etc. *Positive health*	• Environmental hazards • Illness • High working demands • etc. *Ill-health*	*Pathogenesis*

Source: Based on Bauer et al. (2006).

assistance in overcoming disabilities or help recover from disease. Finally, the relative weight of salutogenic resources and pathogenic risk factors may vary throughout someone's career (Bauer et al., 2006; Vaandrager and Koelen, 2013).

In sum, the pathogenic orientation focuses on how risk factors of individuals and their working environment lead to ill-health; the salutogenic perspective examines how resources and the ability to recognize and use these resources in our working life may support developments toward positive health. The pathogenic perspective addresses health matters in terms of ill-health, disorders, sickness, impairment, shortcomings, malfunctioning and disability. The salutogenic perspective on the other hand addresses health matters in terms of mental capital, well-being, physical fitness, functioning, positive quality of life, participation and employability.

Since the pathogenic and salutogenic orientation are complementary, different approaches for what we would like to call workplace health development processes are conceivable. Health protection and prevention of disease and disorder (pathogenetic interventions) include interventions aimed at limiting the risks of disease. On the other hand, health promotion (salutogenic interventions) emphasizes supporting and providing healthy choices for employees. Health development is an integral part of (working) life. In essence, measures from the salutogenic perspective aim to enable employees to increase control over the determinants of health.

A distinction can be made between ongoing upstream[3] health development measures (including attention to possible health consequences of all workplace policies) and intended or specific downstream health interventions. Both general measures and specific interventions are important for workplace health. As such, workplace health development processes take place in an interdisciplinary sphere were efforts aimed at health promotion, protection and safety, prevention and healthcare are equally important. As a matter of fact, workplace health focuses primarily on opportunities for good health. This means, also in the case of ill-health, that upstream efforts are being made that should positively affect an employee's health status. Although measures (only) directed at the individual level (e.g. lifestyle) are of great importance, they will not suffice when it comes to realizing comprehensive change in the workplace in terms of healthy working conditions. Health promotion in the workplace also requires integration with other parts of the organization, as well as interactions in line with the intended purpose and interplay among the various subsystems (Hanson, 2007).

5.2 Innovative parts of workplace health development processes

The above-described comprehensive approach takes into account the complexity and dynamics of health and well-being in the workplace. The approach regards employees not as separate from their environment but as part of it, with explicit attention focused on this particular context. Furthermore, emphasis is on what positively creates health (the salutogenic perspective) within such a context. The effectiveness of measures or interventions will increase when all aspects of workplace health – safety and physical, mental and social aspects – are integrated into a complex whole (Naaldenberg et al., 2009). The comprehensive approach is innovative in three other respects as well: it utilizes upstream and salutogenic opportunities; it comprises, as we will further elaborate below, empowerment of employees; and it yields organizational goals for addressing workplace health. In terms of the multi-level perspective from transition studies (Geels and Schot, 2007), workplace health development may be perceived as a niche practice which, eventually, may develop into a regime practice, embedded in interrelated structures.

Since health is determined by a complex interplay of environmental (social, ecological, economic, organizational) and individual determinants, promoting health goes beyond the current health system and the responsibility of the individual alone. For instance, mental and social health can be strengthened through structural attention to meaningful work, continuous education and training on the job. Ensuring meaningful resources in the workplace, as well as strengthening the capacities of employees to use these resources, is complementary to downstream efforts, such as safety measures or health-protecting equipment. Capacity building and strengthening capacities of employees to recognize the resources at their disposal contributes to managing the everyday challenges resulting from all sorts of stimuli, deadlines and information (Eriksson and Lindström, 2008). Furthermore, improving skills can enhance workability, i.e. the ability of gaining and maintaining physical, mental and emotional fitness for the job (Ilmarinen, 2009).

Employees themselves in particular are often quite capable of indicating what they need in their work situation and what is best for their health. For this reason, the strategy of empowerment – fostering the ability and desire of employees to act in empowered ways and to have the autonomy to take part in decision-making processes – is perhaps the most important prerequisite in promoting workplace health. Empowering employees to control the determinants of their health entails that structures which govern working life are tailored to promote good health. In addition, since the "ownership of health" is distributed over a variety of actors from different disciplines, involving and connecting these actors (such as employees, executive board members, and human resource and occupational health managers) is a crucial element of workplace health development processes. Boosting their knowledge and other capacities is another key step in working toward solutions.

Traditionally, healthcare in the workplace is aimed at the improvement of individual health. But from the broader health development perspective, health promotion becomes a strategy that both presupposes and supports organizational learning, development and performance. Thus, it influences the organization's capacity to carry out its mission (Hanson, 2007). The potential of the workforce and its ability to develop have become the subject of a new understanding of managing workplace health, namely as managing "fit for the job" next to management of absenteeism and applying safety measures to prevent accidents in the workplace. A "fit for the job" policy is important because organizations need their employees' full potential, while the workforce needs skills and health to perform in the best possible way. Within this understanding, the promotion of health becomes a strategic issue that supports organizational development and strengthens business performance (Baart et al., 2003; Raaijmakers et al., 2009).

5.3 System innovation for workplace health development: the experience of three case studies

It is possible to distinguish three "system" levels in workplaces. First, businesses and organizations where people work are systems in themselves, with various stakeholders such as management, human resource management, occupational health workers, individual employees and employee representation. At the same time, these entities are subsystems of the larger environment (Koelen and Van den Ban, 2004), in this case the system of occupational health, with stakeholders such as the labor inspectorate responsible for the enforcement of health and safety law, occupational health services, reintegration services, employers' organizations (including SMEs), unions, universities, management training institutes, lifestyle organizations, insurance companies, as well as various levels of government. Third, these practices are embedded in at least two wider systems: the health system and the work or employment system. Each of these is characterized by a regime which has emerged in the history of our advanced welfare state. We refer to system innovation when changes pertain to this level (as well).

In the context of a study which we conducted, three Dutch companies participated in a three-year research project (2006-2009) on system innovation for workplace health promotion (Vaandrager et al., 2006). These companies were interested in introducing feasible innovations in the workplace in order to contribute to significant structural change in workplace health development (system innovation). In each workplace, the following phases were identified:

- A preliminary phase, to introduce workplaces to the systems approach. It was explained that it was the intention to work with a long-term vision, to learn and experiment through a step-by-step collaborative approach.
- A system and actor analysis phase at the system level of companies themselves, to identify potential opportunities and dysfunctions of the company level system: operational routines, culture and governance mechanisms, incentive structures and legislation; existing knowledge and existing routines for evidence-based decision-making.
- A development phase including workshops and brainstorming meetings to discuss new systems or arrangements.

- An implementation phase: working toward system innovation.
- An evaluation phase.

The main focus was on the system level of the workplaces themselves, but of course there were influences of the wider system as well. We discovered that, despite many efforts, it was difficult to take a salutogenic orientation as point of departure for interventions and actions in the workplace, and the reasons for this will be explored below.

The nature of the research in this project may best be described as participatory action research. Action research is a type of research in which solutions to address certain problems are proposed based on research, after which these solutions are put into practice to see if they work and, subsequently, they are again tested against the theory (Koelen and Van den Ban, 2004; Whyte, 1991). Results of the research were thus immediately fed back into the program. They served as point of departure for the companies involved to decide on how to continue. This research therefore literally aimed to stimulate and guide action, while the researcher collaborated with all the other parties involved. The project began with in-depth interviews with stakeholder representatives from the participating workplaces (system and actor analysis). In this section we briefly describe what happened in selected episodes of the cases, so as to be able to draw some lessons from it in the subsequent section.

TMG

TMG (Telegraaf Media Groep) is one of the largest Dutch media conglomerates (approximately 3,000 employees) with a leadership position in daily newspapers, magazines, online and offline media and radio. Due to rapid developments in the area of new media, TMG developed a portfolio of different types of media companies that complemented print media and/or were innovative in relation to the publishers of print media (internet, digital). Geographical boundaries increasingly played a lesser role, and reducing fixed costs in core operating units was crucial for TMG to be able to adapt to that new reality and to be able to continue to invest in growth in the areas of print, the internet and digital media. Due to the above-mentioned technological innovations in the media sector, the job descriptions and required competencies were changing rapidly and employees needed to keep up with these developments. Thus novel technologies, the emergence of new media and economic globalization implied that TMG as a traditional family company needed to rethink its employment policy. This was also their main driver to collaborate in the project.

As a first step, interviews were carried out and documents studied to explore the company's initiatives and vision on workplace health development. Documents were gathered and analyzed, and semi-structured interviews were held with 27 stakeholders (June to September 2007). People who were interviewed were involved in health or employability issues due to their position (HRM, management board, central works committee) or had expressed ideas to do things differently.

Results of the system analysis

Although the medical/pathogenic perspective of workplace health development being perceived as promoting a healthy lifestyle was also present, the most dominant perspective at TMG was to keep employees employable for the job. As a consequence, workplace health development was mainly seen as the core business of the HRM department. This employability (and essentially salutogenic) perspective varied from supportive to economical: "employability facilitates personal growth and development" versus "employability policy can be cost effective." These economic motives seemed to have the upper hand. Employability policy within TMG therefore mainly concerned the dynamics between employment benefits and the required competencies and skills of employees. This was also expressed in its stated core values:

> TMG is a reliable and committed employer. Employees are offered extensive development opportunities and good income. In exchange, TMG expects its employees to proactively handle changes, to further develop themselves and to contribute to the development of the enterprise in a drastically changing marketplace in a committed, and professional way.
>
> (www.corporate.tmg.nl)

Despite this vision, interviewees expressed their concerns that there was a lack of mobility and a lack of incentives to improve employability within TMG, and this is why TMG was searching for short-term instruments to improve this situation.

Suggested practices for future steps

The central approach in this phase was to organize a new structure for TMG's employability policy because this seemed the best entry point for change. In addition, it was believed that a shift in regimes was needed from seeing change as an opportunity for development, health and well-being, rather than as a threat to being no longer employable. One of the ideas to make a start on this new structure was to present the results of the system analysis to stakeholders within TMG, and to initiate a debate about the existing culture, patterns, communication and possible solutions for workplace health development within TMG.

Experiences during the implementation

Unfortunately, the planned debate was cancelled. As TMG informed us, they did not want to proceed because they were in search of clear, short-term steps and goal-oriented instruments. They also explained that this short cyclic and pragmatic approach was related to the "newspaper" way of thinking: there needs to be a newspaper every day. The approach of the research project, marked as it was by a long-term vision, learning and experimenting in projects and a step-by-step collaborative approach, appeared to be a poor fit. It was therefore decided to halt the project within this company.

TMG continued on its own, however, and developed a special career center for three groups of employees: (1) employees who were redundant, (2) employees who were interested in a career change, and (3) employees with high potential. In 2009, 169 employees participated in this project and the majority (154 employees) decided to continue with career development. The interventions concerned person-fit solutions. Participants were security guards, administrative staff, postroom employees, facility employees, sales assistants, desk-top publishers, designers, managers and drivers. A total of 175 employees participated in workshops in which the "new" employment policy was explained. One hundred and fifty employees had three individual career counseling talks, 86 employees entered special training courses and nine employees managed to find a job outside TMG.

By and large, TMG decided to focus on training and to apply a practical and short-term approach, and, as a result, the issue of health development more or less disappeared from the agenda.

KPN

KPN is a provider of telecommunications and ICT services and has a 125-year track record. Formerly a state company, it privatized in 1989. The organizational structure is built around five different customer segments and is headed by a management board. In 2010, this workplace had about 12,000 employees.

As a first step of the project a system analysis was carried out to gain a deeper understanding of the company's knowledge of workplace health and reasons to participate in the research project on system innovation for workplace health development. Documents related to health and employability were gathered and 11 semi-structured interviews with stakeholders took place (June to October 2007). Interviewees were four people from the corporate center of human resources services, one member of the "works council," two senior advisers, two (external) occupational health professionals and two staff from the security division.

Attention to health in the workplace was not new for KPN. Several research projects around stress and mental health problems had been carried out in the past (Rhenen et al., 2007; Van der Klink et al., 2003). However, it was also believed that attention to health should be based more on a salu-togenic model of health, because the aforementioned initiatives were mainly restricted to being individual-oriented and pathogenic-oriented. Furthermore, stakeholders of KPN felt that this shift fitted well with the company's corpo-rate social responsibility (CSR) policy.

Results of the system analysis

Three different perspectives of workplace health development were found as a result of the system analysis. On the one hand, workplace health develop-ment was seen to promote – mainly by occupational health specialists – an individual healthy lifestyle (including mental health promotion), physical health and the safe working of employees. As such they basically embraced a medical and pathogenic perspective. On the other hand, and partly reflecting the neoliberal turn mentioned above, managers saw workplace health devel-opment primarily as an opportunity to move away from "pampering" workers and to promote another normative principle about the employment relationship: seeing workers as "active human beings in democratic com-munities entitled to human rights." This perspective had an emphasis on indi-vidual responsibility for health. From a more economic angle, finally, workplace health was perceived as a way to promote employability and there-fore these interviewees stressed the idea that it was important to actively encourage employees to continuously develop their skills and thereby take charge of planning their own career path. This last perspective, which may be characterized as the most salutogenic of the three, was mainly put forward by the members of the human resources services. In a special meeting these pre-liminary findings of the system and actor analysis were presented to the stake-holders (including the interviewees). Overall, it was recognized that links between these perspectives were lacking. The stakeholders were given the opportunity to comment on the results and future steps were planned.

Suggested practices for future steps

One of the ideas of KPN was to more proactively organize special health weeks and promote healthy lifestyle activities. Furthermore, an individual lifestyle check (a brief check-up) covering lifestyles and fitness including tips for a healthier lifestyle was planned. A study on employee participation and chronic illness among employees aged 45 and over was also suggested (all three were based on the first perspective presented above).

To combine a career with other ambitions such as childcare or voluntary work, KPN developed a "New Way of Working" strategy. This strategy aimed to make it possible for employees to work for KPN regardless of time and place (based on the second perspective presented above).

Finally, based on the perspective which may be characterized as most salu-togenic, KPN proposed to introduce a personal employability budget of

€1,000 per employee. Employees were free to utilize this budget in accordance with their own views in order to enhance their employability.

It should be noted that none of these ideas resulted from the project only; they might as well have been enforced by the system analysis and the commitment to participate in this project.

Experiences during the implementation

Overall, the strategies at KPN may be categorized as both pathogenic and salutogenic, yet fragmented and only moving slowly forward toward a more integrative approach.

The opportunities for improvement highlighted during the system analysis phase such as better links between occupational health, human resource management and general management were recognized, but follow-up activities were limited in empowering employees and were barely related to an organizational salutogenic development perspective. Managers were still more reactive to health problems rather than taking a proactive approach of creating the conditions for health development. This state of affairs was probably due to the fact that the main emphasis within KPN was on shifting the responsibility for workplace health – in line with the neoliberal paradigm – from the organization to the individual (stop pampering), which was so strong that there was generally less attention paid to providing healthy choices and enabling employees to take control over the determinants of health. Stakeholders also complained that there were still a number of employees favoring the "old model" in which the employer is fully responsible for the care of employees.

Furthermore, although there was recognition that workplace health at KPN was a shared responsibility, it was difficult to get things moving. The HRM department continued to be the main driver of the process (rather than the desired collaborative approach), and at the end of the project period the wish to work in a more interdisciplinary fashion was still expressed, which indicated that attempts in this area had been only partly successful at best.

Deventer Hospital

The third workplace is Deventer Hospital (approximately 2,000 employees). It was set up in 1985 as a result of a merger of two regional hospitals. The hospital had a special training center for medical specialists and nurses, as well as a history in disease prevention activities, such as company fitness, the opportunity to have a preventive consult with a company physician and possibilities for active revalidation. In 2008 the hospital moved to a new location and as part of this move, the hospital organized a project called "Fit into the new building." This was a contest among employees geared to doing exercise, losing weight and eating healthily. Despite these existing health-related activities, the hospital was eager to find new ideas and ways to manage workplace health. A first step in the project (preliminary phase) was to join the already existing health policy steering group meeting and to carry out a document analysis.

Results of the preliminary phase

Employees of Deventer Hospital basically espoused two viewpoints regarding workplace health development. The first, most medical/pathogenic perspective appeared to be largely driven by the hospital's occupational health service. Its staff perceived health development as promoting a healthy lifestyle, physical fitness and safe working conditions for employees. Others within the hospital, on the other hand, saw workplace health development as a core quality dimension of the services provided by the hospital, such as patient safety, clinical effectiveness and people's health in the neighboring communities. Healthy working conditions for employees and investment in capacity building of employees based on this quality management perspective were perceived as a natural part of good care for patients and a pleasant atmosphere for guests. This last perspective in particular clearly belongs to a salutogenic perspective.

During the subsequent period (the development and implementation phase), new health practices were developed at Deventer Hospital.

Suggested practices for future steps

Based on the preliminary phase, the hospital decided to first develop a new vision on workplace health development and to debate whether it was ethical for them as an organization to promote healthy lifestyles. Furthermore, it was proposed to adopt a comprehensive approach and to link health management with human resource management, leadership, training and career planning.

Experiences during the implementation

In a special workshop for employees and various stakeholders of the hospital, chaired by the Board, it was discussed whether and how an employer (the hospital management) could "interfere" with the lifestyle of employees (staff of the hospital). The discussion in the workshop concerned the responsibility for workplace health. The two main parties – staff and management – agreed that a balance was needed between the employer's responsibility for health development and the room afforded to employees to develop their full potential.

In response, the hospital formulated a health development policy and a vision document, closely linked to its general mission. Instead of the term "health management" which had been used in the past, it was decided to subsume all activities and policies related to health development under the slogan "Deventer hospital works healthy." Ensuring employability and increasing commitment and employee satisfaction were formulated as important objectives of the vision paper. Strikingly, in this case, personal development motives, rather than economic motives, largely informed this policy document.

A collaborative approach to promote health was closely linked to the primary process at Deventer Hospital. The basic idea was that when employees are healthy, committed and happy, patient care will improve. This made it easier to interconnect the different disciplines of occupational health, human resource management and general management. As a stakeholder, the occupational health service – a driving force in the process – also decided to shift its emphasis from only promoting healthy lifestyles to a broader integral health development perspective. This certainly contributed to the start of the hospital's implementation of "integrated health management" (Zwetsloot and Pot, 2004).

Despite these promising advances, it was remarkable that employee involvement in policy development was not really an issue at Deventer Hospital. A more active consideration of employees' opinions would have benefitted further developments.

5.4 Regimes and persistent problems in the area of workplace health promotion

The results of the case studies reported on here triggered debates about the meaning of workplace health development, company policy and vision development, and a variety of activities such as health checks and personal health budgets. These developments show a move toward a more salutogenic approach of health in the workplace. In all three cases the "incumbent regime" continued to be the most dominant, although Deventer Hospital may be characterized as the most salutogenic. Many new practices at TMG and KPN were only a "drop in the ocean" and existing structures did not facilitate a salutogenic approach. Aside from the prevailing pathogenic approaches, it appeared to be a struggle to develop and implement practices based on salutogenesis. Interestingly, not only did specific company health policies appear to be enablers or barriers for workplace health, but also policies coming from other fields. For instance, in all three cases employability was an important concern associated with social security and economic policies. Links between these policy areas would be logical but seemed to be difficult in practice (see e.g. TMG).

As we have learned from the case studies, workplace health development strategies did not achieve their full potential. There appeared to be a number of features of the system constraining the change process. These included the dominance of the pathogenic orientation, the downstream focus, medical actors setting the scene, lack of employee involvement (empowerment) and compartmentalization of domains. We will discuss these elements in more detail below.

Enforcement and action is still about care for and preventive ill-health

What transpires from the cases is the fact that none has completely implemented the new health model of salutogenesis. There were attempts to change and apply a more positive model of health which was reflected in the way stakeholders in the system analysis phase talked about work and health. However, in all three case studies it was learned that already in the planning phase there were more prevalent perspectives on the pathogenic side than on the salutogenic one. Thus, while knowledge of workplace health had expanded toward a more positive orientation on health and well-being, enforcement and action still held on to thinking mainly in terms of care for, and prevention of, ill-health. In two of the case studies employees could be medically tested and received medical advice, and this was presented as "health management." This type of health check is focused on the individual employee and his or her health (lose weight, more exercise, etc.). The system hardly facilitated the broader integrated approach of workplace health development. Consequently, routines for decisions on health in the workplace and working procedures of stakeholders were mainly based on the medical paradigm.

Public and occupational health actors set the scene

Main actors involved in workplace health development processes were public and occupational health services, company management (human resources, safety), employees and society (or the social environment). One of the characteristics of the incumbent regime is that society and subsequent company management and employees have learned that public health and occupational health services are responsible for health. Here an imbalance between the different actors becomes visible: within the workplace system, the ownership of health is passed on to only one sector (HRM or occupational health), while it should rather be something shared and interdisciplinary. Health in the workplace more or less became a product that could be delivered by professionals. Over time, public health and occupational health more than once served as a "waste basket" for issues that in fact are socially embedded, such as workability and chronic diseases related to lifestyle. For sure, multi-interventions and commitment from all actors are needed here. Reassigning responsibility is quite difficult, however.

Downstream focus dominates upstream thinking

It appeared that workplace health at KPN and initially also at Deventer Hospital was primarily perceived as promoting a healthy lifestyle, physical health and the safe working of employees (downstream model and focused on the individual). Although various initiatives running in these workplaces were based more on the upstream model such as organizational development, training of management and education of employees, they were not always linked to workplace health promotion. In workshops and discussions, therefore, attention was paid to how to ensure equal attention for positive health and ill-health.

Central role and appreciation of empowerment of employees is missing

In the three case studies, but mainly at TMG, it was clear that the involved workplaces have become quite complex due to scaling up, (medical) technological developments, automation and ICT, as well as growing responsibilities for individual employees. Owing to specialization, employees were dependent on other employees and departments, and their job responsibilities were subject to rapid change. This created interdependence, and employees felt less in control. From a health promotion perspective, this feeling of control or empowerment is central to health and well-being. There were various initiatives to increase this control: KPN made a personal yearly budget available which employees could use for training, personal fitness and retraining. At Deventer Hospital a special brainstorming session was organized to discuss whether personal health is a private concern or a company concern, and at TMG training sessions for employees were organized to discuss their employability. Despite these good intentions, employees themselves also tended to define health development along the lines of the medical paradigm of physical health, instead of mental and social health. It was also found that employees are somewhat afraid to take control. Health development explained along the medical paradigm comes with a risk discourse that goes beyond own responsibility. Health promotion principles demand an active approach and an environment in which the organization and doctors are coaches instead of experts. Here we see a clear need to go beyond the mere "responsibilization" implied in neoliberal policies.

Given the current regime, the continuation of a lead role for public health and occupational health services, and controlling along with standardizing health-related issues close to the disease outcome is much easier. Yet, this directly contradicts the "enabling" and "being in control" part of positive health.

Compartmentalization of domains

Work-based strategies for health require cooperation among different disciplines such as labor, health, economics, social service, health and social insurance, business management, human resource management, and occupational health and safety. This cooperation appears difficult in practice because of different domains, responsibilities and daily routines (Koelen et al., 2008). In order to stimulate the use of resources for health, a better and fairer balance between different actors, their responsibilities and lead roles is needed.

Within the incumbent regime, a gap is present between different domains that act in the field of workplace health development processes. This gap is defined by insufficiencies in the services offered and reinforced by the policies for workplace health. Connections between the domains involved are largely absent in policy and practice because healthcare, protection, prevention and health promotion have evolved separately without a clear link to business management. Each domain offers its own alternatives for taking care of health and health promotion. Since the current structures also require short-term predefined goals in each of these domains, it is hard to work according to an integrated approach for which you need integrated goals. Moreover, choices are made from a specific specialist domain standpoint, instead of a holistic viewpoint including business and business management. This has serious limitations for enforcing workplace health development processes, in which the entrance point for the conceptualization of health should be human beings, the workers in the context of the workplace, not the different specializations. On the other hand, business managers do not view health as an important resource for business, nor is health (promotion) seen as a key performance indicator.

What is lacking in policy and practice alike is a powerful and shared vision, as well as integrated aims that do justice to workplace health development processes.

5.5 What is needed?

Many of the barriers discussed in Section 5.4 are rooted in dominant assumptions of the incumbent regime. Based on transition theory (Elzen et al., 2004; Grin et al., 2010; Rotmans, 2005), it is clear that a number of regime elements need to change as part of a transition that better facilitates workplace health promotion practices that sufficiently reflect the salutogenic orientation. Transitions are regarded here as involving fundamental and interrelated changes in technology, organization, institutions and culture. A salutogenic transition comprises a society-wide change that goes beyond what is currently believed to be the workplace health development structure. Mutual reinforcements and combined action from the sectors of employment, health and safety are required. Synchronicity and interaction of developments in different domains are key.

Transition theory (Elzen et al., 2004; Grin et al., 2010; Rotmans, 2005) suggest that a shared vision (1) may help to redefine assumptions, and (2) may form the functional equivalent of structure where the incumbent regime does not provide proper guidance for novel practices. The so-called multi-level perspective (MLP) (Geels and Schot, 2007; Grin, 2008) provides a dynamic view on innovation. The core of the MLP is that transitions are shaped by interaction among three levels: the socio-technical landscape, the socio-technical regimes and niches.

In the MLP dynamic, system innovations develop as follows. A novelty emerges in a local practice (in this case a workplace) and becomes part of a niche when a network of actors (management, HRM, OSH, employees) is formed who share certain expectations about the future success of the novelty (happy employees, better products, sustainable production), and are willing to fund and work on further development. Niches may emerge and develop partly in response to pressure and serious problems in an existing regime (high levels of stress, aging, health problems), which can be either internal to the regime itself (employees becoming despensable, high sickness figures) or which emerge from the socio-technical landscape (e.g. diabetes, overweight, the fact that people need to work longer and be fit). The further success of niche formation is linked to processes within the niche (micro-level), but also to developments at the level of the existing regime (meso-level) and the socio-technical landscape (macro-level) (see Figure 5.1).

Based on Section 5.4 below, we formulate some crucial elements of a vision that were constraints in the case studies. Each of these elements is a possible step toward workplace health system innovation.

A long-term positive and inspiring vision of workplace health

A long-term positive and inspiring vision of workplace health is a first step in a reorientation. This vision should reflect the ownership of health as interdisciplinary. This requires that open-ended pathways leaving space for learning and new ideas be facilitated. Furthermore, benefits and goals must be comprehensible for business management, employees, occupational health services, public health and society at large. Workplace health development processes have everything to do with ambition and possibilities. This may be translated

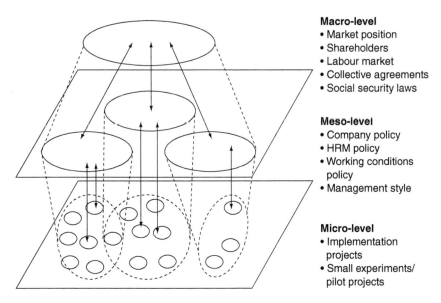

Macro-level
• Market position
• Shareholders
• Labour market
• Collective agreements
• Social security laws

Meso-level
• Company policy
• HRM policy
• Working conditions policy
• Management style

Micro-level
• Implementation projects
• Small experiments/pilot projects

Figure 5.1 Multi-level approach of system innovation: workplace health development

into a company's vision of health, in line with the company's mission and vision in reference to business goals. At Deventer Hospital, for example, salutogenic approaches and necessary skills will follow from such a vision of health. Helping company decision-makers understand how social and physical environments profoundly affect the well-being of employees is a first step toward a system innovation. For example, in terms of strategic direction, does the organization's vision and/or mission statement recognize that employees are an investment, a key element in success? Do the organization's policies recognize the workplace environment as a determinant of employee health? Do the actions and comments of the leadership team reinforce a healthy workplace? Is there a process in place to link employee and workplace health policies/issues to the organization's human resource planning and strategic direction?

Health is a shared responsibility and views of employees are central

In successful health promotion in the workplace, health is characterized by the commitment of the top management, seeing the employee as the most important asset, and by high involvement of (empowered) employees who are challenged *and* enabled to explore improvements in work and health beyond the medical perspective. This aspect tends to be underused because the management of health in workplaces is still the domain of professionals, including occupational health services, rather than that of managers and employees themselves. Linked to this aspect there is also the issue of individual, organizational or social responsibility for the health of employees.

A human focus is central. The health-related behavior of employees is dependent on the organization of the working environment, and policies that underpin social organization (Nutbeam and Harris, 1999). Moreover, the perspective on upstream efforts and the focus on resources for health encompass personal factors such as comprehension, manageability and meaningfulness. Synergy in and between the areas mentioned will lead to the effectiveness of integrated health promotion initiatives.

When an employee focus is in place, a company will invest clear efforts to foster and support an environment that encourages and assists employees to become involved in workplace health policy and activities, as well as contribute to the overall goals of the organization. It is preferable that in the contact between line management and employees there is attention to needs and preferences on both sides, adjusting the work to the employee, resulting in a higher quality of work and working conditions, and therefore good business.

Since every employee possibly has different needs and preferences, a variety of activities is preferred. In this way, joint responsibility for developing healthy work and a healthy workplace is fully acknowledged.

Health promotion is a normal business procedure

Workplace health management is directed not only toward promoting health throughout the company from a system perspective, but also toward increasing good health as part of normal business procedures (such as training in specific skills, career planning, job evaluation, etc.). Both governance streams (health promotion, business procedures) influence each other. Furthermore, sound preconditions for health cannot be delivered quickly by experts but are based on cooperation of all actors involved, and their shared achievements should be rewarded instead of single outcomes. It is therefore necessary to understand and influence human-related or so-called "soft" processes of a company in a suitable way. Health promotion involves a long-term process of change, which is based on learning and collective understanding of the determining factors of health as well as of the company's goal and the conditions under which it operates (Hanson, 2007). Significantly, the same drivers that help produce goods and services also help produce and sustain health. Corporate social responsibility can be an umbrella for sustainable health and workability of people (workers), combined with a "green policy" on planet and profit.

Workplace health is wealth

Aging and future labor shortages urge employers and government to reconsider workplace health measures and instruments. As demonstrated by our case studies, there is no easy way to do so. Assumptions should be redefined and structures replaced in such a way that they actually include health development as a linchpin of the business model, encourage empowerment of employees and stimulate combined action from different disciplines based on the view that "good health is good for workers, is good for business."

Notes

1 We choose to use the concept of "health" here, even though our interpretation of health, as that which makes life good for the individual person living it, could also be referred to as "well-being."
2 The term "ill-health" is used as a collective description of a variety of states which cover injury, illness, dysfunction, feelings of discomfort or other states which fall within this category (Hanson, 2007).
3 Most measures may be described as either "downstream" or "upstream." Interventions are called "downstream" when they are closely linked to diseases and their effects; interventions on a structural level (e.g. higher income or better company management) are termed "upstream."

6 Toward a sustainable welfare and health system in Spain

Experiences with the case management program

Francisco Ródenas and Jorge Garcés

6.1 Introduction

This chapter discusses recent initiatives to deal with the problem of the unsustainability of social protection systems and traditional healthcare in Spain, as an example of a Mediterranean welfare state. Over the past few years, the Spanish government has been stressing the vulnerability of current social protection regimes (Directorate-General for Economic and Financial Affairs, 2002a, 2002b). Many of the attempts to resolve them have not been successful, however.

We will present and discuss an approach to overcome the persistence of this problem (Grin et al., 2010: 2–3), called the "Sustainable Socio-Health Model" (SSHM), which we designed and implemented as researchers at the Polibienestar Research Institute of the University of Valencia (Garcés et al., 2011), with funding and support from the Ministries of Health and Social Welfare of the regional government. It is a new management model of health and social resources that starts from three criteria: proximity, improving efficiency and raising quality of services. Our model proposes the integrated use of the portfolios of health and social services to assist people who need long-term care. Central to this model are case management teams, which define individual pathways based on individual needs. As case management practices transcend the boundaries between the now separate regimes of healthcare and social care, they presuppose structural change as well as cultural changes beyond the basic values nurtured by the welfare state. As a consequence, any proposal for reform is bound to raise considerable dispute, an issue to which we will return in the final section.

In the remainder of this chapter, we will present the SSHM, discuss experiences gained with its implementation and reflect on these experiences from a transition perspective. Before doing so, however, let us briefly review the set of interconnected challenges facing the healthcare and social support systems in Spain.

New challenges facing the healthcare and social support systems
in Spain

As in most countries in Europe and North America, in Spain the most debated problem with respect to healthcare probably concerns its affordability. More specifically, Spain, like other Mediterranean countries, has significantly invested in health systems over the past few decades, above all in care for disabled and dependent people. This has prompted serious doubts as to the sustainability of this system in the medium term. These concerns were further fueled by the financial crisis, which increased the risk for the state to go bankrupt (Jackson and Howe, 2003). In Spain and many other countries, therefore, a need was felt to improve the effectiveness of their social protection systems without increasing the costs to the public sector (Dixon and Mossialos, 2002; Mossialos et al., 2002).

Furthermore, technological and scientific advances in the nineteenth and twentieth centuries in developed nations have led to an increase in life expectancy as well as to a variety of health problems related to lifestyle and the environment. This factor has contributed to a society characterized by an unprecedentedly high share of elderly people and a predominance of particular (chronic) diseases (WHO, 2002a). In Spain, the number of people with some level of dependency is estimated to go up by 50 percent within two decades, from 959,890 dependent people in 2000 to 1,496,226 in 2020 (MTAS, 2005). Elderly people are the group most affected by loss of functional capacity; they have to cope with physical and mental deterioration and are more likely to suffer from chronic diseases and interrelated patterns of multiple health problems (Grundy and Glaser, 2000; Garcés et al., 2004; Singh, 2005).

These trends have at least two crucial implications (García-Armesto et al., 2010). First, in Spain, like in other OECD countries (see Introduction to this volume), the demographic dynamic of population aging (with a spectacular increase of life expectancy) and a low rate of economic growth will significantly contribute to serious problems regarding the financial tenability of pension and health systems. In Spain, pension expenditures will increase to 15.7 percent of the GDP by 2050 (European Commission, 2006). Second, these trends also give rise to other problems. There will not be a sufficiently mature and organized supply of socio-health services to deal with the demand. The health systems that were largely designed in the 1950s and 1960s will not be able to absorb the pressure of socio-health demands, created by a combination of this quantitative increase and the growing diversification of the demand, following on from ongoing processes of individualization and immigration. Moreover, it does not help in resolving these problems that Mediterranean welfare states have less coordination between different social and healthcare resources than one might consider necessary to cover the wide variety of needs of older dependent adults, while modifications in supply and service planning to meet those needs have been limited (Carpenter et al., 1999; Garcés et al., 2003; Fine and Glendinning, 2005). These problems have been exacerbated by attempts to reduce or control public spending (Comas et al., 2006) through imposing zero growth in the supply of public resources and a shift toward private supply and/or family or informal care (Knapp et al., 2001; Field and Peck, 2003).

The latter takes us to a third set of problems, related to changes in Spain's intergenerational solidarity culture. Many elderly people need long-term care to maintain and promote maximum quality of life, well-being, dignity and independence in their functioning in everyday life (WHO, 2002b; Bains, 2003). In providing such care, informal care providers within the family – especially women – play a significant role (OECD, 1998; Havens, 1999; Garcés et al., 2003).

At this level there is a sustainability problem as well. "Natural" and inter-generational solidarity are under pressure due to changes such as the increase of single-parent households and the choice of young people to live alone. This trend is being circumstantially altered by the economic crisis, forcing families with fewer economic resources to share housing and expenses, which increases family stress. In addition, as women are increasingly entering the labor market while maintaining their main role in informal care, the problem of overburdened caregivers will grow larger (National Alliance for Caregiving and AARP, 1997; Family Caregiver Alliance, 2001; MTAS, 2005). The assistance required frequently exceeds the informal carer's physical and mental capability and becomes a chronic stress factor, the so-called informal caregiv-er's burden (Zarit, 1998, 2002; Garcés et al., 2008). In addition, caregivers' stress and emotional distress have serious consequences for the care recipient, principally involving the earlier institutionalization of the dependent person (Logdon et al., 1999) and maltreatment and abuse (McGuire and Fulmer, 1997; Mockus Parks and Novielli, 2000). The social and health repercussions will be perpetuated unless strategic actions are implemented to mitigate them (Garcés et al., 2010a, 2010b). The short-term and long-term consequences of informal carers' stress translate for the government into financial pressure on social protection systems (Carretero et al., 2007).

Tensions occur not only around intergenerational solidarity, but also with regard to solidarity between classes. At present, the systems of protection function on the basis of principles of solidarity in relation to income level and individual wealth, which means that the tax burden falls mainly on the middle class. Especially when faced with an increase of poverty and in times of eco-nomic crisis, the government tends to increase the tax burden on this par-ticular class. But the middle class is reluctant to pay more taxes when receiving fewer quality services in return, which has been described as "the squaring of the circle of welfare" (George and Miller, 1994).[1]

Finally, the effort to deal with non-communicable diseases, which consti-tute an increasing share of health problems (see Introduction to this volume), is badly served by the existing functional differentiation between social ser-vices and health systems. These two levels largely operate in parallel and in an uncoordinated manner with distinct assessment systems, different training and separate professional cultures. This leads to ineffectiveness and inefficiency, having a negative effect on the quality of life of its users and giving rise in addition to missed opportunities to reduce government expenditures on social protection systems.

Against this backdrop, as we concluded, there is a need to restructure social assistance and health systems. We have proposed an orientation for such restructuring, the so-called "Sustainable Socio-Health Model." In this contribution, we will discuss our proposal from a transition studies perspective (Section 6.2). Next, we will present an experiment in Valencia and interpret its proceedings and outcomes in terms of transition theory. The experiment entails a real, albeit partial, application of the proposed model that should not be considered in isolation but as part of a larger process of change that puts forward a reorganization of resources in the health and social systems, focusing on the patient/user who accesses a unique portfolio of services. In isolation, it may be confused with a "standard government efficiency pilot" that only aims to cut costs. The example of Valencia shows that it is possible to put the SSHM into practice, at least on a small scale. As implementation of the SSHM is only possible when making changes to the incumbent regime's structure, culture and practices, the experiences with the experiment will provide relevant insights into what these regime changes entail and the barriers that will be encountered. This provides the basis, finally, for several proposals as to the model's further development.

6.2 The Sustainable Social-Health Model

Against the background of these sets of fundamental problems, a group of researchers at the Polibienestar Research Institute of the University of Valencia have proposed the "Sustainable Socio-Health Model" (SSHM). Essentially, it aims for a joint reorganization of health and social systems into a more integrated, individual client-oriented system, in order to provide an answer to the needs of people requiring long-term care. The model considers the convergence of a social services system and the health system, at the level of individual clients and their needs and possibilities, as a holistic model of attention to people who need long-term care to increase their welfare and quality of life – the latter in the sense of enabling a fulfilling daily life, and, when the time comes, offering opportunities for dying with dignity (Garcés, 2000).

The underlying presumption is that a careful study of the needs and possibilities of each patient can lead to more tailor-made solutions for individuals *and* free up many resources through more tailor-made practices, *if* at least we use such insight to improve efficiency in structures and processes from different systems by (1) decreasing the overlapping work, (2) avoiding unnecessary re-admissions, and (3) improving the patient's quality of life at home. In order to achieve such improvements in structures and processes, a case management methodology with multidisciplinary teamwork was applied, designing personal care pathways supported by social and health services.

In the remainder of this section we will, first, outline the axiological assumptions behind the model and how they are reflected in it. Second, we will argue that the change toward such a model may be fruitfully understood as a transition, i.e. a process of fundamental transformation of practices and structures – more specifically involving, in this instance, a transformation of the structures of two systems while transcending their functional differentiation.

Axiological basis and outline of the Sustainable Socio-Health Model

The model envisages care practices that are affordable and accessible, because professionals and clients seek to use the system to deal with individual needs while respecting the universal principle of welfare state equity (also proposed as one of the ethical principles of sustainable healthcare by Jameton and McGuire (2002) as "justice and equality: everyone should have reasonable access to adequate resources needed for healthfulness"). Quality is promoted by developing an integral understanding of individual needs – social, health-wise, functional, psychological, economic and cultural – and providing an individualized method of planning and managing them (Batalden and Davidoff, 2007). This ensures that appropriate care is tailored to the needs and cultural preferences of the clients. This new system would be supported by three principles: social sustainability, quality of life and dignified death, and social co-responsibility. Each is elaborated below.

Social sustainability

The principle of social sustainability (Garcés, 2000) is defined as the extension of the welfare principle of universality (Fitzpatrick, 1996; Gilbert and Terrell, 2004) in time, in such a way that welfare is a right, not only for current citizens but also for later generations.

From the axiological point of view, the principle of social sustainability takes on the value of solidarity between generations, and is legitimized ethically through a wider and deeper reanalysis of the fundamental social values of freedom and equality: (1) freedom and responsibility, insofar as our present freedom implies the responsibility of taking into account our successors in our actions or the conditions of life we nurture; (2) equality of rights and obligations, for no current or future citizen should have their freedom, their options or their decision capacity impaired as a result of our actions (Garcés et al., 2003). We operationalized this principle on the basis of three elements:

- Reorganization of the portfolios of services, creating streamlined management structures that can make decisions from a unified portfolio of health and social services (Garcés et al., 2013).
- Improving preventive measures linked to specific health and social risks; for example, establishing criteria for identifying patients at high risk of

hospital readmission to activate protocols from primary healthcare to delay or avoid hospitalization (Ródenas et al., 2013).

- Using ICT to improve decision-making on setting up new programs or services during the transition to new protection systems; for example, the design and implementation of simulation tools for improving the care of patients requiring long-term care (Grimaldo et al., 2013, 2014).

Social sustainability is related to the principle of "No-loser constraint with hypothetical compensation"; i.e., that it is legitimate to carry out changes in health policy if (1) the benefits outweigh harmful effects – cost/benefits ratio – as long as (2) there is an offsetting subsequent redistribution of benefits among the population (an increase in equity), such that citizens badly affected by the first phase of change eventually improve their situation into one that is at least not worse than the one prior to the beginning of the change.

Quality of life and dignified death

The quality of life axiom in this model is not confined to establishing a dignified standard of life, but should also be reinterpreted as a subjective right of citizens. On the one hand, a person should be able to improve her or his subjective welfare through remaining at home and with their family for as long as possible. This requires properly helping both the client and the main caregiver through social and emotional support as well as therapies and active rehabilitation. On the other hand, there should be optimal accessibility in the sense that the client obtains the service at the time and place and in the amount they need at a reasonable cost, eliminating physical, geographic, organizational, social and cultural barriers (Garcés et al., 2003). We operationalized this principle as follows:

- *Proximity:* an acceptable distance between clients and service providers. The social care and healthcare model must be able to offer dependent persons the services they require in their immediate surroundings, starting from an interdisciplinary valuation of every situation with a Personalized Care Plan (Davies, 1992; Challis, 1993; Hébert, 2002).
- *Effectiveness of the social and healthcare model:* the degree to which clients manage to improve their health and welfare while remaining in their familiar surroundings (OECD, 2005), boosting resources such as at-home help, phone assistance or medication and home hospitalization.
- *Efficiency:* a good ratio between the real impact of the service and its production cost (Docteur, 2001).

In addition, we have proposed to include in the model the concept of dying with dignity. With the epidemiological and demographic changes and subsequent degenerative processes, the number of years that people have fairly extensive care needs increases. There is an increasing need for bioethical health protocols beyond the sphere of the hospital, as well as for legislation to safeguard individual rights related to the decision when and how one dies. The right to a good death has been unresolved in Spain as of yet. This calls for the need to develop moral and quality standards on dying, and to establish a sense of balance between relevant concerns associated with power, trust, money, hope and integrity.

Social co-responsibility

Co-responsibility deals with the degree of individual or group involvement in the social and financial maintenance of public protection structures. Taking on this principle does not mean a wager on individualism, responsibility and meritocracy leading to a Friedmanian retreat of the state. On the contrary, social co-responsibility means maintaining a state protection structure at the same time as individuals bear own responsibility for welfare. It is crucial that this is not just an attribution of responsibility to citizens by the state – it should at least be as much a matter of increasing people's agency (improved opportunities to live one's life through more autonomy and less dependency) and quality of life (see above).

Financial co-responsibility is understood here as a supportive, active contribution to financing public welfare through partial payment of services in the protection systems used, depending on the income and the tax burden of the user and/or their relatives, so that other people who objectively cannot finance part of their needs also benefit (Garcés et al., 2003). To be sure, financial co-responsibility consists in providing individual solidarity to society through the national state institutions, but the state should find formulas that prevent problems of fiscal refusal and increase its co-responsibility with the middle class; one way would consist in reducing taxes for people who would have made a more efficient use of the social protection system. It deals with the considerable weighted or balanced reward to those that reduce expenditures on social protection systems with the adoption of behaviors and practices marked by less frequent use of public services (for example, health, which is the most expensive) and by the adoption of preventive behaviors and practices associated with health risks.

Key elements of the model

In elaborating these principles into more concrete terms, the research team at the Polibienestar Research Institute could draw upon a set of international experiences. Models reflecting certain similar principles have been proposed and applied in countries such as the UK, Ireland and Canada (Longley, 2004). For example, in relation to our principle of quality of life, the UK health system reform in 1998 (Department of Health, 1998) put special emphasis on the development of the principle of accessibility to the system by improving the proximity of primary and community services (Robinson and Dixon,

1999). This approach was used to operationalize our principle of quality of life. Local administration and national departments jointly guarantee providing care services to senior citizens, maintaining and strengthening their independence, among other measures by the *reduction of preventable hospital admittance*, developing *prevention services* and relief attention, and the provision of additional *help to non-professional carers*.

The Northern Ireland System of Health and Personal Social Services (Northern Ireland Department of Health, Social Services and Public Safety, 2002a) has been able to reduce inequalities, improving access to care and promoting the integrated management of health and social care (Jordan et al., 2006). Of the reforms put forward, this system aimed to improve primary and community care as the first point of contact with the system, suggesting its role in maintaining the chronically ill in the community. With respect to specialized outpatients' departments and hospitalization, it introduced a plan of hospital modernization taking into account the aging of the population and a growing need for medical care, new technologies and new management models, as well as procedural improvements. In addition, the various documents produced throughout the process – on the reform of hospital services and the improved quality of care practices – appeared helpful (Northern Ireland Department of Health, Social Services and Public Safety, 2002b).

6.3 Why the SSHM implies a transition

The SSHM model implies a profound transformation, a transition indeed: new practices and structural change are needed both within and between the systems of social protection and healthcare. Without trying to be exhaustive, it is easy to list several fundamental changes *within* these systems. New distributions of tasks between citizens, society, caregivers and the state imply institutional changes and different cultural assumptions among all those involved on how to understand and realize quality of life and a dignified death. Citizens should change their expectations in this respect. Professional caregivers must scrutinize their professional routines and attitudes in order to help realize a less supply-driven, more tailor-made type of care and to support clients in increasing their agency and sense of own responsibility. These elements of change are known from studies on dealing with persistent problems in other domains, such as energy (Voß, 2007; Truffer et al., 2008; Verbong and Loorbach, 2012; Smith and Raven, 2012), mobility (Geels, 2005; Kemp et al., 2012) or agriculture (Roep et al., 2003; Grin et al., 2004; Bos and Grin, 2008; Spaargaren et al., 2012). As argued in the literature just cited (see also the Introduction to this volume), a transition perspective may provide significant added value for dealing with such problems.

No less important are changes *between* these systems: at the core of the SSHM, as we have seen, is a more integral approach to various kinds of practices. At present, the social and health models in Spain are operating in parallel, as watertight compartments. In addition, Spain has a decentralized health and social system where Regional Ministries of Health and Regional Ministries of Social Welfare are fully responsible for providing healthcare and social care to the population. This welfare model, with separate healthcare and social services and their interventions, has changed under the new national dependency system, which came into force in 2007 and established for the first time specific rights of dependent people and their caregivers.

Our model assumes a much more integral approach. Again, such a need for transcendence of the boundaries between formerly separate systems in order to resolve persistent problems has been observed in other fields as well. Analyses that make this point, and mention the added value of looking into such issues from the perspective of transition theory, discuss, for instance, the borders between energy and agriculture for bio-energy (Raven and Geels, 2010; Ulmanen, 2013) and energy-producing greenhouses (Hoes et al., 2011; Termeer and Dewulf, 2012) or between urban and mobility systems (Switzer et al., 2013). Similarly, novel distributions of tasks between decentralized, autonomous practices and the national state imply a transition.

Following Loorbach and Rotmans (2010), a transition involves fundamental changes to the system structures, culture and practice. In Table 6.1, we have drawn upon this distinction to summarize the transition implied in the SSHM.

6.4 The case management model

We tested the SSHM in the Valencian Community (VC) (Spain), comprising a region of some five million inhabitants (Instituto Nacional de Estadística, 2012), by applying the principles of the sustainable social care and healthcare model in the VC to those in the population in need of long-term care. The model is primarily geared to the needs of dependent people; that is, those with reduced autonomy to carry out the basic activities of daily life (ADL), who need the help of another person, and who find themselves in a situation where they require the use of social and healthcare resources (Owen et al., 2002). The needs of patients constitute a key factor in the sustainability of healthcare. As Andrew Jameton and Catherine McGuire (2002) put it: "the main responsibility of health professionals and institutions is to provide patients with competent, adequate, appropriate and humane care."

To respond to their needs, we apply a case management model as an operationalization of the SSHM, which permits us to design personal welfare itineraries based on a portfolio, social services and health. Case management has been identified as an effective care and services integration strategy (Applebaum et al., 2002), which is geared not only to matching supply and demand for persons in complex situations – with functional impairment and a high risk of institutionalization – through the building up of a network of services over time and across services, but also to empowering patients and their relatives to use it on their own (cf. PROCARE European Project (Billings

Table 6.1 Structural changes in the transitional process

	Characteristics	*Current regime*	*Sustainable socio-health model*
Structure	• Physical (stocks, flows) • Economic (market, production, consumption, budget) • Institutional (actors, individuals and organizations)	• Physical structure with an upset balance of size and without a flow of protocols • Public productivity/ private consumption • Focus on the cost of the production of services, limited evaluation of the investment in prevention • Core: services and programs	• Reduction in size of both and a flow of protocols • Public and private production. Private consumption • Evaluation of the balance between investment in prevention, healthcare and treatment • Core: people who require care
Culture	• Values • Norms • Methodology • Paradigms	• Universality, equality, accessibility • Differentiated norms by the system (health/welfare), multidisciplinary methodology, without connection • Service protocols • Functional paradigm • Ethical debate focused on therapies: life-saving and new technology	• Social sustainability, quality, co-responsibility, common norms for both systems, interdisciplinary methodology • Case management and itineraries of maximum efficiency • Ecosystemic paradigm • Ethical debate focused on humanization and bioethics
Practice	• Productive routines • Conducts	• Management agreements differentiated by services • Cooperation within each service • Obligations with patients and families before concrete problems	• Management agreements for joint intervention (home, community, institutional) • Intersystem and services cooperation of different areas and intervention levels • Long-term obligations

Source: Based on Van Raak's model (unpublished 2008), cited in Loorbach and Rotmans (2010: 110).

and Leichsenring, 2005) and authors such as Scharlach et al. (2001)). The coordination of the care delivery would avoid or reduce the loss of information and double treatments and lead to a decrease in the use of care services (Leichsenring and Alaszewski, 2004). The use of case management applied to social care and healthcare for senior citizens and dependent persons has increased greatly in recent decades in Europe as well as at an international level (Davies, 1994; Challis et al., 2001; Engel and Engels, 2000; Scharlach et al., 2001; WHO, 2002b).

The basis of this model is the sole assessment of cases through internationally valid instruments. To this end, we have elaborated our model in two different ways:

1   We developed proper methodological and technical capacities to identify, for specific individual needs, an integrated services portfolio, which both ensures quality of care for individuals and reduces the overall system burden (Garcés et al., 2004, 2006; Ródenas et al., 2008). We developed tools for:

   •   the multidisciplinary coordination of professional human resource organization in decision-making on the use of the services portfolio by case management;
   •   creating care pathways that cross the boundaries between the social and health systems, based on criteria of maximum efficiency for the welfare of the user;
   •   prediction of individual pathways and their repercussions on the evolution of the entire health system in real time, based on socio-mathematical models (Grimaldo et al., 2014).

   We will discuss these support tools below.
2   We elaborated and experimented with concrete practices of intersystem coordination creating a unique portfolio of services integrated by social and health resources that previously operated separately. At the heart of these practices is case management. We will discuss this issue in the next section.

Outline of a decision-making system for defining integral pathways of services

In order to support case management teams, it is necessary to provide them with a decision system that may help them to decide, in individual cases, what care pathway fit the client's needs, while optimizing quality of life and the use of scarce resources. In this section we will outline the model we have developed for these purposes, focusing on one key aspect: the optimization of hospital use – a high-cost resource – on behalf of the people who require socio-healthcare.

In essence, the model is designed to help the teams use patients' clinical and social data to come to a consensus on the appropriateness and timeliness of admission and/or referral to other resources (Walsh and Clark, 2002; Smith et al., 2000). As a basis we have chosen the internationally recognized tools of assessment, filtering and classification from the Resident Assessment Instrument (RAI), designed by the scientific community InterRAI.

Originally applied to nursing home clients, the RAI instrument has grown into a family of instruments, also covering other services such as mental health, acute care and home care (Bernabei et al., 2008). This approach offered a more detailed evaluation of patient necessities, improvement of care planning, and jointly resulted in the improvement of the quality of attention (Rubenstein et al., 1991; Stuck et al., 1993; McCusker and Verdon, 2006; Beswick et al., 2008). The InterRAI community conducted a variety of evaluations of these instruments,[2] helped ensure that lessons learned around one assessment instrument were taken into account in those developed later, and in 2000 a major update of all instruments was performed, drawing upon all this cross-learning. In this way, a common core of 70 indicators was established for all instruments, while another 100 indicators were common to many of them. Reliability and validity of the resulting instruments were then evaluated in a major cross-country study (Hirdes et al., 2008).

We based our methodology on the interRAI Long-Term Care Facilities Assessment System (we used the "nursing home" version) and the interRAI Home Care Assessment System (HC), which enables comprehensive, standardized evaluation of the needs, strengths and preferences of persons receiving short-term post-acute care in skilled nursing facilities, as well as of persons living in chronic care and nursing home institutional settings or at home. Both tools collect data about physical, cognitive and emotional functions, as well as clinical diagnoses. It also includes information about an extensive group of symptoms, signs, syndromes and administered treatments.

More concretely, our decision support system includes the following information collected through RAI tools:

- Personal data, including identification number within the health system, age, gender, etc.
- Social and health scores extracted from the referral protocol.
- Data on informal care: flag indicating whether the patient has a caregiver or not; type of caregiver (if any): relative, employee, friend, neighbor, etc. caregiver availability: full, nights and weekends, part-time, etc.
- Data on existing treatment, number and type of medicines consumed.
- Health techniques required by the patient (e.g. number, who carries them out (i.e. health or non-health staff), periodicity, etc.).
- Patient constraints on the use of some health or social resources.

Through the patient's identification number, additional historical data may be retrieved from the health system databases using RAI tools (for instance, on the prior utilization of the different health system facilities, their effectiveness, efficiency and other information).

The case management teams, whose mode of operation we will discuss in more detail below, use our system to consider the following aspects when assessing patients in the SSHM:

- Pathology and state of the illness.
- Dependency for activities of daily living.

- Cognitive state.
- Caregiver burden.
- Resources already being used by the patient (e.g. chronic care hospital, home help services, etc.).

6.5 Testing the case management model in Valencia

In 2004, we performed a case management program in primary care in the Valencian Autonomous Region (Spain). This program was designed to reduce the frequency of use of social care and healthcare resources while maintaining, if not improving, quality of care. We set up a pilot case management unit in two primary care centers of the town of Burjassot within the region's health department number 6. Both public and private healthcare and social services took part in the study (Ródenas et al., 2008). The following health and social resources (Garcés et al., 2006) were available for inclusion in the care pathways:

- *Healthcare resources:* primary care center; specialty care center; one home hospitalization unit (at the public hospital Arnau de Vilanova in Valencia); one palliative care unit at the Dr. Moliner Long-Term Care Public Hospital in Valencia; one Public Mental Health unit in Valencia; ambulance service (healthcare-adapted transport), and non-pharmaceutical complementary benefits.
- *Social resources:* two long-term public placements in the "Velluters" nursing home for the older adults (placed in Valencia); ten temporary placements in the "Velluters" nursing home for the older adults (placed in Valencia); six placements at the day center for the older adults in "Burjassot"; remote care, technical aids and removal of architectural barriers.

The direct work with the patients participating in the project was carried out by a multidisciplinary case management team, comprising a physician, a nurse and a social worker who were motivated by the study's concern and voluntarily engaged and trained for the purpose. All the study protocols were approved by the Health Valencian Regional Government Ethics Committee of Health.

In the year 2004, the Ministry of Health estimated that there were 65,000 ill people over the age of 65 in the Valencian Community who required socio-health at home (Generalitat Valenciana, 2004). Of the 152 patients participating in the study, 101 were placed in an intervention group and 51 in a control group for comparison.

Patients potentially eligible to be included in the study were first identified by a doctor, a nurse or a social worker at the primary care centers of Burjassot, after which they were referred to the case management team. At this point, the case management team decided whether the patient would be included by reviewing the total points obtained in the health and social indicators of the derivation protocol. If the patient obtained certain, predefined values, he or she was included in the research and randomly assigned either to the control group or the intervention group. The patients in the control group continued to use the same normal care resources.

With each patient in the intervention group an integral care pathway was defined, sharing the decision-making among the case management team, the patient and the main informal caregiver. Next, the case management team informed the doctor/nurse/social worker previously taking care of the patient. Following the shared agreement of the plan of integral care, the resources were made available and the pathway started. The team monitored the process and took care of all the administrative processes for both the patient and the informal caregiver. The pathway lasted for periods of between six and nine months.

Based on the decision-making system, and when the patient profile so allowed, the case management team would define fair and necessary care to dependent persons in their own home and social and family environment, or in assisted nursing homes (with medical and more or less intensive clinical care) where necessary. Four factors were taken into consideration to determine whether or not dependent persons needed to be attended in facilities outside of hospitals (or for the referral of already admitted social care and healthcare patients):

- *Clinical complexity* was defined according to the needs of care required by patients. Three levels were distinguished: "high," "medium" and "low." For example, patients with enteral or parenteral feeling, assisted breathing or respiratory therapy, transfusion or thoracic-parecenthesis were classified at the highest level.
- The *level of dependence for performing activities of daily life* determined the degree of daily social care required from others by the patient.
- The *sufficient caregiver was* a person under the age of 75 who either belonged to the immediate family of the patient or was independent and employed to look after the patient for as much time as was needed, or at least for six months at the patient's or their own home.
- Finally, the law currently in force in Spain places *limits on the age* of those who can benefit from certain resources such as homes for the elderly (age 60 and over).

Patients should be moved from hospital after they are duly stabilized, unless they are in an acute phase of illness. In particular, our criterion stipulates that patients attended at an STS be referred to a HCLS after being stabilized. In other cases, patients may be assigned.

6.6 Results of the project

The results of the project show a tendency toward the effectiveness of the case management program, but they reach a statistically significant effect in few variables measured. On the one hand, the intervention group needed fewer office visits and hospital admissions by the emergency service than the control group, but there was no significant difference. On the other hand, the case management program significantly reduced the exclusive use of healthcare resources, promoting the use of cheaper resources. Patients involved in the project were more satisfied, especially with the healthcare resources. Thus, 55.5 percent of these patients were very satisfied with the care received and the benefits of the healthcare resources they had used, especially in-home care. The results were similar for the caregivers; they appeared very satisfied with the healthcare resources received by their family members.

Drawing upon this experiment, we could also estimate the total efficiency gain that may be achieved. Here we shall concentrate our analysis on the most expensive resources of the hospital facilities: the Short-Term Stay (STS), the Hospitals Chronically Long Stay (HCLS) and the Units Psychiatric Hospitalization (UPH). The databases and official records of the different hospitals provide annual economic, medical and statistical data on every patient: gender, age, clinical diagnosis, number of stays (nights spent in hospital) for every patient and clinical circumstance entered; and also the total annual cost of each service, as well as the total annual number of stays. This way, we could find out the number of persons attending in a year, the total number of hospital stays in that year and the average cost per stay (see Table 6.2). The high cost of dependence – between 59.86 and 83.03 percent of the total – makes it worthwhile to examine other possible care alternatives. Data from the field research, through direct interviews from a sample of 1,265 dependent persons in the Valencian Autonomous Region (Garcés et al., 2004), could be used to quantify the distribution of patients per type of hospital according to their degree of dependence.

Our proposal implies that the primary care attention team can directly assign the home or community resources, as well as deciding the intensity of care. They can also decide on admission of patients to hospital. Inside the hospitals, other teams must perform monitoring of the status of patients admitted, to decide whether it is appropriate and opportune to refer patients to other resources. Thus we propose that from STS, stabilized patients may be referred to other convalescence, rehabilitation or long-term-stay HCLS units, without a loss in the quality of care. Some patients may also be referred from HCLS and also from UPH following a period of treatment at these centers either to their home or to residences, with adequate medical and social services.

Table 6.3 shows two concrete scenarios, with economic savings and the number and extra percentage of patients that could be treated yearly in these hospital units with no increase in cost.

Table 6.2 Costs of the hospital stays of dependent persons, 2004

	Hospital unit		
	Short-term stay	Hospital for the chronically ill and long-term stay	Units for psychiatric hospitalization
Total patients attended	13,000	6,400	4,000
Total stays	61,043	139,528	87,618
Total cost (euros)	13,886,999.80	20,704,075.00	20,888,815.30
Cost per stay (euros)	227.50	148.39	238.41
Dependent persons attended	7,774	4,339	1,360
Dependent persons as % of total persons	59.80	67.80	34.00
Total annual stays of dependent persons	36,537.80	115,856.64	57,528.00
Annual dependent persons' stays as % of total stays	59.86	83.03	65.66
Average annual dependent persons' stays	4.70	26.70	42.30
Average annual stays of independent persons	4.69	11.49	11.40
Annual cost per dependent person (euros)	1,069.23	3,961.92	10,084.65
Annual cost per independent person (euros)	1,066.75	1,704.44	2,717.31
Ratio: annual cost per dependent person versus independent person	1.00	2.32	3.71
Annual cost of dependent persons (euros)	8,312,180.29	17,191,564.16	7,219,248.85
Percentage of total annual cost of dependent persons	59.86	83.03	71.60

Sources: Polibienestar, University of Valencia (2009). Records of the hospitals in the Valencian Autonomous Region, economic database of the Health Department.

The baseline scenario considers a reduction of 10 percent of the average time of stay in each hospital unit. It shows that for every 10 percent reduction in the average number of hospital stays of dependent people, 4 percent more might be provided with care without any additional cost. Of course, there is a theoretical limit in the possible reduction of the average stay which would be very important to estimate, and this can only be done on the basis of the management of socio-health resources. Using this scenario as a baseline, the benefits can be calculated for the percentages of reduction of average stays.

In sum, our findings show that the case management program and RAI tools are crucial for being able to design new welfare itineraries, with the end result of boosting the efficiency of social and health attention for people who

Table 6.3 Cost of the alternative care proposal and savings. Number of extra dependent persons who could be treated in hospitals at the current cost and with the current length of stay, 2004

Scenarios		Short-term stay	Hospital for the chronically ill and long-term stay	Units for psychiatric hospitalization	Total
Present	Average stay	4.70	26.70	42.30	–
	Cost total (euros/year)	8,312,180.29	17,191,564.16	7,219,248.85	32,722,993.30
Baseline scenario	Average stay reduced by 10%	4.23	24.03	38.07	–
	Saving (euros/year)	289,014.00	760,534.81	963,375.77	2,012,924.59
	Total cost (euros/year)	8,023,166.29	16,431,029.35	6,255,873.08	30,710,068.71
	Number of extra dependent persons who could be treated (year)	270	192	96	558
	% extra versus total dependent persons treated (year)	3.48	4.42	7.02	4.14

Source: Polibienestar, University of Valencia (2009).

require LTC, while also improving their quality of life. The care benefits for these people can be increased if the following parameters are optimized:

- *Adaptation* of the resources and services to the specific needs of each dependent person (Brown et al., 2003). It is possible to define the health and social care profile of each service and establish which of them, or which combination, should be applied in a particular case in order to maximize the patient's quality of life. For example, almost a quarter (24.6 percent) of patients admitted to Hospitals for the Chronically ill and Long Stay (HCLS) have profiles similar to those of patients who end up in nursing homes (temporary stays), Units of Home Hospitalization (UHH) and the Home Help Service (HHS), implying that they could perhaps receive care through these services (Garcés et al., 2006).
- Increasing the *opportunity to use* resources for the population as a whole through adequate management of services in patients' referral itineraries (Kane et al., 2000).

That the gains are still limited is precisely because these conditions run up against difficulties which from the perspective of transition theory we may interpret as expressions of the incumbent regime that imply inertia or resistance against the transformation pursued. In terms of Table 6.1, a problem implied in the incumbent *structure* concerns the wide differences in budget size, as well as in the organization and number of resources, between social and health systems. In the health system, access to resources and services is both an individual right and free, while the social system is linked to individual income, which complicates the management of a unique portfolio of resources. In addition, the absence of inter-system structures limits opportunities for coordination while increasing the compartmentalization of the functionality of resources.

In terms of *culture*, the second area of system change depicted in Table 6.1, we have observed important issues as to the societal acceptability of the axiological principles implied in the SSHM. A case in point concerns the principle of co-responsibility, which is based on rights; this complicates instant implementation. In addition, the concept of co-responsibility may be perceived as referring to a meritocracy of good health, social and economic practices, and this perverts the meaning we want to give to the term. For us, "co-responsibility" entails that the user of protective systems achieves more autonomy and at the same time influences the system by interacting with it. We do not want to suggest that those who do not use those social protection systems responsibly would somehow be discriminated against when accessing the system.

A second cultural barrier concerns the principle of dignified death, as this conflicts with religious traditional values of Mediterranean societies as well as more conservative political ideologies. These cultural inclinations have also translated into legal rules. This may hinder implementation of the model. For example, active euthanasia in Spain is illegal, and governments in these societies are still consolidating health and social protection systems. Should they approach the management of the quality of death as a matter of individual choice, as a value associated with an excessively liberal or progressive society?

Finally, there are barriers pertaining to the transformation of *practices*. In our testing of the model we identified certain barriers that will have to be resolved to make a transition of the model possible. The first has to do with internal corporatism of professionals in both the social and health systems. This is shown by a reciprocal ignorance of inter-system professionals who seem to distrust the legal scope of professional duties. In a pilot management case, for example, the case management team is likely to meet with hostility from colleagues in primary health and specialized care in health and social centers. It is evident in such a case that a cultural change and a change of professional attitudes are necessary, with an acknowledgment of the added value of team and interdisciplinary work, as well as a need for training in the values and methodology of the socio-health model.

6.7 Conclusions

Is the socio-health model a viable and adequate alternative to confront the unsustainability of health systems in Southern Europe? By testing the model on real portfolio socio-health resources, we established that the model is basically adequate. Patients and informal caregivers in the Valencia experiment appeared to be really positive about the care provided, as well as about the increased autonomy and opportunities for patients to receive care at home. Model calculations, informed by data from Valencia, suggest that this increased quality may go hand in hand with more efficient use of resources. However, it is evident that there are important problems that have yet to be resolved if the system is to be scaled up.

First and foremost, it is important to overcome the structural and cultural problems that stand in the way of more integrated approaches: differences in funding between the health system and the social support system, the lack of structure for inter-system coordination and a reluctance among some professionals to work in a more client-oriented way, beyond disciplinary boundaries.

A second major problem is related to cultural inertia. Expectations about the welfare state, a reluctance to accept death and the potential misunderstanding of co-responsibility as an emphasis on meritocracy, rather than on increased autonomy of patients and caregivers, may all make introduction of the system more difficult. This too may be understood as a barrier, firmly embedded in the current regime.

Ironically, this underscores the persistence of the problems discussed in the first section. We see again that fragmentation and discontinuity are constant factors in our health and social care systems, while the expectations that undermine the tenability of the welfare state also complicate transformative efforts to resolve these problems. Taking a transition perspective on the experiences with the SSHM model reveals how reforms are limited in scope and effectiveness in a regime that tends to reproduce itself.

Yet, from a transition perspective we also see opportunities for further change. While transitions are slow and cumbersome processes of change, they may proceed when new practices and structural change inform and reinforce each other (Grin, 2006, 2010: 265–284; Geels and Schot, 2010: 47–53). First, our experiment may be understood as a niche experiment in the sense that it has helped to further elaborate and legitimate a socio-technical vision, which may provide orientation to the collective. Drawing upon integrated models (Kodner and Spreeuwenberg, 2002; Gröne and Garcia-Barbero, 2002; Gallud et al., 2004) and organizational tools (Terraza et al., 2006; Colin-Thomé and Belfield, 2004), we created two new professional positions, the so-called "management nurses" and "nurses of continuity," and they apply case management methodology from a primary care health service and hospitals, connecting both spheres with each other and with social resources.

Second, we derive from the experiences in Valencia a new regime element, the "socio-health agencies," which may help to create more coordination between the social assistance system and the health system, and provide some leverage for overcoming cultural inertia. Small and dynamic structures may be created as strategic key assets for a decentralized public administration. These agencies could contract socio-health services and manage access to them by providing an answer to the needs of a person requiring long-term care and offering sustained assistance through social and health resources. In this way, they could help raise public support, and thus legitimacy, for a more integral, client-focused approach as taken by the case management teams. Through rules for decision-making and resource allocation they could counteract tendencies to maintain the boundaries between the two systems and support more integrated care pathways.

Third, those agencies and other proponents of the transition might explicitly link their efforts to various "landscape" tendencies. Our proposal fits well with current tendencies in welfare states, in Spain as much as elsewhere, toward devolution of governance and a shift from generic provisions to customized service for individuals.

More crucially, we mention here the increasing cultural inclination toward autonomy. As a consequence of emancipation and individualization, starting with the middle class, people will increasingly attach value to their independence and freedom to shape their own lives. They do not simply like to be treated or "taken care of" as patients anymore; rather, they seek support for their own life plans. In the same vein, care professionals increasingly favor autonomous, client-focused professional judgment and action over merely following highly protocolized discipline or management-driven instructions. Our system should be further developed from that perspective, as a way to capitalize on the legitimizing power of this cultural tendency. This will also contribute to promoting the idea of co-responsibility as an important cultural value.

Notes

1 The theory of "squaring the circle of welfare," put forward by George and Miller (1994), may be applied to countries such as Spain by analyzing the political and economic equilibrium to which some states are subject when aiming to level the resources with the need for: (1) satisfying the growing public demand for the provision of top-quality welfare, (2) satisfying the public demand in parallel to the limitation of the tax levels, (3) maintaining and increasing the levels of economic growth, and (4) maintaining and improving the opportunity of choice.
2 Assessment studies were published in 12 countries: Australia, Canada, Czech Republic, France, Iceland, Italy, Japan, Korea, Holland, Norway, United States and Spain (see Hirdes et al., 2008).

7 The making of a Transition Program in the Dutch care sector[1]

Suzanne Van den Bosch and Jord Neuteboom

7.1 Introduction

This chapter describes the experiences with and lessons from developing and managing a Transition Program in the Dutch care sector (2007–2010). This program encompassed two rounds of 26 transition experiments in actual care practices that were conducted to explore radically new ways of meeting the need for long-term care among the Dutch population. This chapter focuses on how this portfolio of transition experiments was developed and managed, including how they were selected, how room was created to set up the selected experiments, how learning was facilitated and how the experiments were monitored. In addition, we describe initial experiences and lessons regarding scaling up successful transition experiments in healthcare.

From the onset, the Transition Program in Long-term Care (TPLC) employed transition management (TM) as its central approach. Contrary to other cases of transition management in practice (as described in Loorbach, 2007), however, this Transition Program immediately started with a first round of transition experiments, instead of first setting up a transition arena and developing a sustainability vision.

Aside from the transition experiments, the program itself had an experimental character, which allowed for a *learning-by-doing* and *doing-by-learning* approach. This implied that the Transition Program provided space to experiment in practice with concrete examples of how *sustainable* care could be provided to the Dutch population, while at the same time providing a "learning environment" to both TM practitioners and TM researchers. The Program Team running the Transition Program consisted of three organizations, including DRIFT (Dutch Research Institute For Transitions based at the Erasmus University Rotterdam), where TM was first conceived. This concerted effort made it possible to apply and further develop TM as a transition governance concept, in co-production with the other actors involved in the Transition Program. As such it provided an ideal context to develop and test new conceptual "steering notions" on transition experiments, such as the *substantive* notion that transition experiments by their nature influence the dominant structure, culture and practices involved, and the *process* notion that experiments may contribute to transitions through the mechanisms of deepening, broadening and scaling up. These notions became part and parcel of the program discourse and practice, which in turn enabled further theoretical development of managing a portfolio of transition experiments.

This chapter discusses the TPLC chronologically. Section 7.2 describes the background and introduces the program. Sections 7.3, 7.4 and 7.5 include a detailed empirical analysis of the first three phases of this Transition Program (2006–2008), describing its initial development (phase I), the first round of transition experiments (phase II) and the selection of the second round of experiments (phase III). Parallel to phase III, a so-called "transition arena" was set up as well (phase IV), with the aim of providing guidance with regard to the portfolio of experiments. For each phase we discuss the specific goals and approach, the barriers as they were encountered and perceived, as well as the ways in which they were tackled and partly overcome. The chapter concludes with a general wrap-up of the whole program, the results that were achieved and the lessons learned.

7.2 Transition Program in Long-term Care: background and introduction

Persistent problems in the care system

The basic assumption of this program is that the societal system for long-term care in the Netherlands is largely unsustainable (Transition Arena Long-term Care, 2009).[2] The increasing rigidity in the care system's *structure, culture* and *practices* severely limits adequate and flexible adaptation to societal developments and needs. From the 1970s, as discussed elsewhere in this book (cf. Chapter 1.1), major exogenous changes implied an array of new demands on the care system. This should be understood as a *tension* between the care system (*regime*) and its environment (*landscape*) (De Haan and Rotmans, 2011). In addition, "the response of the care system was aimed at excessive command and control and mechanisation, by applying the mechanism of financial accountability" (Transition Arena Long-term Care, 2009). This may be understood as *stress* (De Haan and Rotmans, 2011) within the care regime that makes it challenging if not impossible to meet the increasing demand for long-term care. This combination of tension and stress in the care system has contributed to the following *symptoms of unsustainability*: low level of internal cooperation, lack of external societal integration (e.g. with other societal domains in which care needs may also be addressed or prevented), increasing and uncontrollable costs (due to lack of control over industry and medical specialists, a spiral effect between health system performance and the expectations it generated, and patients being influenced by professional rationality as well as by their portrayal as consumers through neoliberal policies since the 1980s), dissatisfied care professionals (especially because freedom and autonomy to provide high-quality care were replaced by management on the basis of rules, standards and protocols that came with, first, governmental regulation to control professional patronage, in response to social movements in the 1970s, and second, neoliberal New Public Management policies since the 1980s (Tonkens, 2008; Newman and Tonkens, 2011), increasing shortages of qualified professionals (partly related to the previous point, partly a demographic problem) and a pressure on relevant human values (such as attention, care and trust), due to trends like individualization, the decline of traditional institutions, the reconstruction of the patient as consumer and an increasing reliance on professionals. These symptoms are systemic in nature for three reasons: they are highly interrelated, transcend individuals, organizations and sub-sectors within the care system, and, as we briefly and admittedly incompletely outlined above, have a structural and cultural basis (Transition Arena Long-term Care, 2009: 13–17).

Underlying these symptoms are *persistent problems* such as the healthcare financing mechanisms that finance "production" instead of prevention, and the standardization and specialization of a care system that neglects individual human needs and values (Transition Arena Long-term Care, 2009). Without fundamental changes, it will be impossible to realize the care system's sustainability. Because of their systemic nature, these symptoms and underlying persistent problems in the care system cannot be solved by conventional policy measures. Addressing these problems requires an approach that acknowledges the complexity and uncertainty and makes space for experimenting with radically new ways of providing care.

Transition management

Transition management (TM) is a new mode of governance, aiming at enabling, facilitating and guiding transitions toward sustainability (Loorbach, 2002; Kemp and Loorbach, 2003; Rotmans, 2005; Loorbach, 2007). The underlying assumption is that even if full control and management of transitions is impossible, *it is possible* to influence the direction and pace of transitions in subtle ways through a series of interventions at different levels using different instruments (Rotmans and Loorbach, 2010).

Empirically, the TM approach is the outcome of a *co-production* process between TM researchers and practitioners in several policy domains, including the energy domain, the waste management domain and the sustainable housing domain (Loorbach, 2007). Theoretically, the TM concept is grounded in two scientific disciplines: complex systems science and governance studies (extensively described in Loorbach, 2007). Based on a combination of deducing concepts from complex systems theory and new forms of governance and inducing new concepts and practical guidelines from case studies, transition experts developed a *practical management framework* (Rotmans and Loorbach, 2001; Loorbach, 2002; Loorbach and Rotmans, 2006).

The TM framework encompasses a portfolio of systemic instruments: a complex systems analysis, sustainability visions, a transition arena and transition pathways, a transition agenda, transition experiments, monitoring and evaluation, and transition coalitions and networks. The TM cycle integrates and structures the different TM instruments in four activity clusters (Loorbach, 2002; Rotmans, 2003; Loorbach, 2007; Loorbach and Rotmans, 2006): (1) structuring the problem in question, establishing the transition arena and envisioning; (2) developing coalitions and transition agendas (transition images and related transition paths); (3) establishing and carrying out transition experiments and mobilizing the resulting transition networks; (4) monitoring, evaluating and learning lessons from the transition experiments and, based on all these, adjusting the vision, agenda and coalitions. Most examples of the application of TM in actual practices, such as in Parkstad Limburg and Flanders (Loorbach, 2007), the Energy Transition (Kern and Smith, 2008) and in Zeeland (Henneman, 2008), start at the "top" of the TM cycle: first, a *transition arena* is set up, which allows one to develop a long-term sustainability vision and interrelated transition pathways, and only later in the process particular transition experiments are selected. According to Loorbach (2007: 115), however, there is no fixed sequence of steps in transition management, while their significance may vary from one cycle to the next: "In practice the transition management activities are carried out partially and completely in sequence, in parallel and in a random sequence."

Predevelopment of the Transition Program in Long-term Care (TPLC)

The TPLC was initiated by the Dutch Ministry of Health, Welfare and Sports and the Dutch care sector associations in the wake of the AWBZ covenant. The AWBZ[3] is the nationwide insurance scheme for long-term care, which is intended to provide the insured with chronic and continuous care, and this may involve considerable financial consequences, such as in care for disabled people with congenital physical or mental disorders. As a result of rising AWBZ expenditures and a projected short-term growth in the demand for long-term care, in August 2004 the Dutch government and care sector associations established the "AWBZ Covenant 2005–2007." The main point agreed upon was that AWBZ expenditures could only grow within the budgetary framework set by the governmental parties at the inception of the then government coalition. To partially compensate for this limited budget, the covenant parties agreed that they would cooperate to improve the entire AWBZ and provide additional incentives for innovation. The total resources for innovation in long-term care that were agreed upon in the covenant included 80 million euros. One part of these innovation resources was allocated to the ZonMw program (focused on implementing existing innovations in long-term care). After a long and cumbersome process another substantial part of the innovation resources was allocated to the TPLC (focused on experimenting with radical innovations in long-term care). These resources were subtracted from the AWBZ premiums (collected through income tax).

However, two years after the completion of the covenant, the resources for innovation in care had not yet been allocated, because the Working Group Innovation in Care (WGI) was still searching for an adequate approach for making recommendations on implementing the covenant to a Board of Directors from the Ministry of Health, Welfare and Sports and the care sector associations. In September 2006, the potential of a transition management approach in the care sector was presented by DRIFT at a meeting organized by the WGI. The WGI and several innovative care institutions, which also attended the AWBZ meeting, recognized the potential of transition management for the long-term care sector (see Box 7.1).

Following this meeting, a consortium of ErnstandYoung (EandY), CC care advisers (CC) and DRIFT was commissioned to develop an action plan for a TPLC. The consortium was a compromise between the Ministry (which preferred the financial expertise of EandY) and the care sector organizations (which had a first interest in CC). It was finally decided by the WGI to include both organizations, and to enrich this consortium with the methodological TM expertise of DRIFT. It was agreed that transition management would be used as a central steering approach. Within DRIFT, Jord Neuteboom (second author) gave direction to the intensive process of preparing the program action plan. He cooperated with the other consultants and the WGI members while continuously involving different researchers at DRIFT, engaged in researching and testing TM concepts and tools (in a variety of policy domains).

Initially, the WGI asked the two consortium partners EandY and CC to elaborate the new approach, while inviting DRIFT to monitor this process and to evaluate it from a transition perspective. The three organizations, however, took the initiative and proposed to the WGI that they would jointly develop an integrated transition management approach, whereby DRIFT was to provide the methodological TM tools and instruments. This proposal, accepted by the WGI, created a conceptual and organizational framework for the three organizations to work together throughout the

---

Box 7.1 Possibilities of transition management in the care sector (DRIFT presentation, AWBZ meeting, September 4, 2006)

The core of the transition management approach:

- a new approach for steering (not a trick or panacea)
- changing the care sector from within using outside support: small, sheltered experiments
- with visionary thinking and practical acting
- in small steps with a long-term focus
- resulting in a societal movement

program, including its implementation phases. It also helped the persons working in the three different organizations to get to know each other, while sharing and combining their different expertise (about TM processes, care content and financial and organizational aspects) and elaborating it into a tailored TM approach for the care sector program. However, the translation of these different fields of expertise into a shared TM approach obviously differed from the straightforward application of TM per se. This partly contingent consortium, then, was indeed unique, representing an experiment in its own right.

In sum, the realization of the TPLC was the result of both contingency and strategic action (from the WGI and the consortium, including DRIFT).

7.3 Developing the Transition Program in Long-term Care (2006)

Preparing the program action plan (September to December 2006)

During the preparation of the program action plan, numerous decisions were taken on how to apply the transition management approach in the long-term care sector. Three important decisions were: (1) to start with transition experiments instead of developing a vision in a transition arena, (2) to select a limited number of experiments, and (3) to focus on transition experiments instead of different types of experiments.

Initially, DRIFT suggested a double-track approach in which a transition arena would be a starting point for formulating a project portfolio and transition experiments. It was explained that starting with a transition arena (Loorbach, 2007) was seen to be important for thoroughly analyzing the persistent problems in the care sector, developing a strong vision of a sustainable care sector, building up trust and belief in change, and strategically influencing existing societal and administrative/political networks. As a follow-up for the transition arena, DRIFT suggested that transition experiments could be set up to provide practical "transition spaces" (i.e. *niches*), which were characterized as:

- Aiming at societal challenges/paths.
- High potential contributions to transition processes.
- High risk (in terms of chance of failure) regarding their applicability in the current situation.
- Ideally consisting of a mix of innovation types (cf. Table 7.1).
- Involving different perceptions: (societal) experiment versus project (participants).

During the process of preparing the program action plan, it was decided that the first priority was to set up transition experiments. This decision was strongly influenced by the Ministry of Health, Welfare and Sports and the care sector associations, which felt pressure to quickly spend the 80 million euros on innovations, which was agreed in the AWBZ covenant 2005 to 2007. Because the budget had to be spent within a few years, a conventional transition management approach that starts with a transition arena and visioning process would have taken up too much time. Furthermore, the Ministry had already defined the main problems (such as future employment problems) and had already developed a vision (including four innovation themes). In view of the delayed implementation of this covenant, the Ministry sought to give an immediate impulse to innovations in care, by "developing good ideas, implementing innovations and rewarding innovative care institutions." The suggested transition arena process did not meet its short-term wants, nor did the Ministry wish to see another "steering group." The consortium lacked not only support for developing a transition arena, but also capacity and funding.

Regarding the allocation of resources to experiments in long-term care, the care sector associations initially proposed to support the institutions they represented with a relatively small amount of money. However, the consortium convinced them that this would be a waste of money, leading only to incremental innovations without stimulating fundamental changes. Thus the program focused on selecting a limited number of experiments, which fitted the idea of supporting front-runner care institutions with initiatives that could really make a difference.

While the first draft of the action plan distinguished between various types of experiments, proposing that "transition experiments" would cover only a small portion (see Table 7.1), eventually the program leaders decided that all experiments would be supported under the heading of "transition experiments" because "optimization experiments" and "innovation experiments" were already supported by a similar ZonMw program, called "Care for better."

Action plan of TPLC (January 2007)

In December 2006, the consortium swiftly produced the final action plan of the TPLC. Partly due to the involvement of DRIFT, the focus in this program evolved from "innovation" (with labor productivity as a central *innovation theme*) to a transition to "sustainable care" as illustrated by a quote from the Ministry (Presentation, instruction meeting, April 2, 2007):

> The program originated from the necessity to address the future employment problems. For this purpose innovation is an important instrument. The theme of this program has further evolved to sustainable care, a term that better covers the scope. Since it is not only about providing more quantitative care with the same amount of labour, but also about qualitatively better (sustainable) care.

The action plan contained many explicit TM concepts (e.g. persistent problems, societal transition challenge, transition arena, deepening, broadening and scaling up) and stated that: "The core of the program encompasses the

Table 7.1 Three different types of experiments in long-term care

Types: aspects	Optimization	Innovation	Transition
Starting point	Working more effective and efficient: realizing and diffusing optimizations	Realizing same objectives in different way. Initiating innovations and making ready for market	Societal challenge: demonstrating fundamentally different structure and culture
Nature of problem	Practical/technological and diffusion	Different domains, inter-organizational, institutional barriers	Uncertain and complex: end goals and pathways are changing, part of societal debate
Perspective	Short term: 1 to 2 years	Short and medium term: 5 to 10 years	Long term: 10 to 20 years
Method	Solutions-driven, applying	Testing and demonstration	Exploring, searching and learning
Learning	First-order learning about single applications	First-order learning (individual)	Second-order learning (collective)
Involved disciplines	One or a few	A few	Many
Actors	Professionals, managers, end-users	Professionals, managers, end-users, engineers, etc.	Multi-actor alliance (across society)
Management context	Conventional project management	Program management	Transition management (visions, arenas, paths)

Source: Draft action plan TPLC (September 27, 2006).

development and execution of *transition experiments*, executed by front runners and innovative parties, which are selectively and directly supported in such a way that the entire care sector can learn from this." Because of the failed previous attempts to implement the AWBZ Covenant 2005 to 2007, the action plan strongly recommended keeping up the current speed and starting with the Transition Program before a final political decision about the portfolio of transition experiments would have been made. The action plan suggested starting immediately in February 2007 with:

- a pilot phase to build up the project organization and start the first transition experiments (recruited and selected based on a "push" strategy);
- a follow-up phase to prepare a broad tender open to all AWBZ care institutions ("pull" strategy).

The underlying idea of the pilot phase was to start off a minimum of three to five "pilot" transition experiments, to demonstrate to the Ministry and care sector associations that a transition management approach was possible, i.e. transition experiments could be selected, experimentation space created and learning and monitoring facilitated.

Indeed, in early February 2007, the Ministry and directors of the care sector associations formally agreed upon the action plan, which kicked off the TPLC. Officially responsible for the program was the WGI, consisting of representatives from the Ministry of Health, Welfare and Sports and various care sector organizations (GGZ Nederland, Actiz, BTN, VGN).[4] A Program Team, consisting of about eight advisers from EandY, CC and DRIFT, was charged with the operational management of the program.

In early spring 2007, ten care institutions were given ample room and financial support to start the first round of ten transition experiments to explore new and often still unknown pathways in long-term care. In March 2008, following the launch of the transition experiments, a *transition arena* was also set up. The front runners who participated in this arena developed a problem definition, sustainability vision and transition pathways for long-term care (Transition Arena Long-term Care, 2009). These front runners did not participate directly in the transition experiments, but the Transition Program connected the various learning experiences from the transition experiments with the strategic outcomes of the transition arena. The second round of another 16 transition experiments started in September. These also involved exploring and learning about radical innovations in practice, in a real-life context in which the end-user is central. The front-runner care institutions engaged in these experiments were found all over the Netherlands and included all sectors of long-term care: care for the elderly, nursing and care, homecare, and healthcare for physically or mentally disabled persons.

7.4 First round of ten transition experiments (2007)

This section will discuss the first round of experiments: the selection strategy, procedure and criteria, the development of the final project plans and the first joint learning session on transition experiments, as well as the many barriers that had to be overcome to finance them; the eventual establishment of funding and the way in which learning and monitoring within the "start-up phase" was facilitated; and the political impact of this first round of experiments.

Pilot phase: selecting first round of transition experiments (February to April 2007)

The selection process of the first round of transition experiments, as conducted by the Program Team, included: (1) the development of a shortlist, (2) extensive visits to shortlisted care institutions, (3) supporting the care institutions with preparing adequate project proposals, (4) informing them about the Transition Program (including financing the transition experiments), and (5) assessing submitted project proposals based on eight selection criteria.

Selection strategy and procedure

The selection strategy may be characterized as a "push strategy" rather than a broad, open tender. A shortlist was put together (mainly based on a balanced portfolio, e.g. distribution among sectors and themes) of 11 potential transition experiments and as many care institutions where these experiments could be carried out. It included front runners already known to or engaged in the Transition Program. The remarkably low number of potential transition experiments in the long-term care sector may be explained by the fact that the Dutch care sector did not have a tradition or culture of radical innovation and was also suffering from cost reductions, limiting the financial and mental space for innovation.

Further selection started in March 2007, with extensive visits to the shortlisted care institutions, followed up by two reports and a tailor-made letter of advice to increase the quality of the project proposal. All care institutions were invited to submit a "free format" project proposal and were requested to add a *transition explanation*, which specifically had to describe the transition aspects of the project (e.g. the societal challenge and potential to scale up the experiment).

Instruction meeting

An instruction meeting was held on April 2, 2007, to inform the 11 participating care institutions about the Transition Program. This was also the first joint meeting of all actors involved in the transition program (the care institutions, the Ministry of Health, Welfare and Sports, the care sector associations and the Program Team). A crucial underlying objective of this meeting was to provide clarity with regard to the financing of the first round of experiments.

Despite the preparations and efforts of the Program Team, however, the representatives of the Ministry did not provide a clear message with regard to the available financial resources and administrative funding procedures. During the meeting it was stated that:

> At this moment the Ministry, in cooperation with the NZa [Dutch Healthcare Authority], is exploring possible ways for financial contributions and/or how an extra policy regulation can/should be created such as a policy regulation for innovation in care. Next to this, additional support is anticipated.[5]

Thus, the instruction meeting exposed a discrepancy between the objective of the Ministry to provide space for experimentation, and a lack of readiness to make available allocated resources.

Final selection based on selection criteria

Despite this uncertainty, reinforced by the instruction meeting, all shortlisted care institutions submitted a project proposal. This reflected their serious commitment and was also due to the active and supportive involvement of the Program Team. The 11 submitted project proposals were discussed and assessed by the Program Team, based on eight selection criteria (cf. Table 7.2), an aggregation of some 35 criteria put forward by the Program Team and the WGI. This was an important step in integrating the different objectives and perspectives of the three organizations represented on the Program Team.

Only one project proposal was put aside because of the limited ability of the care institution and its direct environment to provide sufficient support to this experiment. All the other project proposals were assessed with a *go* based on their scores on the eight criteria. Their high scores hardly came as a surprise, as the selection strategy had centered on inviting only known and engaged front runners to submit a project proposal (*push strategy*), while the Program Team had also provided advice about improving their proposals from a transition perspective. In fact, it may well be regarded as a "transitioning process," whereby the various participating care institutions successfully translated the transition perspective to their specific project context.

The resulting number of ten (instead of the initial idea of four to eight) transition experiments (Table 7.3) was considered appropriate by the Program Team, because the distribution of the innovation themes, learning opportunities and budgets was well balanced. Therefore, the Program Team advised the WGI to give its support to them.

This selection process was also a learning process for the Program Team. Regarding the selection strategy, the "push" strategy was successful in quickly

Table 7.2 Selection criteria applied to one of the selected transition experiments

Selection criteria	Example of selected transition experiment: Neighborhood Care (Buurtzorg)
1 Connection to persistent problem	Persistent problem: increasing costs and decreasing quality of homecare
2 Connection to themes and solution directions	Efficient management (+ prevention and social support)
3 Plausible and well substantiated	Project plan is well considered, solid and convincing
4 Motivation	Entrepreneur with high personal drive
5 Ability	Own investment
6 Radical innovative	Providing high-quality, low-cost homecare outside existing organizations
7 Growth and learning potential	High ambition to grow and share learning experiences
8 Added value, program ↔ project	High added value: only entrepreneur, high-risk project in need of support

Table 7.3 First round of transition experiments in healthcare

Project	Description
1 Assertive Community Treatment (ACT) for youth in Rotterdam	Multidisciplinary and outreaching ACT teams support youngsters with psychiatric problems
2 Transmural network STEM	Starting up a societal dialog about dying
3 WEIS in the neighborhood	Improving quality of life in districts
4 Neighborhood care ("Buurtzorg")	Innovative autonomous teams of community nurses
5 Permanently better	Providing care to long-term psychiatric patients in own environment (with FACT method)
6 Case manager dementia	Case managers who support people with dementia to live at home for as long as possible
7 At home with dementia	One point of support for treatment and counseling in all phases and aspects of dementia
8 Smart Caring Community (*Omkeer 2.0*)	Developing an ideal social support system in a city district and rural area
9 Video networks – a plan for scaling up	Further developing and scaling up "telecare"
10 Meeting place Prinsenhof	A self-organized community meeting place for seniors and disabled people

engaging front runners to start off a transition process in the care sector. This active engagement preceding an actual political decision resulted in a high commitment of the participating care institutions toward the Transition Program (and vice versa). From a TM perspective this was positive in terms of mobilizing front runners and starting up projects. However, because a transition perspective had already been brought into the projects by the Program Team before the selection started, the actual selection may have partly been in the decision to advise on particular projects. Furthermore, while transition management emphasizes the importance of variation and selection, no selection moments after the start-up phase took place. Thus, even when DRIFT suggested discontinuing particular projects, the Program Team did not make use of its competence to discontinue experiments that did not meet expectations.

Pilot phase: final project plans and first learning session (June to July 2007)

Final project plans

The selection advice for the first round was not immediately adopted by the Ministry's representatives. After several weeks of uncertainty, they demanded that ten care institutions would be requested to "submit a final project plan to strengthen their project proposals and lay the foundations of a business case." The Program Team emphasized to the care institutions that they should hold on to their original project proposals, and that these final project plans aimed primarily to "speed up the process of contracting and financing and to stimulate a positive outcome of this process." ErnstandYoung provided a format for the final project plans, mainly comprising general project management aspects (e.g. project goals, results, regulatory and financial conditions, activities and planning and budget), and several TM outcome measures (e.g. learning goals, transition goals, transition effects in terms of different cultures, structures and practices). In addition, the care institutions were requested to describe their project proposal as SMART (Specific, Measurable, Acceptable, Realistic and Time restricted) as possible. This would raise conventional "project management" to the level of transition experiment management. At the same time, this also created a major tension with the Transition Management approach, which is about experimenting, searching and learning about unknown pathways, whereas the SMART approach assumes that the outcome of a transition experiment can be predicted a priori. This contradiction caused several care institutions to complain about the new request, as they were convinced that a SMART approach could not be applied to their projects and would rather limit their creativity. Eventually, all care institutions completed their project plans (with support from the Program Team). The requested SMART formulation did not strongly influence the content of the transition experiments: the original project proposals continued to serve as a starting point.

First learning session

A week after completion of the final project plans, the Program Team organized the program's first learning session. This session was attended by all selected care institutions, several representatives from the Ministry and the care sector associations, and the NZa (Dutch Healthcare Authority). The learning goals were:

1   To provide a shared thinking and working framework for the Transition Program: the policies and intentions of the Ministry and a first exploration of the system barriers in long-term care.
2   To exhibit the unique main aspects of the different transition experiments (to inspire, synchronize and exchange).
3   Letting policy and practice meet each other, by inspiring contacts between actors involved in the program.

Coming after the "failed" instruction meeting, an important underlying process goal of this first learning session was to inspire and put positive pressure on the Ministry to financially support the transition experiments.

Therefore, the Program Team had specifically requested the care institutions to present the essence of their transition experiment with "heart and soul."

The ten presentations were very authentic, and exceptionally creative, personal and persuasive. For example, the "heart and soul" presentation about *STEM* (the Dutch abbreviation for *"Dying In Your Own Way"*) involved a live interview with Corrie, a woman suffering from cancer who made a strong personal plea for a more dignified and humanized type of care system, with a focus on the personal wishes of clients.

Several shared ideas emerged from these "heart and soul" presentations, such as returning power to the client and the care professional and making use of the capacities of relatives and neighborhoods to take care of each other in social networks. Together, these presentations had a profound personal impact and underlined that the end-user truly was at the heart of the program.

The presentations about the transition experiments were preceded by a speech from a representative of the Ministry's director of care, Arnold Moerkamp, about the policies and intentions of the Ministry. It was exemplary in revealing the complexities, tensions and ambiguities surrounding governmental support of the transition experiments:

- On the one hand, the Ministry stated that no decision on the financing of the experiments had yet been made and, on the other hand, it stated that the Ministry wanted to start as quickly as possible.
- As a reason for the complicated financing procedure, the Ministry claimed it wanted to get rid of "pilotitis," referring to the observation that many subsidized experiments never overcome the status of experiment and never became structurally embedded (after completion of the experiment).
- Contrary to only providing subsidy grants, the Ministry wanted to involve the current financing system (e.g. care insurers and care offices) in the experiments right from the start. An advantage of this approach, according to the Ministry, was that this enabled learning about how the system is working – or not working.

The Ministry valued the commitment of the ten selected care institutions, illustrated by the quote: "In fact you offer us your contribution to the transition." But the Ministry did not make any long-term promise to support the ten transition experiments. To reduce the perceived risks for the care institutions, the Ministry did make a short-term financial promise to compensate for the extra activities that were conducted in the context of the Transition Program – as had been strongly recommended by the Program Team – to build trust among the participating care institutions.

Start-up phase of the transition experiments (August to December 2007)

Creating (financial) space for the transition experiments

Even though the Transition Program had originated from the AWBZ Covenant 2005 to 2007, which included a sizable budget of 80 million euros for innovation, in the pilot phase of the Transition Program it had become apparent that this money was a paper tiger. Shortly before the *start-up phase* of the transition experiments, concrete agreements about if and how the transition experiments would be financed were still lacking. As the Ministry learned, the Program Team was right about its expectation that the existing regulations and procedures would provide insufficient room for funding the transition experiments. This resulted in *tensions* between the Ministry and the Dutch Healthcare Authority NZa, which also followed from a feared decrease in power of the NZa and the Care Offices, and a fundamental disagreement about the decision of the Ministry to allocate the innovation resources to preselected transition experiments (instead of giving all care institutions access to the innovation resources).

Eventually, on August 17, 2007, the Ministry sent a letter to the NZa, instructing it to change the policy regulation on "Contractual space 2007." The letter announced that the resources from the AWBZ covenant would be allocated to the ten transition experiments, specifying for each experiment the total amount allocated. Following up this letter, the NZa modified the policy regulation (including a one-time raise of the contractual space in 2007), which enabled the Care Offices to finance the start-up phase of the transition experiments as of September 1, 2007.

To create this financial and legal space for transition experiments, the Program Team had to deal with a lot of tensions within the "regime" (e.g. those between the Ministry, the NZa and the Care Offices). As a result, the management process evolved into a compromise between the aims of the Ministry and the TM aims. Examples of TM notions that were successfully translated to the TPLC included: the selection criteria, the learning sessions and the monitoring framework. On the other hand, the SMART format for the project proposals, which was related to the cumbersome effort to finance the transition experiments, ran counter to the TM principles.

During the pilot phase and start-up phase of the Transition Program, the Program Team thus had to deal with three main challenges: (1) integrating the different objectives and perspectives within the Program Team into a shared management approach, (2) overcoming the barriers in the regime through a sustained, collaborative effort, and (3) providing support and encouragement to the transition experiments (including the necessary financial, juridical, organizational, geographical and mental space). The Program Team was successful in providing enough space to front-runner care institutions to experiment with radically new care practices that deviated from the care "regime" (the dominant structure, culture and practices in the care sector). However, because of the focus on promoting experiments and overcoming regime barriers, the Program Team was not always successful in involving and engaging key "regime players" (e.g. the Ministry) in a supportive way.

Learning sessions and program monitoring

To support the care institutions with starting up and further developing their transition experiments, and to enable maximum cross-learning, the Program Team organized monthly learning sessions with all project leaders. The second and third learning session focused on discussing the most important problems (and possible solutions) that the care institutions encountered in their daily practice and in realizing their societal challenge. The aim of these discussions was to deepen the insight into the persistent problems that were identified in the first learning session.

The start-up phase also allowed the Program Team to gain experience in monitoring the transition experiments. A "Transition Monitoring Handbook" was put together, in which the mechanisms of deepening, broadening and scaling up (see Box 7.2; Van den Bosch, 2010) and three transition monitoring indicators (Taanman, 2014) were translated into a matrix with nine central monitoring questions (see Figure 7.1).

The handbook was applied as a basic monitoring instrument within the TPLC. The nine central questions had to be answered in the annual reports to be submitted by the project leaders. Furthermore, the monitoring matrix was applied in monitoring meetings between the project leaders and the Program Team; these meetings were regularly held so as to gain insight into the progress of the transition experiments, feeding the (re-)definition of management priorities on that basis (Van den Bosch, 2010: 210).

Political impact of the Transition Program in Long-term Care

At the end of the start-up phase of the TPLC, the first round of transition experiments became the subject of parliamentary deliberations, following a letter from the State Secretary of Health, Welfare and Sports, Jet Bussemaker, in which she informed both chambers of Parliament about experiments in the AWBZ care.[6] This letter referred to previous debates, stating that "Stimulating innovation is an important ambition of the AWBZ sector, as agreed upon in the AWBZ covenant 2005–2007." The letter was followed up by written answers[7] to questions from members of the permanent parliamentary committee on Health, Welfare and Sports.

This parliamentary discussion is interesting for three reasons: it illustrates what *issues* politicians emphasized; it gives insight into the *changes* to which the Transition Program contributed; and it reflects different *transition patterns* that were (implicitly) anticipated by the Ministry.

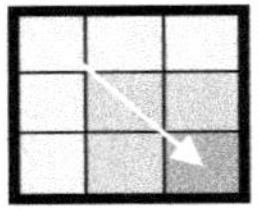

ACTIONS →

INDICATORS →

	DEEPENING	BROADENING	SCALING UP
	Actions aimed at learning as much as possible from the experiment in the specific context	Actions aimed at repeating the experiment in different contexts or linking it to other functions and domains	Actions aimed at embedding the experiment at a higher scale level
DIRECTION — Indicators aimed at the long-term vision on the problem, future image and pathway	In which way is the vision of the experiment on the problem, future image and pathway changed and why?	In which way is the experiment vision brought into line with and stimulated within the own organization, peer groups or similar projects?	In which way is the vision of the experiment brought into notice or embedded at sector level?
CHANGE — Indicators aimed at dealing with opportunities and barriers in daily practice	In which way were new possibilities and barriers utilized within the specific context of experiment?	In which way did cooperation with similar projects take place, to make use of the possibilities and barriers in a broader context?	In which way does the experiment take away institutional barriers at sector level and what support is needed for this?
SUSTAINABILITY — Indicators aimed at testing future image and results of sustainability ambition	In which way are lasting benefits realized in the experiment and how is evidence provided?	In which way do the lasting benefits apply to other contexts and what does the experiment do to research and improve this?	In which way are lasting benefits diffused at sector level and negative side-effects prevented?

Figure 7.1 Transition monitoring matrix

Source: *Transition Monitoring Handbook*, TPLC, August 2007.

Box 7.2 Lessons learned regarding the scaling up of Neighborhood Care (*Buurtzorg*)

Neighborhood Care was the only first-round transition experiment that had already started to scale up. With regard to deepening, broadening and scaling up, the following lessons learned may be directly derived from the annual report (2007) of Neighborhood Care:

1 Open search and learning process (deepening)

- Giving freedom to the Neighborhood Care teams to be entrepreneurs.
- Stimulating the creation of standards "owned by" the professionals (instead of the organization).
- Conducting (and spreading) research to evaluate the results regarding care content and development of the organization.

2 Repeating and connecting (broadening)

- Incorporating a large number of new teams in the Neighborhood Care practice.
- Expanding and reinforcing connections with essential partners and stake-holders (e.g. general practitioners, specialists, health insurers, knowledge and education institutes, organizations of volunteers, etc.), which creates sustainable networks.

3 Embedding in the regime (scaling up)

- Bringing the vision of Neighborhood Care to the attention of "regime players" (e.g. the Ministry, political parties, Innovation Platform, care insurers). From this, various activities emerged (e.g. working visits, workshops and TV shows), and this speeded up the process of allowing Neighborhood Care in all Care Office regions.
- Realizing necessary production agreements with the Care Offices.
- Providing a standard plan of action to new Neighborhood Care teams (balancing between giving freedom to work and standardization).
- Designing and realizing adequate ICT support.

The *issues* that were mentioned in these parliamentary questions mainly included the results, monitoring and evaluation of the transition experiments. The parliamentary committee was specifically interested in being periodically informed about the transition experiments' progress. One question addressed the issue of whether *the amount of 13 million euros for experiments in 2008 was substantial enough to expect quick and positive results.* In her reply, the State Secretary claimed that through setting up the various separate transition experiments the necessary room for experimenting within the care sector had already been created, and that the additional amount of 13 million euros would provide the sector with an extra opportunity to utilize the existing innovative

potential, while it could simultaneously keep an eye on the financial accountability. This exchange reflects, again, the tension between creating room for
experimentation so as to resolve long-standing, persistent problems that raise
significant political concern on the one hand, and the short-term, result-driven
political expectations on the other. Yet this tension was resolved, as additional
resources for short-term small-scale experiments in healthcare could fulfil the
political need for positive results in the short term. More general issues
involved the follow-up and structural implementation of experiments in
healthcare and the relation to the persistent job market problems.

The parliamentary paper also reflected several *changes* that had been influenced by the Transition Program. The most concrete changes involved not
only modifications of existing policy regulations and procedures to make
room for the transition experiments, but also, indirectly, the creation of a
new policy regulation with regard to experimentation in healthcare. Interestingly, the parliamentary paper reflected a different perspective (or discourse)
regarding innovation in healthcare, perceiving small-scale experiments as an
important means to change the existing care system. The discourse used in
this parliamentary paper included phrases such as "innovating means experimenting," "these small-scale experiments are about innovation that cannot be
financed within the existing rules," "making available lessons learned," "creating room," "structural implementation," "in principle new types of care
will replace the old ones" and "a successful innovation can be incorporated
into the regular system."

In terms of the transition *patterns* distinguished by De Haan and Rotmans
(2011), the State Secretary's replies correspond with a preference for an
adaptation pattern, in which new innovations are incorporated into the existing care system. This may be inferred from such measures as the modification
of existing policy regulations, the adoption of successful innovations in the
regular (financing) system and the principle that innovations in healthcare will
replace old practices. Another type of pattern that was (implicitly) stimulated
by the Ministry is an *empowerment* pattern, which creates space for innovations
(in niches) outside the regime. An example is the focus on small-scale experiments and, more specifically, the allocation of resources to experiments that
cannot or can only partly or with considerable administrative difficulty be
financed by the present system.

7.5 Selecting the second round of 16 transition experiments (January to April 2008)

At the end of the start-up phase of the first ten transition experiments in
healthcare, the selection of the second round of 16 transition experiments
began. This section will analyze this selection process, and compare it with
the selection process of the first round of transition experiments. The section
ends with an analysis of the final selection of the second round, and a portfolio analysis of all 26 transition experiments.

Selection strategy, procedure and criteria

The selection process of the first and second rounds of transition experiments differed in several ways (see Table 7.4).

These differences reflect different selection strategies, which again are due to their contextualization in the pilot and start-up phase and the "growth" phase of the Transition Program, respectively. Following up the "push strategy" of the first round, the selection process of the second round of transition experiments was characterized by a "pull strategy." In a broad tender, all AWBZ acknowledged care institutions were invited to submit project proposals. Furthermore, the criteria to select the second round of transition experiments were optimized by the Program Team (see Table 7.5). The selection criteria had originated from the earlier defined aims, innovation themes and starting-points of the transition program. However, the optimized criteria resulted in a better integration of the key TM elements that were applied in this transition program. The optimized selection criteria included three TM criteria:

- *Connection to persistent problem/societal challenge.* This criterion made explicit that a societal challenge (one that is related to overcoming a persistent problem) is a starting point of transition experiments.
- *Radically changing the structure, culture and practices.* This criterion further defined the original criterion "radically innovative" and explicitly distinguished the innovativeness of a project from common practices (and the interrelated structure and culture).
- *Learning, growing and changing potential (deepening, broadening and scaling up).* It was explained to the care institutions that "The project should have a high *transition potential*: the potential of solutions, within three years, to (a) learn from it, (b) be repeated in a different context within the care sector and (c) be able to influence the structure, culture and practices in the sector."

Final selection of project proposals

The selection criteria (see Table 7.5) provided a basis for assessing and discussing the submitted project proposals (42 in total) for the second round of the TPLC. Each project proposal was assessed by a team of two or three Program Team members who assigned a green, orange or red score to each criterion. This resulted in the following portfolio of selected second round proposals (see Table 7.6).

Portfolio analysis

The selection of individual experiments for the second round of the TPLC was supplemented with a portfolio analysis. This portfolio analysis was

Table 7.4 Comparison between selection process of first- and second-round transition experiments in healthcare

	Selection of first round	*Selection of second round*
Selection strategy	"Push-strategy," starting with *shortlist* of known potential transition experiments and related care institutions	"Pull-strategy," broad tender open to all AWBZ acknowledged care institutions
Procedure to increase quality of submitted project proposals	Highly personal procedure with extensive visits to all (11) shortlist care institutions, followed up by two reports and a personal letter of advice (to increase the quality of project proposals)	Formal procedure that started with assessment of pre-applications (129 in total), followed up by a letter of advice (100 standardized negative advices and 29 personal positive advices to increase the quality of project proposals)
Format for project proposal	Free format + transition explanation (+ after the selection by the Program Team a *final project plan* was requested to speed up the financing and contracting procedure)	Standardized format, similar to format of *final project plans* in the first round (added with one extra question to specify project activities in terms of deepening, broadening and/or scaling up)
Number of submitted project proposals	11	42
Number of selected experiments	10	16
Selection criteria	Eight criteria (derived from 35 criteria brought in by the separate organizations of the Program Team) → Table 7.2	Nine optimized criteria (that integrated the three perspectives: transition management, a broad care approach and an organizational perspective) → Table 7.5
Duration of selection process (from project proposal invitations to the selection by the Program Team)	1.5 months	Four months (caused by the round of pre-applications, a meeting day and the extra involvement of the care sector organizations during the last phase)
Time between selection by the Program Team and start of the transition experiments	Four months (caused by a complex contracting and financing procedure)	Four months (caused by necessary time to "transition" and improve the quality of project plans)

Table 7.5 Optimized selection criteria applied at one of the selected transition experiments

Optimized selection criteria	Example of selected transition experiment: imagination as a working method
Innovation themes	
• Connection to innovation themes	• Social support systems
Transition management	
• Connection to persistent problem/ societal challenge	• Poor communication between elderly people with memory problems and their environment
• Radically changing the structure, culture and practices	• Changing the prevailing way of thinking and communicating with elderly people
• Learning, growing and changing potential (deepening, broadening and scaling up)	• Aimed at transferring new working method (based on imagination) to 200 care locations and embedding this in daily practices
Care broad approach	
• Focus on end-user	• Elderly people and their direct environment
• Involving other actors from within and outside of the care sector	• Cooperation between different care institutions and a theater production agency
Motivation and ability	
• Intrinsic motivation (track record, supportive environment, space for unorthodox approach)	• High motivation to "use experiment as a catalyst in the care sector"
• Thorough and plausible business case	• Needs to be further specified
Quality of the proposal	
• To the point, clear and SMART formulation	• Clear proposal

conducted by DRIFT to gain insight into the diversity and coherence between the transition experiments of both the first and second rounds. The analysis demonstrated that:

- In terms of *variety*, the portfolio showed a good spread across target groups, innovation themes and new practices.
- In terms of *coherence* (in problems, target groups and practices), different clusters of experiments could be recognized. Based on coherence in problems addressed, the 26 transition experiments could be clustered in three main problems: "lack of diversity in care," "not able to continue living at home comfortably" and "lack of human contact." Clustering based on coherence in the target group or new practices resulted in a large number of clusters, in which most experiments were part of more than one cluster.

Table 7.6 Second round of transition experiments in healthcare

Project	Description
1 From harness to summer dress/doing less ... achieving more	Realizing a breakthrough in dominant mindset and working practices of care professionals
2 "Dementia coach"	Providing support (by telephone coaching) to informal care providers of people with dementia
3 Village health center	Introducing community nurses to realize small-scale 24-hour homecare in a village
4 Giving meaning as business	Developing a new business model to support clients with fundamental questions about life
5 Tailor-made care through lifestyle monitoring	Developing new care arrangements based on the monitoring of activity patterns of elderly at home
6 Work for experiential experts	Integrating the knowledge and experience of former psychiatric patients in mental care teams
7 The free rein	Creating a challenging and inspiring learning/ working/care environment
8 Presence (radical connection from zero to 100)	Learning communities of "present" care providers with attention and commitment to their clients
9 Telecare for new target groups	Applying telecare technology to support migrants, mentally disabled and psychiatric clients
10 Good neighbors wanted	Developing individual living arrangements for mentally disabled people in new district in Almere
11 Early, continuous and integral	Developing care chains for integrated support of disabled or chronically ill children and parents
12 Twente approach "well-cared-for" living	Developing new sustainable business models to improve care for elderly and physically disabled
13 Societal learning places	Enabling clients with psychiatric background to provide (housing) services in care for the elderly
14 Care home for (Islamic) Turkish and Moroccan elderly	Developing an expertise center and multicultural home for Islamic Turkish and Moroccan elderly
15 Own director with schizophrenia	Developing a care program for people with schizophrenia that stimulates self-management
16 Imagination as working method	Transferring imagination method to improve communication with elderly with memory problems

- In terms of *scope*, the analysis provided preliminary insights into the extent to which the transition experiments together contributed to a transition in healthcare. The scope had been defined by the Ministry and care sector associations in four "guiding" innovation themes: (1) prevention and redefining care demand, (2) social and societal support systems, (3) remote care, and (4) efficient management.

The portfolio analysis was used to support the selection of the second round of transition experiments in healthcare (but it did not change the outcome of the selection process).

Reflection on selecting the second round of 16 transition experiments (2008)

In terms of selection criteria, the selection process of the second round of transition experiments in healthcare involved an optimization of the first round. At the same time, however, it required a different procedure, as the selection strategy was different (pull instead of push strategy). The Program Team learned that even though the pull strategy did not allow enough time to visit the participating care institutions, meetings with several potential transition experiments were crucial to gain insight into motivation and ability.

The TM approach could not be fully integrated into the selection process; for instance, the portfolio analysis was added to the selection process but not fully integrated because the other organizations did not immediately see the short-term value of this analysis. Another reason was that the often "last-minute" and ad hoc interventions of DRIFT did not match the strict procedures of the Ministry (which were mainly managed by ErnstandYoung).

Furthermore, the presence of different objectives and perspectives within the Program Team did not always correspond to the objectives of TM. The different perspectives within the Program Team ranged from aiming for short-term results, strictly within the framework of the four innovation themes provided by the Ministry, to a more open search and learning process outside the boundaries of the existing care sector.

One Program Team member characterized his role as a "regime player" that sometimes (consciously) opposed the alternative approach of DRIFT. If these different roles within the Program Team enabled a critical perspective on the added value of TM concepts and tools, it also made it more difficult to implement the TM approach to an extent that enabled a complete test of its application to the care sector.

7.6 Transition arena

As noted above, contrary to the approach in earlier transition management programs (Rotmans and Loorbach, 2010), the program started with a portfolio of experiments, rather than with the establishment of a so-called transition arena, to develop a joint vision as well as transition pathways, including experiments. Yet, also within the TPLC, a transition arena was eventually established. This occurred in spite of initial reluctance on the side of especially the Ministry, and owing to the strong support of all other actors involved in the program: initially especially the care sector organizations in the Working Group Innovation, and later on also various individuals who took part in the transition arena. In this section we discuss this process and its outcomes.

The initiative to conduct a transition arena process after all was taken by DRIFT and motivated as an essential and integral part of a full-fledged transition management approach. It was put forward on several occasions as being essential to the governing bodies of the transition program, and for that reason it was also included in the officially approved program proposal that provided the basis for all later actions and activities. Yet, when it came to formally supporting and funding an elaboration of the transition arena, the formal steering bodies declined concrete support. In particular, the Ministry of Health, Welfare and Sports put forward several objections to actually develop a transition arena for this program: the fear of losing focus within the program on experimenting; dispute on the role and function of a transition arena next to the existing formal steering structure; no need for another policy document or a new vision; lack of financial means available, etc. After a prolonged and painstaking process (lasting more than a year) of putting forward proposals, giving presentations and heated debates within the Working Group Innovation (the operational governing body), the formal start-up of the transition arena was approved by the Ministry in early 2008. This was mainly due to the strong support and pressure from the care sector associations involved. The transition arena began in March 2008, when the selection process of the second round was already well under way. For this reason, the transition arena did not play a role in the selection processes of the first round of transition experiments, and it had a marginal part, and only indirectly so, in the second round of transition experiments.

In order not to lose further momentum, DRIFT on its own initiative had already begun several preliminary activities: elaborating the approach, drafting a long list of potential participants, making general problem analyses, collecting visionary documents, etc. Eventually, the Ministry granted DRIFT a subsidy, ensuring the necessary free "room for maneuver" to conduct the further arena process according to TM standard operating practice, safeguarding it against further regime interference.

Following an intensive process of interviewing potential participants, a selection was made of 13 arena participants, representing a strong diversity in background (from within and from outside of the healthcare sector), operating level and perspective. Following the transition management approach (Loorbach, 2007), in the course of 18 months six so-called "transition arena" meetings were held with mediation and scientific support from DRIFT and many supporting activities in between these meetings. This resulted in a

breakthrough document which was endorsed by all participants: "Human(s')
care: a transition movement" (Transition Arena Long-term Care, 2009). The
transition experiments were presented to the arena, and all experiments were
included in the vision document, providing illustrations of sustainable future
care. In this way the experiments were used to enrich the vision document
and the experiments could include the arena findings in further shaping their
experiments (e.g. connecting the experiment to a broader vision). The final
document provided an in-depth analysis of the persistent and structural problems in Dutch healthcare and their underlying root causes. It furthermore
provided a first outline of new development principles for sustainable healthcare: (1) centering on human life, (2) providing economic value, and (3)
integrating care into society.

These principles were combined into a sustainability vision composed of
six aspirational sketches. Succinctly put, these covered the following concerns: (1) future care will first of all empower people in self-management and
inner directedness, and (2) will also support the societal care fabric, coined as
"Together-Care." Furthermore, future care will enable other societal sectors
(living and housing, working, education, lifestyle, etc.) to (4) create healthy
conditions which prevent people from needing formal care or help them
cope better with their chronic illnesses or ailments. (5) Care professionals will
be provided with more room to use and develop their craftwomanship and
they will be supported by much broader societal organizations that provide a
whole range of integral services including care. (6) This development will be
supported by a sustainable system that facilitates, rather than obstructs, the
realization of these transitional changes.

This vision document concluded with an outline of concrete actions that
might further spark and speed up the transition movement. Many drew upon
the experiences gained in the 26 experiments. Regarding the final point,
namely a sustainable health system, several paths of action were proposed:

- Room for experimentation: more mental and regulatory space for, and
  political patience regarding, experiments.
- Power shift: from the care system toward primary (professional and
  informal) caregivers and patients, who should gain more agency over care
  practices and resource allocation.
- Deregulation: more generic, patient- and practice-oriented rules, including funding rules – the current system is still centered around providing
  (given) services and products, rather than meeting needs tailored to specific patients and contexts.
- Quality control should better facilitate experimenting by becoming more
  dialogic as a process and taking the creation of societal value, rather than
  narrowly defined cost-effectiveness, as a guiding principle.

7.6 Conclusions

The TPLC (2007–2010) may be regarded as a "milestone" in the scientific and practical development of Transition Management (TM), and specifically the TM instrument transition experiments: the program started with experiments and only later established an arena. This occurred due to the state of the care sector, which did not have a history of radical innovation. That a transition program could nevertheless be established was because the sector was also characterized by some persistent problems, as well as by a number of innovators interested in experiments to deal with these problems. The Program Team managed to overcome the inertia against radical change, which was to a large extent through strategic operating, drawing upon these innovators and the legitimacy generated through the transition experiments.

This had at least three important consequences for managing a portfolio of transition experiments regarding the selection, creation of space and interaction with a transition arena. The experience gained on these topics is of interest for further transition efforts in healthcare, as well as for the further development of TM more generally.

Selection of experiments

When it comes to selection, the most crucial issue, as we have seen, is to ensure a sustained focus on radical innovation, regardless of regime influences that may run counter to it. From this perspective in particular, several lessons are important. First, because a sustainability vision and transition pathways were initially lacking, the portfolio of experiments could not be developed based on an existing "transition agenda." Instead, a selection procedure and specific selection criteria were developed (see sections 7.4 and 7.5). The *selection procedure* included both a "push" and a "pull" strategy with the underlying aim to build upon the existing, bottom-up initiatives within the care sector, by selecting front runners (niche players) that are in need of financial, legislative or mental space. The developed *selection criteria* (Table 7.5) included three TM criteria: (1) the extent to which the desired outcome of the experiment radically changed structure, culture and practices (*radical innovation criterion*); (2) the potential of the experiment to learn, grow and change the existing care sector (*deepening, broadening and scaling-up criterion*), and (3) the connection of the experiment to a persistent problem and related societal challenge (*sustainability criterion*). All three criteria – above all the first one – have proven to have crucial distinctive value.

Another key lesson has been that the selection process should focus on how an experiment fits the total portfolio, especially in cases with a larger portfolio of transition experiments (>10–20). In such situations, future images and transition pathways, developed by a transition arena (partly based on lessons from earlier experiments) could help to define a balanced portfolio.

Third, we have seen how the regime influenced the selection process and, thus, the definition of the selected projects. On the other hand, we have seen that, in addition to the innovators, patients and primary caregivers are also important allies in maintaining a transition orientation. Therefore, future selection procedures could stimulate end-users to be actively involved in developing transition experiments. Role-play, "storytelling" and other techniques to demonstrate what is involved may be of help here.

Fourth, it is crucial that regime players have no decisive influence on selection; and ideally, the set of regime actors close to the selection process should be diverse enough to allow for checks and balances between them.

Finally, a strong focus on radical innovations also implies room for failure. It is even crucial that some experiments may be discontinued – this is the idea behind the TM's principle of continuous variation and selection (Rotmans and Loorbach, 2010). We therefore recommend including and, when necessary, using, the possibility that transition experiments that fail to meet expectations can be stopped before the end of the Transition Program. Based on our experiences we warn against adding *formal* selection moments, because this decreases the *mental space* to experiment and "learn by failure" (implying that learning experiences are more important than short-term results).

Creating space for transition experiments

A second consequence of the fact that a transition arena was established only late in the process was that it became less easy to have front runners (help) provide the space for setting up the transition experiments. Instead, the financial and legislative space for the selected transition experiments was created by the regime (the covenant between the Ministry and the care sector associations). As a result, the regime was directly involved and could influence the transition experiments, which, as we have seen, resulted in many tensions in terms of managing the transition experiments (e.g. keeping up the speed versus slow financial procedures, open search and learning process versus SMART project plans, and radically changing the regime versus involving regime interests). However, the direct involvement of regime players also provided opportunities (e.g. financial support, knowledge about the care sector and mobilizing a large number of care institutions). One lesson is that, with hindsight, it can be stated that the agreements in the covenant should have been more precise with regard to how the resources could be allocated.

Second, it was a strong point that the transition experiments in healthcare were financed by modifications in existing financial structures (policy regulations) rather than by a subsidy. Interestingly, the Ministry stated that this provided opportunities to learn about these financial structures. However, the modified policy regulations concerned only *temporary* measures to support small-scale experimentation. This did not allow the actors to learn much about the changes that are necessary to *structurally* finance radically new practices in long-term care. Therefore, learning about structural financing should always be an explicit goal in a transition experiment (Grin, 2008, 2010; Schuitmaker and ter Haar, Chapter 4, this volume).[8]

Scaling up successful transition experiments

A third consequence of the relatively late establishment of a transition arena pertained to the limited interaction between the first round of transition experiments and the transition arena. In the first phase of the TPLC, the transition experiments were not supported by a shared vision on a sustainable care sector, nor were they connected by transition pathways.

In the TM approach followed, learning experiences in the transition experiments were used to gain insight into the persistent problems in the care sector and to provide *building blocks* for developing a shared sustainability vision. The management of the transition experiments was determined less by a normative guidance developed a priori (problem analysis, vision, pathways) than by an open search and learning process, with a strong shared drive to change the existing *structure, culture and practices* in the care sector and influence the *deepening, broadening and scaling up* of transition experiments (Box 7.2). These concepts, then, served as important steering notions that were translated to the context of the TPLC.

One key lesson in this regard has been that in order to support the scaling up of successful transition experiments the Program Team did well to (1) pay attention to coaching project leaders, (2) conduct supportive analyses and create conditions to remove regime barriers (e.g. with regard to procedures, financing structures), (3) extend the links with regime players, and (4) connect the transition experiments to strategic activities in a transition arena (sustainability vision, transition pathways).

A second lesson concerns the first experiences with setting up a "scaling-up" team with a selection of project leaders and, ideally, different experts on scaling up (juridical, socio-cultural, institutional, etc.) who could formulate explicit scaling-up objectives and strategies.

Third, and perhaps most fundamentally, this case study also illustrates how niche actors can be *empowered* to exercise "innovative power,"[9] but are also linked to actions by regime actors (Grin, 2010: 265–266, 282–284) who may exercise "constitutive" power (Avelino and Rotmans, 2009). Follow-up research, drawing in particular upon the work by Avelino (2010), should specifically elaborate on the consequences of different types of TM approaches (vision-driven versus experiment-driven) in relation to different contexts and in relation to different types (e.g. Grin, 2012a) of "niche/regime interactions."

Finally, this case study has shown that an experiment-driven TM approach in healthcare was the result of a specific context in which the care regime enabled space (niches) for innovation but also caused barriers. A crucial question for follow-up (action) research is to what extent the transition experiments will be able to scale up and influence the care regime, and how

Transition Management can support this scaling-up process. If anything, this case study has taught us regarding such future attempts at TM in healthcare that each approach should always be sensitive to the specific contexts of these experiments.

Notes

1 This chapter is largely based on the PhD thesis by Suzanne Van den Bosch (2010).
2 Because sustainability is a normative topic, this explanation of the unsustainability of the Dutch care system is based on the shared problem analysis of the transition arena in healthcare (Transition Arena Long-term Care, 2009).
3 The AWBZ resources are collected through the income and payroll tax systems, along with the contributions for the other national insurance schemes. Regional Care Offices are responsible for the allocation of the AWBZ resources to the care providers by means of contracting. Each year a policy measure on "contractual space" determines the maximum annual budget care offices can use to contract out healthcare.
4 As of November 2007, the national client advisory body LOC-LPR and Zorgverzekeraars Nederland (association for healthcare insurance organizations) have also participated in the WGI.
5 Internal report of the instruction meeting April 2, 2007, TPLC, April 5, 2007.
6 Letter from State Secretary of Health, Welfare and Sports to the chambers of Parliament, December 4, 2007. KST113399, 30186, Nr. 64 (www.europa-nu.nl/id/vi3jbk13o5vb/brief_staatssecretaris_over).
7 Letter from State Secretary of Health, Welfare and Sports, "Experiments with AWBZ-care," February 12, 2008 (www.rijksoverheid.nl/documenten-en-publicaties/kamerstukken/2008/02/12/brief-experimenten-met-awbz-zorg.html).
8 In mid-2008 the TPLC started to support each first-round transition experiment with developing a "societal business case." For each experiment the (societal) costs and benefits were calculated by ErnstandYoung, and solutions for structural financing were explored.
9 Avelino and Rotmans (2009: 11) define *innovative power* as the capacity of actors to create or discover new resources and define *constitutive power* as the capacity to constitute the distribution of resources. To "constitute" something means to establish, institute or enact it.

8   Trying to transform structure, culture and practice

Comparing two innovation projects
of the Transition Program in
Long-term Care

Erica ter Haar-van Twillert and
Suzanne Van den Bosch

8.1 Introduction

> Some societal problems ask for radical solutions because of their persistency. Examples are problems in the field of climate change, energy supply and mobility. There are comparable problems in healthcare. Due to the ageing of the population, increasing costs and labour shortage our health system is endangered. With this the quality and accessibility of healthcare come into play. Besides that, clients as well as care professionals experience the health system as a maze of fragmentation, office windows and financial sections. This impedes innovation and asks for radical changes in our health system.

As argued in the above quote from the introduction of the brochure of the Dutch Transition Program in Long-term Care (2008), a transition in healthcare is needed for several reasons. Developments and trends in the *landscape*, such as demographic and economic developments, are pressing upon the incumbent care *regime*, on its dominant structures, culture and practices. For example, the aging of the population increases the demand for long-term care, while at the same time the workforce in healthcare is decreasing. The current health system seems unable to deal with new societal challenges. Part I of this volume showed that negative side-effects and challenges evolved alongside the development of appreciated health systems. The problems pertaining to the Dutch care system – such as fragmentation and too much specialization – have also been known for sometime (Schrijvers, 1997). To address societal challenges and overcome persistent problems, the dominant structure, culture and practices in health systems need to be transformed.

This chapter is about how working on system innovation and transition takes place in actual practice, and, more specifically, about efforts to overcome the persistent problems in the Dutch care system. Our argument concentrates on the analysis and comparison of two projects involving innovative practices in healthcare, which are both supported by the Transition Program in Long-term Care (hereafter called the Transition Program) (cf. Van den Bosch and Neuteboom, Chapter 7, this volume). The core of the program is a portfolio of 26 transition experiments: innovation projects that are focused on identifying, exploring and learning about radically new ways to meet societal needs. The experiments are geared toward transforming prevailing practices and their interrelated structure and culture within particular domains of the health system devoted to long-term care, which encompasses care for the elderly, nursing and care, homecare, and care for physically or mentally disabled persons. The transition experiments explore and generate insight into promising radical innovations in practice. Concrete experiences have to stimulate new solutions for the persistent problems in the care sector. The experiments address four common innovation themes: (1) prevention and redefinition of the care demand; (2) social and societal support systems; (3) telecare (remote care), and (4) efficient management.

This chapter presents the results and lessons learned from two case studies on two projects of the Transition Program. The first project we discuss is ACT-Youth, an Assertive Community Treatment (ACT) project aimed at young people in Rotterdam which was initiated by a large mental healthcare institution. It aimed to address the social challenges of young individuals who suffer from complex psychosocial and psychiatric problems which were not dealt with by existing care providers. The experiment involved five multidisciplinary and outreaching ACT teams at various locations in Rotterdam, which provided integrated mental healthcare to youth in a fundamentally different way. The transition goals of this experiment included changes in structure (e.g. changing power structure between professionals and youth), culture (e.g. changing organizational culture and meeting youth culture) and practices (e.g. an integrated and outreaching approach). The Transition Program supported the management of ACT-Youth, following a "transition experiment" approach aimed at learning about societal challenges and realizing specific changes in structure, culture and practices.

The second project pertains to "telecare for elderly and chronically ill people." The Transition Program supported this transition experiment at different levels: at the level of a network of facilities actively involved in video care pilots and at the level of two of the care institutions involved. The ambition of the project was to develop a way of care providing whereby control is returned to the client and caregiver, while also offering room for professionals to provide personalized care. The project aimed to slow down, if not reverse, two trends: the growing demand for care and the decreasing number of people who want to work in the care sector. Significantly, the project has been arranged as a process of learning, whereby the pioneering actors constantly develop and adjust their views and interventions while also encouraging each other to reflect on the issues involved.

Although both projects sought to work on the quality of care to stimulate integration and positive changes in the balance of power and responsibility between clients and professionals, they started from different viewpoints and approaches. For one thing, they addressed different segments of the health system (mental healthcare system for youngsters versus telecare in the home-care system) and zoomed in on different client groups (young people versus the elderly and chronically ill). Moreover, the telecare project included an obvious technological component which was absent in the ACT-Youth project. Furthermore, if the latter may be regarded as one specific transition experiment, the telecare project involved a program in its own right, which initially covered ten projects but which will be expanded to include as many as 17 projects.

The main questions of this chapter center on how these innovative practices developed within their context and how this influenced changes in established practices and the interrelated structure and culture. We explore these concerns by comparing the two projects with regards not only to the approach followed to influence the dominant structure, culture and practices, but also the resistance and barriers encountered, and how these were dealt with.

The following sections include an elaboration of the two projects and a comparative analysis, which focuses on the differences and distinctions between the two projects (including the different approaches adopted to system innovation). The chapter ends with a discussion and conclusion regarding how the two projects influenced prevailing structures, cultures and practices of the health system.

8.2 Act-Youth Rotterdam

The ACT-Youth project originated in the context of persistent problems within the Dutch long-term care system. In "mental healthcare for young-sters," a subsystem within the overall care system, these problems led to the following symptoms of unsustainability: an increasing number of (often homeless) youngsters with multiple complex problems (associated with emotional, behavioral, financial, social and/or school drop-out issues) and a failure on the part of care providers to give adequate support to these youngsters, if they managed to reach them at all. Evidently, a situation like this may possibly lead to increasing problems in society at large (such as higher school drop-out rate, crime, vandalism, etc.). Researchers from the Netherlands Court of Audit (2004) concluded that the number of "homeless youngsters" was on the rise, while the care facilities were insufficient, too fragmented and difficult to find. Moreover, there was not enough coordination among the various care providers and facilities, and their services needed to be brought in line with the care demand among youngsters.

In 2004 the City of Rotterdam wanted to address these problems by stimulating specialized care to youngsters with multiple problems between the ages of 14 and 23. Two mental healthcare facilities in Rotterdam, namely GGZ Group Europoort and Bavo RNO Group (which would later merge into one mental healthcare institute) took up this challenge. They first asked their innovation manager to conduct a field and literature study (Zimmermann, 2004). It was found that a substantial group of about 600 youngsters between the ages of 12 and 24 who suffer from complex psychosocial and psychiatric problems were not reached by the then available care providers and services. These youngsters were in urgent need of mental healthcare in order to prevent an increase of their specific problems *and* an increase in social problems and the interrelated costs. It was concluded that these youngsters needed a care provider who would be able to hook up with their way of life.

To this end, the Rotterdam mental healthcare services adopted the Assertive Community Treatment (ACT) model, which was developed in the USA for adults suffering from serious psychiatric problems and which at the time was gaining increasing attention in the Netherlands (Mulder and Kroon, 2005). Inspired by the ACT model, they developed the so-called ACT-Youth approach, which aimed specifically at addressing the mental health problems of youngsters, including emotional and behavioral problems, autism, mental retardation, psychoses and post-traumatic stress disorders. These problems have often been linked to domestic violence or problematic family situations, war violence, sexual abuse, mistreatment or neglect (Van Dijk et al., 2006). The objective of the ACT-Youth approach was defined as "offering specialist mental healthcare to youngsters who cannot find their way, or cannot hold on, to the regular care providers" (ACT-Youth, 2005). The ACT-Youth approach includes the following key characteristics: outreaching (searching for and approaching youngsters with problems in their own environment), multidisciplinary team composition based on problems of the target group, shared caseload, low client–professional ratio, independent and flexible treatments and support, no limits in the duration of a treatment and the number of contacts, 24-hour availability and an "unorthodox" approach. A key aspect of ACT-Youth is that integrated care is offered in different domains of life at the same time and by the same ACT team. As one youngster commented in this respect:

> I receive support from ACT-Youth in all areas... I don't have to go anywhere [to different organizations], or ACT-Youth will go with me. Also at moments when I don't feel like it or don't dare to, they always keep on coming and supporting me.... I receive comprehensible support from one team and one facility who help me out with everything.

The first ACT-Youth team in Rotterdam was set up in January 2005. The ambulant ACT teams proactively looked for youngsters with complex problems and provided integral support, diagnosis and treatment. The first two years of ACT-Youth may be regarded as a "pioneering phase" (2005–2007), characterized by improvisation and flexibility, a lack of organizational embedding, and structured management and rapid "organic" growth of the number of teams (five in total). In 2006 ACT-Youth was selected as a transition experiment for the Transition Program (Van den Bosch and Neuteboom, Chapter 7, this volume). From that moment, the innovation manager of ACT-Youth received support in further developing and managing ACT-Youth as a transition experiment. This support was mainly provided by two team members of the Transition Program: a transition researcher (the second author of this chapter) and an adviser from DRIFT. The transition researcher followed an action research approach (Greenwood and Levin, 1998; Dick, 2004), thereby combining a researcher role and a Program Team member role during 2007 and 2008 (Van den Bosch, 2010). The researcher role involved several tasks: conducting interviews, analyzing and reflecting on how ACT-Youth was set up and managed, participating in strategic sessions with the actors involved, and giving presentations and putting forward theoretical knowledge about transition experiments. The Program Team member role comprised: supporting the innovation manager of ACT-Youth with various management activities (e.g. writing the project plan, contracting, reporting), participating in a number of informal and formal meetings with the innovation manager and general manager of ACT-Youth, and participating in meetings to monitor the transition experiment's progress.

When selected for the Transition Program, ACT-Youth had already been experimenting for two years, but an explicit long-term perspective was lacking. Based on a first interview with the actors involved, the existing goals of ACT-Youth were reframed in terms of desired changes in structure (e.g. changing power structures between professionals and youth), culture (e.g. changing organizational culture and meeting youth culture) and practices (e.g. an integrated and outreaching approach). During the process of further developing ACT-Youth as a "transition experiment," a strategy was developed to work toward a future image of 20 ACT teams in Rotterdam. Different types of ACT teams could then cover various levels of psychological and psychiatric problems within the estimated target group in Rotterdam (approximately 2,000 youngsters with problems of various degrees of complexity). However, to realize this vision many barriers had to be overcome (cf. the next section). The reports about ACT-Youth drafted for the Transition Program, as well as the regular learning meetings, played an important role in making these barriers explicit. Furthermore, the monitoring activities conducted as part of the Transition Program supported ACT-Youth in structuring and prioritizing their strategic activities (Van den Bosch, 2010).

In general, the approach to system innovation followed in ACT-Youth may be characterized as learning-by-doing, a process which was accompanied in part by protection from mainstream pressure (provided by the director of the mental healthcare facility involved, while the Transition Program also created "space for experimentation"), and this stimulated pioneering and trial-and-error. While ACT-Youth was initiated by one mental healthcare institution in Rotterdam, during the process ACT-Youth cooperated with other youth-related organizations as well (e.g. schools, a Rebound Centre, social services). Their shared aim was to provide a balanced care chain which was centered around youngsters. The learning process may be characterized as "second order" (Hall, 1993), because the existing institutions were questioned and new practices were developed based on a different frame of reference (e.g. the youngster involved is center-stage, not the institution). When ACT-Youth was supported by the Transition Program, more attention was paid to structuring the learning, evaluation and monitoring processes. This included defining explicit learning objectives, facilitating regular "transition meetings" (of the innovation manager, the general manager of ACT-Youth and two Program Team members) to discuss the progress in the transition experiment, facilitating meetings with the managers of the five ACT-Youth teams and with the ACT professionals, and a monitoring meeting took place every few months to discuss and report on the learning experiences and (re)define management priorities. In addition, the ACT-Youth innovation manager participated in the monthly learning sessions held with participants of the other transition experiments of the Transition Program.

The interaction between ACT-Youth and the Transition Program may be characterized as a process in which the two were mutually dependent. The latter needed the former because this transition experiment had a high appeal and high sense of urgency and could be used to learn about and stimulate a transition in long-term care. In addition, ACT-Youth needed the support of the Transition Program to obtain enough "space" for further development, change and learning within the ACT-Youth teams. The support it provided is best characterized in terms of different types of space for experimentation: "financial space" (e.g. subsidies), "organizational space" (e.g. commitment of powerful actors in the organization), "(transition) management space" (e.g. instruments and expertise on managing transition experiments), "mental space" (e.g. an inspiring environment that stimulates out-of-the-box thinking), "juridical space" (e.g. exemptions from rules and legislation) and "geographical space" (e.g. geographical flexibility in providing care) (Van den Bosch, 2010). This space was enabled by different resources of the Transition Program, including money, knowledge and expertise (e.g. regarding organizational management and Transition Management), language (e.g. transition discourse) and connections with regime actors (such as the ministry involved and various care facilities). The interaction with the Transition Program mainly created "mental space" for the various participants of ACT-Youth – space that was important in reinforcing the special (experimental) status of ACT-Youth and to broaden the perspective on ACT-Youth by connecting it to a transition that transcends its own organization.

Especially during the Transition Program's start-up phase (August to December 2007), ACT-Youth encountered many barriers, which could be related to the dominant structure, culture and practices of the Dutch health system. The ACT teams were set up within the institutional context of the mental healthcare system in the Netherlands (the Dutch abbreviation for this system is GGZ). In the 2007 annual report of ACT-Youth this system was characterized as follows:

The mental healthcare system is primarily aimed at (and is funded for) diagnosis and, related to this, treatment of psychiatric problems. If a specific indication for mental health problems is lacking or the youngster does not want to be helped, the usual practice is that nothing is done. The mental health system for young people is organized in this way: supply-driven, long waiting lists and institutionally organized around specific problem areas. The current system lacks incentives for creating a new integrated supply (as the current supply is under pressure already), which is only partially funded and which provides aid to youngsters without first diagnosing their mental problems according to the protocols (DSM-4 diagnostic criteria). In fact, ACT-Youth cannot become successful within the boundaries of the current mental healthcare system.

(ACT-Youth, 2008)

Within the context of this system, it was very difficult for ACT-Youth to contribute to a transition process. The vision of its innovation manager was to move the ACT approach outside of the Rotterdam mental healthcare services (since the demand for mental healthcare for youngsters was much greater than the available supply). Keeping ACT-Youth within its institutional boundaries, after all, would limit further growth in meeting the needs of youngsters. However, this was not the main priority of the mental healthcare institution involved; because the current Dutch care sector is market-driven, its main priority was economic survival and continuation.

Because the ACT approach deviated from the prevailing mental healthcare system, many activities of the ACT teams, such as visits to clients with more than one care professional or more than one contact moment a day, could in fact not be funded. This threatened the continuation of the ACT teams and led to budgetary shortfalls. The project plan of ACT-Youth estimated that each ACT team needed an annual budget of 300,000 euros to cover all activities not covered by the present (AWBZ) financing system. This shortage was temporarily compensated by the financial support of the Transition Program. However, searching for structural financing was explicitly defined as a learning objective in the ACT-Youth project plan.

In 2007 important developments in the organizational context of ACT-Youth took place as well, including austerity measures and a merger with another large mental healthcare institution. This resulted in a downscaling of the organizational budget, a limit to further growth and waiting lists for the ACT teams (ACT-Youth, 2008). By the end of 2007 ACT-Youth had grown out of its "pioneering phase" and was in need of organizational restructuring. The Transition Program supported this process by conducting an experiment scan (Demoulin and Felius, 2007). This led to the conclusion that ACT-Youth had grown too rapidly, leaving insufficient time to allow its primary processes and management structure to crystallize and to organize the interrelated governance (Demoulin and Felius, 2007). The organizational barriers also resulted in a loss of confidence in the ACT approach, both external (other care institutions and network partners) and internal (the directors and other departments of the umbrella organization), which may be regarded as *"mental barriers"* that limited the successful development of ACT-Youth.

Strategies

To overcome the obstacles encountered and to contribute to a transition process, the general manager and innovation manager of ACT-Youth conducted several "management activities" that may be understood in terms of "deepening," "broadening" and "scaling up" (Van den Bosch and Rotmans, 2008).

Deepening (learning as much as possible in a specific context; e.g. Kemp et al., 1989; Loeber et al., 2007; Röling, 2002; Van den Bosch and Taanman, 2006) was stimulated by structuring the learning process, which resulted in explicit learning objectives, learning about all relevant aspects of a societal challenge (e.g. financial aspects, institutional aspects), regular learning meetings and reporting on learning experiences. In addition, different types of actors were involved in the learning process; so-called "product groups" were set up in which the ACT professionals could further develop and improve their approach. And the youngsters themselves were provided with a virtual platform (the web paper Active Youngsters Rotterdam, www.transitieprogramma.nl) to stimulate participation and online dialogue. The learning results were fed back as much as possible to strategic actors, including directors and policy-makers.

Broadening (repeating the experiment in different contexts and linking it to other functions and domains; see e.g. Rotmans and Loorbach, 2006; Van den Bosch and Rotmans, 2008; Van den Bosch, 2010) was stimulated by experimenting with the ACT approach on a new target group (youngsters instead of adults) and implementing ACT teams at different locations in Rotterdam. ACT-Youth was also connected to similar innovations with a different function (e.g. the Rebound Center in Rotterdam) and in 2008 a function was added to its existing teams: the Mobile Diagnosis, Consultation and Expertise team. This increased the flexibility and accessibility of specialized mental healthcare in Rotterdam. Furthermore, ACT-Youth was involved in setting up similar ACT teams within other organizations and regions (e.g. Tender Youth Care in the Province of Brabant and De Jutters in The Hague).

Scaling up (embedding the experiment in – new – dominant structures, cultures and practices at a higher scale level; see e.g. Geels and Raven, 2006; Rotmans and Loorbach, 2006; Van den Bosch and Rotmans, 2008) was stimulated by embedding ACT-Youth in the dominant structure and related practices and culture of the Rotterdam mental healthcare organization (e.g. ACT-Youth was incorporated into a new independent care company, called Child and Youth Psychiatry). ACT-Youth also cooperated in the "Every Child Wins" regional program, which aimed to realize a breakthrough in the current mismatch between the "supply" of the youth-related organizations in Rotterdam and the "demands" of youngsters with developmental or behavioral problems. In general, an important result of ACT-Youth was that it occupied a strong position in Rotterdam. The project allowed the Rotterdam mental healthcare institution to leave its ivory tower and establish connections with other organizations dealing with youngsters in Rotterdam (such as the Youth Care Bureau, youth care providers, educational institutions, the Rotterdam Public Health Service). Outside Rotterdam, ACT-Youth was brought to the attention of important national media and policy-makers (who are part of the "regime").

Changes in structure, culture and practices

Looking back at the initial goals of ACT-Youth with regard to transforming the structure, culture and practices of the mental healthcare system, it is possible to describe the first results of the transition experiment. As such, ACT-Youth was set up to influence the dominant structure, culture and practices regarding mental healthcare provisions to youngsters in Rotterdam and eventually the Netherlands. Its project plan, drafted for the Transition Program, formulated the following desired (interrelated) changes in structure, culture and practices:

Structure:
*   The target group of young people is not subdivided into groups receiving either care or psychiatric help: rather, care is offered in an integrated way, centered around the youngster involved.
*   Different roles for care professionals: youngsters are central and are approached in their own environment (rather than in the care professionals' institutional environment).
*   Different way of financing: preferably, ACT-Youth Rotterdam wants to work with a lump-sum amount (15,000 euros) for each youngster per year.

Culture:
*   Establishing a connection with the attitude of youngsters (respect for their territory, dress codes, behavioral codes, etc.) in relation to their cultural context.
*   Rather than starting from the notion of providing no care if the youngster involved does not want it or is unable able to handle it, care should start from imagining the problems at hand and connecting to what the youngster *does* want or can handle.

Practices:
*   Providing care does not start with research and diagnosis, but with offering practical help (this enables building up trust and swift breaking of vicious circles, after which it is easier to set a correct diagnosis and to prevent further problems from developing).

- Various specialists work together on location (e.g. a district) and when necessary will visit a youngster together (this potentially raises insight into the problems while the professionals may also learn from each other).

On a small scale, most of these desired changes in structures, cultures and practices were successfully realized by the five ACT teams operating at different locations in Rotterdam. An important concrete result of the transition experiment's first two years (2007 and 2008) was that during these years the ACT teams provided integrated mental healthcare to about 400 youngsters (with a marginal drop-out rate and no incidents or suicides). The launch of similar initiatives in The Hague and Brabant was one specific result of the ACT-Youth project's expansion. With regard to scaling up, the actors involved succeeded in embedding a radically new approach at different scale levels, including their own organization, a (regional) network and, to a lesser extent, the (national) mental healthcare system (Van den Bosch, 2010). By 2008, however, ACT-Youth had not yet managed to receive structural funding (meaning for a period of at least five years). With the support of the Transition Program, ACT-Youth had meanwhile begun to develop a *Social Business Case* to calculate and demonstrate its costs and benefits to society.

8.3 Telecare

The telecare project originates from the opportunities of new technologies for providing care. With the spread of the internet and the development of the information society, several homecare organizations have sought to use new communication technologies to support the care process. From the start, the focus has been on video communication between the client at home and the health professional (nurse), to facilitate, for example, daily contact to verify if everything is all right, the control or coaching of crucial medication administered, and camera surveillance at night when there is a risk of clients wandering and falling. Another example involves tele-monitoring (coaching and early intervention based on measurements performed by clients) of chronic diseases such as diabetics, Chronic Obstructive Pulmonary Disease (COPD) and heart failure. The aim of this technology is to increase clients' safety and self-management opportunities; the screen may help them to find services they need (care, welfare, fun and comfort), but it may also facilitate early intervention and coaching to prevent their condition from worsening.

The first initiatives in the Netherlands to use video-conferencing between client and nurse via television or screen in homecare started in around 2000/2001. There were a lot of technical problems, which even led to the bankruptcy of several technology companies involved. Based on this experience, several care providers took up the initiative to cooperate in this development in around 2003/2004. This cooperation initiated the telecare network. In this arrangement, the participating homecare organizations – supported by the sector organization Actiz – shared experiences from their telecare experiments and worked together on shared interests. In July 2005 the funding for experiments became available. The experimental regulation for screen-to-screen care (NZa, CA-123/197), temporarily set up for a period of five years, made it possible to have telecare reimbursed by the care administration office and also receive compensation for the investments. Care organizations that made use of this regulation had to take part in monitoring research to investigate the effects of telecare (Bos et al., 2005; Bos and Francke, 2006; Peeters et al., 2007, 2009). Moreover, ties were established between the project coordinator and a professor in system innovation at the University of Amsterdam. Together they developed a program plan aimed at fundamental change, following the approach of reflexive design (Grin, 2004), and a set-up of the project that aligns the regime with the innovative practices. In addition, qualitative monitoring was included (Grin and Weterings, 2005; Actiz, 2007). In 2006 the Transition Program provided opportunities for two of the participating organizations to submit a project proposal. One proposal was about using video-networks for a broad service arrangement[1] and the other was about telecare for specific target groups (e.g. diabetics, heart failure or COPD patients). Furthermore, the telecare-network, as an experiment in its own right, could also be part of the Transition Program. With its support, the "telecare-network" obtained a more formal status and developed into an official program within the sector organization (Actiz, 2007). The different telecare experiments have been tracked continuously, to adjust them or improve external conditions. Consisting of several interrelated parts, the program has been centered around the network, where project managers discuss and deliberate about the development of telecare. Together with the support of experts and scientists, deepening was realized regarding problems, solutions, opportunities and strategy. In addition, a so-called national consultation has been put in place, which through the program organizes meetings with policy organizations involved in telecare.[2] This national consultation functions also as a guiding commission of the research monitor. Within the context of the program, meetings have also been organized for monitor researchers involved in telecare. The project coordinator together with the program leader of the sector organization organizes and chairs all three kinds of meetings and reports on the developments in the different parts of the program to each other. They steer both the content and the process, and play a central role in network building, in the learning process and in the ongoing dynamics of change (Grin and Van Staveren, 2007). The process may be characterized as an interactive, reflexive learning process to design options for joint action. Project managers, policy-makers, experts and scientists have contributed to the process. The method should be seen as the next (reflexive) generation of the interactive assessment method elaborated and described by Grin and Van Staveren (2007).

The homecare sector has been faced with financial problems, however; the decrease in the number of qualified professionals and a projected increase in the demand for care in the decades ahead, due to aging, pose challenges as well. Most project managers motivate their start with telecare in terms of the search for an innovation that can help close that gap (Grin et al., 2008). They also mention a more positive reason, suggesting that this innovation supports clients' sustained independent living at home. To improve the benefits of telecare it is important to change the process of providing care, but the new practice of telecare can also help break down old structures and stimulate the development of a new care process.

> More of the same will not work out; it has to be different. This calls for great demands on the part of policymakers, financiers and care providers – for crossing boundaries and reconsidering the role of discussing conventional parties and domains.
>
> (Actiz, 2007)

Since the program was implemented, there have been learning processes that reflect how the existing structure, culture and practices hamper the development of telecare, as well as the strategies and actions performed to overcome structural barriers. Below we will discuss a few representative examples.

In the beginning, the convergence of the care system and the technical domain gave rise to particular barriers. The actors in fact ran into a lot of technical problems and challenges (e.g. Stevens, 2005; Grin et al., 2008; Nouws, 2008). There seemed to be an enduring expectation about technical opportunities – the notion that "everything is possible" – but no ready-to-use technology was actually available. Some technology companies promised more than they delivered. Care organizations, on the other hand, were not always clear about the specific care demands, such as those related to issues of privacy, safety, reliability, picture quality, and user-friendliness. In addition, different care situations require different demands; monitoring at night needs other camera qualities than social talk to check whether things are going well. To tackle these problems, a strategic checklist was developed to support the choices which care organizations had to make (Van Fulpen, 2008). Eventually, by 2008 at least three telecare systems had been established that seemed reasonably reliable. The role and responsibility of care organizations regarding technical developments changed during the project. If in the first years of the project the focus was on technology and control over the technical system, later it shifted to the meaning of telecare for the care process. The role of the care organization regarding technology could be changed because of the newly available reliable systems, but there was also another side to the matter. General forces and developments in society, such as the virtual all-out liberalization of the past decades, have also had particular effects on healthcare (Harrison, 2004). The introduction of market forces in the care sector stimulated competition, which at the beginning of the project hampered cooperation among the different care organizations. Some organizations were eager to invent their own telecare system and to be the first to have an edge over other homecare organizations. As the project unfolded, however, the actors seemed to become more open; the project managers grew aware of the many structural changes needed to provide qualitative telecare, and that these could only be realized through mutual cooperation and learning from each other. Their focus shifted toward learning and integration in the organization and stimulating fundamental change in care. They learned to handle competition in more positive ways: to make distinctions based on the quality of care instead of on technology. They formed coalitions of care organizations to develop content and purchase technology. At the same time, some barriers and challenges continued to linger, such as issues concerning the integration of technologies, the openness of the technical system, technical standards, (public) infrastructure, and the further development of content and techniques.

When reliable video contact became possible, the resistance among professionals proved to be an important barrier. Most care professionals seemed to have little interest in technology. At first sight, they viewed telecare as a potential reduction of their professionalism and yet another factor leading to budget cuts. Seeing the new technology largely as a threat, they left no mental space for innovation, an attitude also fueled by ongoing changes and the increasing number of rules, financial problems and organizational restructurings as a result of mergers of care organizations. Furthermore, professionals have been dissatisfied with the increase of management control, planning and paperwork, leaving less room for their professionalism (Freidson, 2001; Tonkens, 2008). The strategy of the telecare program was changed to a focus on the professional and to show telecare as an opportunity for presence and coaching. The professor of system innovation involved in the project drew a connection between the discussion about professionalism in society at large (Stichting Beroepseer) and the decreasing workforce. Arguing that the effect of the decreasing workforce cannot be reduced by more efficiency only, he suggested that one can also try to break the trend by making the job more interesting. This logic, visually represented in Figure 8.1, underscored how telecare can be an answer to particular social challenges: by breaking the trend of the ever-growing care demand, as well as the trend of an ever-decreasing workforce.

In trying to curb the falling number of working health professionals in general, telecare in fact offers particular opportunities for strengthening professionalism and providing room to the very soul of giving care. It is argued that it is important to use telecare in this way if it is to be most effective. Learning takes place through experience with telecare and through involvement in the developmental process of how telecare could support the professionals in personalized care. During the project it became clear that once professionals were involved in telecare[3] they learned to see telecare as an opportunity for improving care and they developed a lot of creative ideas about specific applications. This learning process was bolstered through placing the development of telecare in a long historical development of using new technologies in care and how this has influenced the care process.[4] When looking closely at a change of

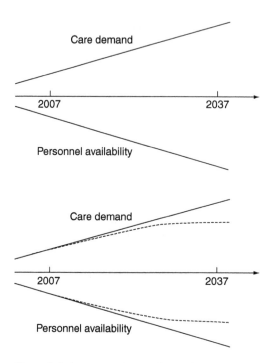

Figure 8.1 Autonomous trends in the demand of care and the workforce: the possible contribution of telecare

discourse about telecare as making the job more interesting rather than more efficient, this change is not just another interpretation of the effect of telecare but of how telecare should be used and what it should aim to achieve. It is a matter of strategically searching for how telecare could contribute to the care process and adhere to a societal force such as a decrease of the healthcare workforce and existing professional discontent.

To decouple the connection between more elderly people and a proportional increase in the demand for care (the other trend in Figure 8.1), it is important to point to social forces such as growing individualism and self-management (Beck and Beck-Gernsheim, 2002), as well as to the significance of well-being and offering opportunities for early intervention and proper attention, which in the long run will decrease the demand for care. The advantages of telecare will be maximized if the way of care providing changes toward client-centered integral care (Grin et al., 2008). This means that the way of providing care is an agreement between professional and client, which requires professional steering, self-planning and flexibility. In the current situation there is top-down management with a focus on production. The development of care is supply-driven; care organizations, professionals and clients are structured by this development and have to learn new practices.

To develop a broad arrangement with comfort services and care requires an integration of domains like care and well-being and close cooperation between professional and informal care (see Figure 8.2). Tele-monitoring decreases admissions to hospitals or care homes and visits by (para)medics. This challenges the division between primary and secondary care and requires intensive cooperation between professions and institutes.[5] Integration and cooperation is needed on several levels. The fragmentation – caused by specialization – between functions and institutions of the health system is hampering this integration and cooperation. In the experiments it also became clear that it is important to start offering services for well-being, fun and comfort,[6] prior to there being a need for care. To label this as care deters people; cooperation with community actors is needed to set up these arrangements. While developing the experiments, there was a continuing discussion about who takes the lead, who is responsible and where the costs and the benefits occur.

That the existing health system does not support client-centered integral care at home becomes clearly visible in the official rules. To start with, the number of rules and the contradictions among existing rules do not support living at home for as long as possible (see Box 8.1, example a). Financial regulations and reimbursement rules are linked with the institutional division in care (see Box 8.1, example b).

To create financial space, the telecare program, in cooperation with the NZa (the Dutch Healthcare Authority, the financial supervisor of Dutch care markets), realized a temporary experimental regulation for screen-to-screen

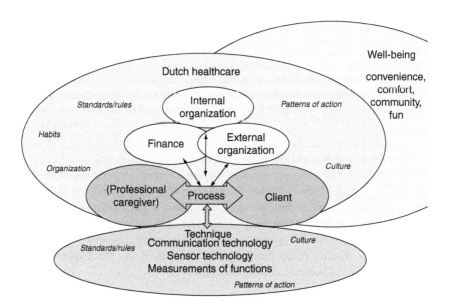

Figure 8.2 Conditions for telecare

Box 8.1 Examples of rules

a Indication

When a client has an indication for permanent stay in a care home, this person is assigned a certain number of hours for the provision of homecare until there is a space available in a care home in the region. If this client refuses to go into a care home and the homecare organization can manage – with telecare – sufficient care at home, this person loses his or her right to a permanent place in a care home (otherwise he or she must accept the care home place offered). As a consequence of this refusal, this person will be assigned many fewer hours of homecare, to the extent that there is too little time to provide adequate care.

b Division of financial flows

When a client is less hospitalized due to tele-monitoring, the homecare organization sees an increase in costs (owing to extra monitoring activities) and the hospital sees a corresponding decrease in costs. The financial flows are separate; the costs and the benefits do not end up in the same place, nor are they compensated. Besides that the hospital benefits from a high occupancy rate, which determines the budget for the following year.

---

care (from 2005 to 2010).[7] This regulation certainly stimulated the development of telecare at the beginning, but it became less effective because of the production limit.[8] Care administration offices in fact dealt differently with the regulation; some care administration offices did not count the compensation hours as production limit and did not need personalized information, while others did. The experiments in which one searches for latitude between the rules to create space for learning were more developed than those which strictly followed the rules (depending on the culture of the care organization, its financial situation, the support of the board, the project manager and the handling of the care administration office). In addition, this regulation was meant for clients with an AWBZ indication, while half of the telecare clients did not have such an indication. The compensation from the AWBZ clients was also used to develop "telecare/service" for stimulating well-being among pre-care clients, but this rule in itself stimulates a focus on care instead of pre-care/prevention. The strategy adopted by the network was mixed. On the one hand, it accepted the uncertainty and used the latitude offered by some care administration offices, but, on the other hand, it pursued more certainty and more fitting rules for the long term. The telecare project managed to prolong the experimental regulation to develop a fitting financial structure in 2011. Up until that time, no new organizations could use the experimental regulation, while the restrictions were the same.

Strategies

The telecare project's aim has been to strengthen the local projects and improve their conditions. In general, the strategy focused on stimulating alignment between the innovative practice, policies (governmental as well as NGOs) and social-historical forces. The program's organizational set-up reflects this strategy. Furthermore, actors involved in deliberations reflect on the development of the practices, their structural conditions and exogenous processes of structural change. As our examples show, this has led, for instance, to new coalitions (technical cooperation), specific discourses (adherence to societal debates about professionalism), new rules (see the financial section) and new practices (learning from the experiments). Such a reflexive approach contributes significantly toward creating mental space and empowering actors (intrinsic motivation) (Avelino, 2009), while it also fosters a continuous search for further development. In addition, the quantitative monitor allows one to track the effect of telecare. Because results may be used in the strategic process, reflexive design may impact upon the strategy adopted. If this strategy rules out barriers and creates space for experimenting, this has to be followed by strategic action for embedding. In innovative practices, great effort goes into fleshing out new visions, insights and discourses, which in turn inform the strategic process. The examples also underscore that the system "fights back": other regulations may again reduce the financial space created, long-term efficiency measures may hamper the mental space for innovation, while the separation of particular functions and funding may get in the way of integration and cooperation between domains, institutes and practitioners. But also with regard to innovative practices, managers may be obliged to follow the existing registration rules, or the cost–reduction motive may still be leading in decision-making (on account of the poor financial state of homecare).

Aside from reflexive monitoring at the intersection of policy, science and practices, monitoring is needed among practices, practitioners and clients. The further development of views about the potential of telecare and how this agrees with clients' needs appears to be the next step in the process, together with realizing structural funding. Although the policy-makers involved are convinced of the legitimacy of telecare, political aspects play a significant role in structural change. Hard evidence about cost-efficiency is articulated as indispensable for persuading political actors. The process of finding trust, legitimization and transformative power has to take place on a national level as well as on a local level. During the project there was an ongoing discussion about when to keep using space in between the rules and when to insist on a more explicit demand for structural change. Currently, telecare arrangements are being developed in close connection with financial structures.

To be sure, the Transition Program provided financial space for deepening activities (learning sessions, advice, workshops and so on). The project coordinator also benefitted from learning from other transition experiments and reflecting on transition in a collaborative fashion, taking up a discourse geared toward deepening, broadening and scaling up. If he welcomed the focus on finding a business case that incorporates societal effects, he regretted that unlike the telecare project, the visioning process conducted by the Transition Arena was not linked to the practices of the transition experiments.

Change of structures, cultures and practices

The need for changes in structures, cultures and practices is fully in line with the project's aims of implementing new technology and changing the dominant way of providing care. Below we discuss these changes in relation to the situation at the start of the project.

Practice:

- Telecare has to be part of the care process. Care professionals provide care at home and from a distance, which increases presence and flexibility. During the project the number of care organizations providing telecare was growing (from ten in 2006 to 17 in 2009). By the end of 2008, 1,021 clients had received telecare. In the research monitor of December 2007 at least three-quarters of the clients perceived an increased quality of life, most of the clients reported that they felt safer, and four out of ten clients reported that they were able to do things more independently (Peeters et al., 2009). Care professionals experienced increased communication opportunities, as well as a better quality and safety of care for their clients.
- Changes needed in the care process pertain to more prevention, more opportunities for surveillance and contacts, and more flexibility. At the start there was a focus on video contact between client and nurse. The options for telecare/services became more varied, and at this point the aim is to work toward the integration of telecare into the overall care process.
- Supporting people's well-being before there is a demand for a specific new mode of care requires coalitions with new partners, such as other care organizations, municipalities, housing corporations and welfare organizations. As a result of experiments, local coalitions have been formed.

Structure:

- Integral financing is needed, which suits client-centered care. Currently, new financial rules are being developed to continue the existing telecare practices, while new subsidies are being looked at to expand this mode of care. The extra financial support of the Transition Program was useful as a resource for extra learning activities and developing practical materials (e.g. expert advice, extra research, workshops, training and information material such as brochures and DVDs). To ensure a sustainable solution, new kinds of business models have to be found for financing healthcare. The support and expertise of the Transition Program in Long-term Care regarding the development of societal business cases was welcomed. In addition to the societal business case, ideas related to business model innovation are inspiring (Christensen et al., 2009).

- There is a need for structures of cooperation and integration among professionals, (care) institutions, social domains and informal caregivers around a client. Local agreements are in place in some projects. Moreover, developments in chains of care have great potential in this context (Ahgren and Axelson, 2007).
- Management and registration rules have to change (raise flexibility and autonomy for client and professional). In the current situation, things are too heavily determined by supply and controlled by the care administration office and the care organization, instead of by the caregiver and the client. Some teams have already organized self-planning and unscheduled care provision.
- The technological infrastructure needs to be open, available and reliable. At the start there was no decent hardware, but a few reliable systems are now in place. Furthermore, coalitions between care organizations have been set up for technological and content development.

Culture:
- From segregation to integration; managers, professionals and clients are used to the structures formed around segregation. They will have to change their internal structures (attitudes, habits and ways of thinking) to cross borders. This is closely linked to change in financial rules and rethinking responsibilities and the value of functions.
- People have to take responsibility for their own well-being and health. The strong notion of the desire to "receive the best care," which has evolved alongside the development of care, gives rise to problems with prevention, integration and financing. The experiments revealed that telecare supports independence (Peeters et al., 2009). On account of ongoing individualization, self-management seems to be more appreciated in general. It is a question, however, of whether healthcare will be able to keep pace with this social trend.
- Professionals will have to change their ideas about technology and need to try out to what extent video contact or other technologies could support clients' health and bring back professionalism. As the experiments underlined, experience with telecare and showing opportunities for increasing the presence of the professional will contribute to changing this culture. There have been contacts with educational institutions that are interested in integrating telecare into their curriculum.

These structures, cultures and practices are strongly interrelated of course, as well as influenced by social-historical forces (Stones, 2005), also called "landscape elements" (Rip and Kemp, 1998). Specialization in medicine has caused fragmentation, which influences structures and culture and hampers integral care. But, conversely, whether or not profound changes in structures, cultures and practices will occur also depends on the development of land-scape elements, such as the information society and individualization, and whether linkages were realized with such development to promote telecare and client-centered integral care. Aside from this dynamic, it will certainly help if more experiments promote change in the same direction. Along this line, contacts have been established with actors who pursue a similar develop-ment in mental healthcare.

In our case study, there is a development from technology push via the organization of care toward client-centered care. Right now, patient organi-zations and organizations of client councils and of voluntary caregivers seem to realize that telecare has become more widely known and that they them-selves may play a more active role in the development of telecare. Hopefully this will contribute to more understanding of the ways in which telecare can support the specific needs of clients (Nouws, 2008).

8.4 Comparison

To compare the ACT-Youth and Telecare projects, Table 8.1 presents a brief overview of the transition experiment characteristics of these two projects. Below, we elaborate the similarities and differences in the development of the two projects in relation to the desired transition in the care system.

The projects differ of course in the types of problems addressed: the incumbent mental healthcare providers fail to meet the demands of young-sters with complex problems (tension within the regime), while the homecare providers are faced with increasing care demands with a decreasing workforce (pressure from landscape developments). Despite this difference, the two pro-jects meet the same persistent barriers grounded in the underlying structures, culture and practices. The first barrier pertains to segregation between profes-sions and institutions, or distance between healthcare and other social domains. Both projects require close *cooperation* with other professionals and organizations within and outside of care to realize client-centered care and to support clients (youngsters, the elderly and the chronically ill) in independent living. Many health systems face fragmentation that threatens the accessibility and quality of care (WHO, 2008; De Brantes et al., 2009). This fragmenta-tion follows on from and is consolidated by financial rules and specialization. This is related to the second persistent barrier: the dominant practice of "complaint-diagnosis-treatment" (Transition Arena Long-term Care, 2009). In both projects, prevention is stimulated by providing support even when an explicit demand for care is lacking. The cases show the importance of flex-ibility and frequent attention to quality and accessibility improvement. Even-tually these features may prevent an increase in the demand (and costs) for healthcare. The ongoing cost-containment policy in healthcare has reduced

Table 8.1 Comparison of characteristics of ACT-Youth and telecare

Characteristics	ACT-Youth	Telecare
Starting point	*Societal challenge:* a substantial group of youngsters who suffer from complex psychosocial and psychiatric problems are not reached by current care providers	*Technical possibilities (video-conferencing) and societal challenge:* a substantial growth of the number of people who need care and fewer possibilities for care organizations (financial and employees) to meet this demand
Nature of problem	*Complex* and *uncertain:* persistent problems in mental healthcare system (tensions in regime)	Complex persistent problems in care in combination with social and demographic development (pressure from the landscape)
Objective	*Contributing to societal change:* influencing the dominant way of organizing, thinking and doing regarding mental healthcare provision to youngsters in Rotterdam and eventually the Netherlands	Contributing to a fundamental change in the homecare process, focusing on client-centered integrated services and care to improve the quality of life and the quality of the professional process
Perspective	Did not start with explicit *long-term* perspective (long-term vision was developed during the experiment)	Evolves during the process of the project. Continuous reflection on the developments in practice and what is strived for
Method	*Open search and learning process:* learning-by-doing, (partly) protected from mainstream pressure, stimulating pioneering, trial-and-error (no explicit method was used, but the Transition Program contributed to structuring the learning process)	*Learning process:* where pioneers together adjust and enrich their thinking and doing and encourage each other to reflect, using the interactive method described by Grin and Van Staveren (2007)
Learning	*Second order* (based on different frame of reference), *collective level* (including managers, professionals, youngsters), *multiple domains* (e.g. mental healthcare institutes, schools, youth care)	*Second order learning:* reflexive, in interaction with practice, policy and science. Domains were broadened during the development of the project from only homecare to a combination of care, comfort and well-being
Actors	*Multi-actor alliance (across society):* initiated by mental healthcare institute in Rotterdam, cooperating with other youth-related organizations to provide a balanced care chain, which is centered around the youngster	Started with technology companies and care organizations but evolved to provinces, municipalities, housing corporations and welfare organizations to provide integral services and care for improving the quality of life

continued

Table 8.1 Continued

Characteristics	ACT-Youth	Telecare
Experiment context	*Real-life societal context*: five ACT teams were set up at different locations in Rotterdam (schools, rebound center, district center, cultural center)	Started with ten organizations which try to develop videoconferencing and telecare for their care clients at home. In 2008 1,021 clients received telecare and the network broadened to 17 organizations
Management context	*Transition Management (TM)*, with a "bottom-up" character (starting with experiments instead of long-term vision and transition arena)	Started bottom up, with a developmental, pragmatic process to design, learn and make strategic choices, reflected against the background of basic care values

Source: Based on Van den Bosch and Rotmans (2008).

these basic features of providing care. This becomes visible in the barrier of the initial perception of nurses regarding telecare. Their first impression was that technology further destroys their profession, rather than that they saw opportunities for boosting the quality of care. The professionals in the ACT teams were highly motivated and they believed in the ACT-Youth approach because it meets those features.

Both projects had already begun before the Transition Program provided a grant. Their start was characterized by tension in and pressure on the existing regime. People in need of long-term care are poorly served through the existing medical rationale. Landscape developments such as aging, a decreasing workforce and the liberalization of healthcare call for another way of providing care, while the development of the information and network society creates new opportunities. If both projects were provided with initial space or protection (a "niche") by the existing care regime, there was also a difference in that ACT-Youth was initiated and implemented by a single mental health-care institution and that it can be marked as one transition experiment taking place at different locations. In contrast, the telecare project involves an intermediate platform that stimulates prolonged interaction between changes in structures and novel practices (Grin, 2010) and in which several telecare practices take part.

Moreover, different approaches to system innovation were adopted in and around the projects. ACT-Youth started out without relying on any explicit method, but the Transition Management (TM) approach adopted by the Transition Program pushed its development toward a transition experiment. The managers of ACT-Youth searched continuously for opportunities to learn more about the ACT-Youth approach within its context ("deepening"), and by applying the ACT-Youth approach in other contexts ("broadening"), as well as embedding it in structures, culture and practices at higher scale levels ("scaling up"). ACT-Youth may be viewed as a niche within the mental healthcare system for youngsters. However, in order to contribute to a transition this niche should grow into a niche regime that is able to fulfill a substantial part of the need for mental healthcare. The issue of how niches can be empowered and grow into niche regimes should be studied in follow-up case study research. A suitable case for follow-up research would be Neighborhood Care ("Buurtzorg"), which is one of the experiments in the Transition Program in Long-term Care that successfully scaled up to a niche regime (see Chapter 7, this volume).

The reflexive design approach couples the niche with the regime and explores how to profit from landscape elements. This is visible in the projects' organizational set-up. The telecare project is an intermediate platform (Grin, 2010), which promotes reflexive learning and visioning in an ongoing deliberative process between project managers, policy-makers, advisers and scientists. Interaction among the three levels of niche, regime and landscape contributed to creating mental space for new patterns of actions, and new storylines tied to exogenous trends and finding new structures.

Both Transition Management and Reflexive Design stimulate reflexive learning. This is why both projects question underlying assumptions in the health system (such as the need for further specialization) and both projects learn about structural barriers (such as fragmentation). The two methods can complement each other (which partly happened in telecare). The way TM was used in the ACT-Youth project stimulates the development of the transition experiment, enhancing learning about radical new ways to fulfill a societal need in a specific context. The reflexive design method was more focused on the overall development and strategy of telecare, stimulating the collective structural changes needed, instead of supporting specific single projects.

8.5 Discussion and conclusion

ACT-Youth and telecare represent promising real-life examples of how radical changes in the care system might be realized. As regards the telecare project, the number of participating care institutions continues to increase. Its experimental financial regulation made it possible for care organizations to launch new initiatives and join the project, but telecare has also been promoted by coalitions between care organizations in technology purchase and content development. In addition, more varied telecare arrangements are meanwhile being provided, and we also observed first signs of integration and change in the care process. The monitor research also established that telecare has indeed increased feelings of safety and independence. Due to the described barriers and the overall problems in homecare, the number of clients who received telecare did not rise sharply. In this respect, scaling up is not just a matter of numbers, but a result of the fact that telecare has evolved into a normal way of providing care. Although the ACT-Youth experiment was limited to one mental healthcare institution, there was a continuous search for opportunities to broaden the approach to new contexts (e.g. new target groups, partners and locations). ACT-Youth was successfully applied as a radically new approach by setting up five ACT teams in Rotterdam, embedding the approach in the Rotterdam region and setting up similar teams in other organizations and regions. To overcome the persistent problems in the care system, a transition process is needed. It may be concluded that both ACT-Youth and telecare could provide a potential contribution to a transition process, because both projects challenge current barriers in healthcare, such as fragmentation and the medical rationale. Based on these findings, the focus of the transition process in healthcare should be to empower patients or clients and to provide care in an integrated way without losing specialized knowledge. This requires crossing borders between social domains, formal and informal care, healthcare institutions and functions, promoting the self-capacity of people and their environment to organize their life, supporting their well-being and taking responsibility for their own health, and stimulating professional judgment and early intervention. Financial structures have to follow these developments; only using – and making more efficient – solution shop models (Christensen et al., 2009) is not an answer.

The scaling up of successful experiments needs to be actively stimulated and requires broad support. The Transition Arena, which was launched following the transition experiments, developed an inspiring future vision – sustainable healthcare is "human-centered" (around the people who need care and the professionals), financially sustainable and socially embedded (Transition Arena Long-term Care, 2009) – and transition pathways, and it may well play a role in mobilizing more actors and supporting more experiments. The telecare project provides an example of how cooperation between different pilot projects together with policy-makers, advisers and scientists can enhance learning effects and strategic action, as well as increase the number of pilot projects and stimulate structural and cultural change. The development of ACT-Youth and telecare shows evidence of the mutual adaptation between the niches and the regime; work in the niche is interpreted, adapted and accommodated within the context of the incumbent regime (Smith, 2007). In addition, the telecare project has revealed how the structural power of societal forces (Arts and Van Tatenhove, 2004) can be mobilized in favor of the innovative practice. Whether fundamental change takes place will depend on whether telecare and ACT-Youth can join and strategically use societal forces to create legitimacy. In this process, reflexive learning will be crucial to understanding the barriers and opportunities. This chapter has shown that transition management and reflexive design can support transition experiments. However, within the field of transition studies, follow-up research is needed to further develop the existing approaches to system innovation, by elaborating on how the interaction among niches, regimes and the landscape may be strategically used to influence processes of broadening and scaling up.

Notes

1 A combination of information, communication, comfort, welfare services and, when needed, care services for citizens in a specific region.
2 For example, the Ministry (VWS), the Dutch Healthcare Authority (NZa), the Council for Health Insurance (CVZ), the Dutch Patient and Consumers Federation (NPCF), the National Organization of Healthcare Client boards (LOC), the national association for people who provide voluntary care (Mezzo) and the care sector organization for health insurers (ZN).
3 Workshops were organized with professionals to brainstorm about the opportunities of telecare and how it can support their professional capacity. A toolkit was developed as learning aids for organizations that provide telecare, including material to include nurses in the development process of telecare.
4 This involved a perspective on telecare as something that will occur due to the information society and that now there was the opportunity to think about how new technologies may be used to improve the quality of the care process and the quality of life of the elderly and chronically ill. In information materials, the development of telecare was couched as the next logical step of using new technologies in care, instead of as something completely new.
5 To have broad service arrangements, cooperation is needed with organizations such as housing corporations, municipalities or service providers (welfare organizations, shopping services, banks, etc.). For tele-monitoring concerning specific diseases, cooperation with other care institutions and professionals is needed.
6 For example, video communication with family and friends, games, local news, shopping services, dinner services and online ordering of services at home.
7 Two other existing regulations were also used, one (CA-259) for infrastructural investments and the other about primary care (CA-289) for reimbursement of the actually delivered care.
8 Extra hours that can be registered for compensation can be counted as production, which is problematic with a tight production limit. If organizations – through an innovation like telecare – can provide more people with care, there is no production space to put it into effect.

9 Contextualizing evidence in Canadian healthcare

The EXTRA program

David Clements and Dirk Essink

9.1 The transition

As much as relationships have been developed across nations, and an international "transition management" community may be observed, it must be acknowledged that transition management is largely a European phenomenon. At the same time, there is certainly no shortage of international experiments in the governance and management of system innovation in other countries outside the European Union, including those that have system-level change as a goal. In this chapter, we discuss Canada's Executive Training for Research Application (EXTRA) program, which can in some ways be seen as a Transition Program *avant la lettre*. This program is an effort initiated by the Canadian government to build capacity for the creation and explicit application of knowledge to innovate the Canadian health system, in the conviction that this contributes to a more sustainable health system. The system currently has limited capacity to apply, contextualize, generate and translate evidence that may be used by practitioners in their settings. The system innovation, the transition, implies a broader and *contextualized* use of "evidence" by healthcare professionals and leaders, which in a reflexive manner and a sustained fashion contributes to improving the health system performance − "a culture of evidence-informed decision-making" (EIDM), in the EXTRA parlance. In contrast to evidence-based medicine (EBM), which has often been criticized for creating obstacles for professionals and neglecting the need for contextualization (Clements, 2004; Brown et al., 2005; Pawson, 2002a), the nature of evidence that is taken into account in EIDM emphasizes the generation (and tailoring) of evidence in deliberative interaction among a variety of actors in their work settings (e.g. hospitals), including both research knowledge (e.g. RCTs) and informal, experiential and tacit knowledge. EIDM focuses on processes for the consideration of scientific forms of evidence within an organizational or systems context, as well as building capacity for non-clinical decision-makers (including policy-makers) to know when and how to include and contextualize research in their own decision-making (Clements, 2004; Culyer and Lomas, 2006). The innovation presented and discussed in this chapter thus entails the transformation of intervention development and implementation in health organizations, challenging both the "trial-and-error" approach of many health practices as well as the "evidence-based medicine" (EBM) approach of the knowledge production system.

The EXTRA program aims to help health system leaders, also called change agents, develop the competencies to use research – through in-person and distance learning, as well as a series of practical "intervention projects" (IPs). In the long term, the program is designed to improve the transfer and uptake of EIDM by healthcare professionals and organizations, by supporting the development of the skills necessary to understand and apply research, collaborate across healthcare professions, integrate different types of knowledge and bring about organizational change. Three major outcomes are expected from the program (progress on these outcomes serving as indicators for success in this chapter): (1) fellows apply the skills learned and use research evidence to bring about organizational change; (2) the skills needed for improved use of research in management are spread beyond those formally enrolled as fellows in EXTRA; and (3) fellows improve their capacity to collaborate as evidence-informed decision-makers between professional streams.

The program is of interest to those concerned with innovation within large and complex systems because of its (1) innovative design, (2) focus on both experimentation (the IPs) and building competence, and (3) overarching goal of contributing to system-wide improvements. As with transition management, EXTRA thus offers an opportunity to understand the dynamics involved in the governance of system innovation.

Our aim is to describe the EXTRA program and to derive lessons from the program regarding the management of system innovation and vice versa, with a specific focus on whether we can train and support change agents. To begin with, we describe the context in which the EXTRA program and its sponsoring organization, the Canadian Health Services Research Foundation (CHSRF),[1] were created. In so doing, we highlight the broad structure of the Canadian health system and its challenges, and provide specific insight into components of the Canadian health system which are closely linked to the long-term objective on change: publicly funded innovation, healthcare professionalism and evidence-informed decision-making (EIDM), In regard to the latter, it is important to draw a distinction between EIDM and traditional conceptions of "evidence-based medicine" (EBM). Thereafter we will try to shed light on the EXTRA program, which builds capacity for EIDM, its structure and results. Finally, we turn to a discussion of what those engaged in the theory and management of system innovation and transitions could learn from the practical experience in Canada, as well as what transition management theory might offer governments wishing to support long-term transformative change in healthcare. Data in this chapter were obtained via published and unpublished data from the EXTRA program, evaluation documentation of the EXTRA program, scientific literature, and personal observations from one of the authors (DC), who has been involved in the program for a number of years as faculty, as well as in the administration and governance of the program.

9.2 The context of the EXTRA program

Canada's health system: structure and financing

Canada is the second-largest country in the world but also one of the world's most sparsely populated, with the vast majority of its 33 million citizens living in urban centers in the south. The country is divided into ten southern provinces and three northern territories, whose governments hold responsibility for the delivery of healthcare services. As such, there is considerable variation among provinces and territories in terms of the services that are publicly funded and delivered.

The government of Canada is a significant funder of healthcare, through transfer payments to the provinces. The Canada Health Act lays down five criteria that must be met by provinces and territories in order to receive federal funding: public administration, comprehensiveness (in terms of coverage for hospital and medical services), universality (all citizens must be eligible), portability (governments must provide care to patients from other provinces), and accessibility (Canada Health Act). The federal government also commits significant funding in the area of public health, as well as health research and innovation, and funds or delivers health services for some select groups, such as First Nations and Inuit persons, the military, veterans and prison inmates.

Canada's sustainability debate

Canadians report overall positive experiences with the health system. Nonetheless, an exhaustive review of more than 15 years of newspaper coverage and public opinion polls has found that they voice concerns about the "sustainability" of the system. They experience frustration when they are unable to access the services they would like to receive in a prompt manner, and members of the broader Canadian public also express a more generalized anxiety about whether services will be available to them when they need it, specifically access to physicians (Soroka, 2011). Even though Canadians rate the system positively, they believe the system requires major changes in order to become sustainable (in the sense that good-quality services will be there when they are needed, now and in the future). As across the OECD, increases in healthcare spending are a concern, as they have outpaced increases in gross domestic product (GDP). In Canada between 1970 and 2002, GDP per capita increased by an average of 2.0 percent annually, while healthcare growth was 3.1 percent per capita annually (Kotlikoff and Hagist, 2005). This causes some concern about the sustainability of healthcare, in terms of its affordability for public funders, particularly when past trends are extrapolated into future projections (Kotlikoff and Hagist, 2005: 7).

The causes of these increases in spending, and the likely trajectory of future spending, have been the subject of considerable analysis, including by the Canadian Institute for Health Information (CIHI), a publicly funded agency responsible for Canada's health data. The reports by the CIHI focus on a number of primary "cost drivers" which may be seen as representing challenges to sustainability (CIHI, 2011a, 2011b): human resources, technology and specialization.

Human resources

The most significant cost driver in the Canadian health system during the past two decades has been the cost of physicians. About half of this cost has been related to increased utilization by patients, with half of that amount being attributable to increased incomes for physicians, which have grown faster than the incomes of other providers of health and social services. In addition, compensation for other healthcare professions (more than half of the budget of a typical Canadian hospital) has also outpaced compensation outside healthcare during this time (CIHI, 2011a: vii) Through the lens of sustainability, the likelihood that governments are paying more for the same service, and paying more for services that could be provided by other providers at a lower cost, are both causes for concern.

Technology

The increasing use of high-cost interventions has increased the cost of healthcare substantially. While few would argue that patients should be denied access to new technologies that represent the potential to improve or extend life, there are a number of examples where healthcare spending has increased, without major benefit to patients:

- *Variations in care* – Research in the United States has indicated clearly that there is not necessarily a link between the amount that governments spend on healthcare and the outcomes for patients. In fact, Fisher et al. (2003a, 2003b) indicated that in many cases, spending more on high-cost, high-technology healthcare tends to lead to worse outcomes for patients, because they are more likely to be subject to invasive procedures, and may be less likely to have access to preventive and non-medical care.
- *Drug "breakthroughs"* – Approximately 5 percent of new prescription medications introduced in Canada between 1990 and 2003 could be classified as "breakthroughs" (PMPRB, 2004). This finding is in keeping with research in other countries (*La Revue Prescrire*, 2005). About 80 percent of increases in drug budgets are due to what have been called "me too" drugs – new and more expensive formulations of existing medications, which often represent no therapeutic benefit (Morgan et al., 2005).

- *End-of-life care* – Research has shown that more than 10 percent of healthcare budgets are devoted to patients who are in their last year of life. This raises questions about inappropriate and high-cost expenditures for patients who cannot benefit, and might be directed to more appropriate non-medical interventions to alleviate their pain and improve their quality of life (Emanuel, 1996; Stooker, 2001).

Specialization

Another factor in the "unsustainability" equation has been the tendency to provide care in more specialized settings. Conversely, increasing the comprehensiveness of primary healthcare is seen as a strategy to help control the growth of hospital costs (Bindman et al., 1996; Delnoij et al., 2000; Macinko et al., 2003). Strengthening the delivery of primary care is seen as a way to reduce costs and promote greater productivity/effectiveness (Macinko et al., 2003). A large body of research concluded that investing in the reform of primary healthcare is a relatively sure way to improve the health of the population – particularly in comparison to investments in specialized care, where the benefits are far less certain. In particular, the inherent benefits of improved continuity of patient care have been shown to result in fewer hospitalizations for preventable health problems, as well as improved functioning of the system as a whole (Casanova and Starfield, 1995; Starfield, 1998).

Growth in healthcare spending becomes problematic when it does not lead to improved health outcomes. The Canadian government has taken up the challenge to ensure that health systems provide services to citizens that improve health, while taking steps to limit services that appear of marginal benefit to patients. This has required investments in the knowledge base about the effectiveness and efficiency of health interventions. Even more critically, it requires nurturing the capacity of decision-makers in the Canadian health system to be able to use this knowledge to improve both health and healthcare.

Change components: building on public funding, evidence and professionalism

Successive Canadian governments, in the context of this "sustainability peril," have launched a number of initiatives to increase the knowledge base about healthcare effectiveness. Among these, the CHSRF is unique, as it had a specific mandate to induce system-wide change. CHSRF did this by building upon values entrenched in the Canadian health system regime: (1) a publicly funded health system, (2) professionalism, and (3) evidence-based medicine (EBM). While all of these values are contested within the Canadian health sphere, they have been seen as the building blocks for solutions to the sustainability problem: publicly funded innovation by professionals to stimulate local and system-wide evidence-informed decision-making (EIDM). Below we highlight these components of change and how these are entrenched and contested in the Canadian health system.

Publicly funded health system

In Canada, the debate about the "sustainability" of the health system has centered around the affordability of the current structure of public financing for health programs. The global financial crisis of recent years, and the subsequent squeeze on government budgets, is only the latest incarnation of the sustainability/affordability debate, which has been called "the national pastime" (Hoey, 2000). Free market proponents and physician groups have long argued that sustainability is a problem of inefficiency that is caused (or at least exacerbated) by Canada's (largely) single-payer (governmental, tax-based) system of financing. In addition to lowering taxes, these critics charge that Canada increase the use of private payment. They also call for Canada to allow a private market for healthcare to flourish, in order to stimulate competition and reduce costs (Skinner and Rovere, 2011).

Opponents of healthcare privatization also acknowledge inefficiency within the publicly funded system, but point out that this is exacerbated by perverse financial incentives (Rachlis et al., 2001). Supporters of the single-payer model argue that Canada's system of financing has little bearing on the growth of healthcare costs, and point to the administrative efficiency and savings of Canadian public health insurance schemes, which have slowed the pace of healthcare spending, in comparison with the USA (Woolhandler et al., 2003). Proponents of the public system even argue for the expansion of public financing to areas beyond hospital and medical care to encompass pharmaceuticals and homecare, and suggest that the power of a single purchaser could allow Canada to better control costs in these areas (Deber, 2003).

The sustainability debate reached fever pitch in the early 2000s, when the Prime Minister's Office appointed Roy Romanow to lead a commission to look at the future of healthcare in Canada. The Romanow Commission, among others, made a number of recommendations aimed at ensuring the sustainability of the health system, while acknowledging that much more is needed to encourage innovation within the system (Romanow, 2003). It is this grounding of faith in publicly funded support for innovation within a publicly funded and administered health system that provided the roots for the creation of CHSRF and the EXTRA program.

Professionalism

In healthcare, governments have generally provided for independent systems of self-regulation for healthcare professionals, particularly physicians, in the belief that clinical expertise makes them the most suitable arbiters of what is best for their patients (Tuohy and Wolfson, 1977). As a result, Harrison and Pollitt (1994: 2) noted that:

> [H]ealth professionals constitute a potential problem for management either because (as in medicine) of their claim to non-managed status or because (as in most of the other professions) of their claim to be managed exclusively by members of their own profession.

Nonetheless, most industrialized nations have struck a so-called "founding bargain" between physicians and the state, where the government's role is generally limited to funder of health services, while healthcare professionals maintain control over clinical matters (Tuohy, 1999). These professional silos (particularly in the case of physicians) have been strong and rather resistant to change, tending to bend interest toward more "narrow" interests (Buse et al., 2008).

In some countries, governments have experimented with "top-down" control mechanisms to be put in place to break the power of professionals, in mechanisms to increase standardization, set clinical guidelines (based on EBM), and shift power from health professionals to health managers (Brown et al., 2005; Schuitmaker, 2010; Van den Bosch, 2010). Canada is perhaps unique in this regard, in the degree to which it has resisted intrusion into this area, and preserving a high degree of independence for healthcare professionals, particularly physicians (Macinko et al., 2003). EXTRA builds on these factors in a number of important ways, including:

- By encouraging healthcare improvement through inter-professional and interdisciplinary teams, which help facilitate the understanding (and reconsidering) of professional and institutional cultures.
- By involving healthcare professionals and their associations in the selection of fellows. This includes getting the time and efforts of EXTRA experience recognized in a number of important ways, including required Continuing Medical Education (CME) credits, and similar credits for the other professions.
- By stimulating healthcare professionals to develop interventions that are adapted to the context in which they work, in particular by involving them in the assessment and improvement of organizational processes that they may not normally have a role in designing or improving.

Evidence-based medicine

Canada has been at the forefront of the development of EBM, described by Sackett and colleagues at McMaster University as "the conscientious and judicious use of current best evidence from clinical care research in the management of individual patients" (Sackett et al., 1996: 71–72). The past decade's advances in information technology and bibliographic tools made it easier for researchers to produce tools to support EBM (such as systematic reviews) and for the diffusion of these tools (Chalmers, 1995; Walshe and Rundall, 2001). EBM has been elaborated by its founders as:

rooted in five linked ideas: firstly, clinical decisions should be based on the best available scientific evidence; secondly, the clinical problem – rather than habits or protocols – should determine the type of evidence to be sought; thirdly, identifying the best evidence means using epidemiological and biostatistical ways of thinking; fourthly, conclusions derived from identifying and critically appraising evidence are useful only if put into action in managing patients or making healthcare decisions; and, finally, performance should be constantly evaluated.

(Davidoff et al., 1995: 1085–1086)

Even though evidence-based medicine dates back to the 1970s, its appeal and the resulting criticism (see Box 9.1) grew rapidly in the 1990s. However, if "evidence" has been contested ground in the healthcare professions, perhaps an even more formidable battleground may be found within the fields of healthcare management and policy, where the use of evidence has been labeled "evidence-informed decision-making," or EIDM (Clements, 2004; Nutley et al., 2007). Scholars of public policy have argued for caution in adapting EBM into EIDM with a recognition of the complexity of the decision-making process and the need to acknowledge many forms of evidence – not only scientific, but also experiential practical knowledge, which is often critical in informing the applicability of technical and scientific evidence within a particular organization, system or culture (Pawson, 2002a). Yanow found that in the application of evidence, managers "denigrate local knowledge, which contributes further to organizational processes that are patronizing and demeaning, and which ultimately do not serve the organization, or its employees" (Yanow, 2004: S23). Pawson (2002a) examines a variety of methods for evidence-based policy (his idiom of EIDM). At one extreme he

---

Box 9.1 Common criticisms of evidence-based medicine

- *It is a poor philosophic base for medicine:* Even though it claims to be a "new paradigm," it ignores some of the basics of the philosophy of science, overemphasizing empiricism and under-recognizing the interplay between theory and observation.
- *It takes too narrow a view of evidence:* Critics claim that EBM places too much emphasis on the RCT and on other quantitative forms of evidence.
- *It is not evidence-based:* In that the theory itself has not been tested, so it cannot be shown that EBM adherents practice better medicine than detractors.
- *The usefulness of applying EBM to individual patients is limited:* Because something has been shown to be effective for a population is not an indication of its effectiveness for an individual patient.
- *EBM reduces the autonomy of the doctor–patient relationship – and is a tool of cost-cutters within the system.*

places over-contextualized narratives as a method, and, at the other, totally decontexutalized meta-analysis (similar to EBM). He proposes the realist synthesis, to bridge the merits of both: "an approach that is sensitive to local conditions ... but renders such observations into transferable lessons" (Pawson, 2002a: 179). Others have advocated well-designed and explicit "deliberative processes" that allow for the integration of so-called "context-free," or scientific, evidence with "contextualized evidence," local and organizational knowledge (Culyer and Loma, 2006). As will come about in the following sections, the EXTRA program advocates such a middle-ground approach, recommending the use of formal evidence, as well as to contextualize and generate evidence and disseminate contextualized evidence among peers. The EXTRA program thus intends to apply a "transdisciplinary" approach to innovation.

9.3 The EXTRA program

In this section we describe the approach embodied in the EXTRA program, and how it builds upon the entrenched elements of the Canadian health system: (1) to stimulate publicly funded innovation, (2) through evidence-informed decision-making, and (3) professionals experiment through applied research in their own setting. By training current leaders, who conduct multiple experiments in their organizations, the Canadian government induces system innovation via pathways of adaptation (see Chapter 3, this volume). The EXTRA program uses EIDM as a decision-making framework and knowledge base but, rather than challenging professional power, it attempts to build upon the strengths embedded in the entrenched power of healthcare professions, by promoting adaptation and experimentation with evidence by professionals themselves within their own settings. The EXTRA program deals explicitly with the many contrasting aspects of EIDM and EBM: EBM focuses on formal knowledge, whereas EIDM incorporates experiential and tacit knowledge; EBM aims for standardization and application of knowledge, whereas EIDM aims for contextualization and generation of knowledge (emphasizing the relations between professionals and users). It is expected that the diffusion of the culture of EIDM and required changes in organizational structures to accommodate contextualization and generation of evidence will promote the health of the Canadian population and imply a radical change in the use and production of knowledge in the health system.

The Canadian Health Services Research Foundation (CHSRF)

The Canadian government created the CHSRF in 1996, one initiative of many in an enhanced agenda to promote health research and innovation in Canada. Specifically, the creation of the CHSRF acknowledged a need for applied research that could benefit healthcare managers and policy-makers;

the organization was given an explicit mandate to focus on these two audiences. Using an overriding philosophy of "linkage and exchange" between these decision-makers and those producing health services research, the CHSRF incorporated both communities into the organization's governance (a Board of Trustees with representation from both communities), priority-setting (through active consultation with healthcare managers and policy-makers), funding decisions (an expanded "merit review" selection process that considers both scientific merit and potential impact on decision-making), the conduct of research (research teams that include both producers and users of research), and communication of results, such as plain-language reports and reader-friendly summaries of research (Lomas, 2000). The CHSRF's founding CEO has referred to the organization as an "in-between" organization that sits between the complex worlds of research and management/policy decision-making, and works to facilitate the development of social networks that can serve as a bridge between these communities, building understanding and facilitating the use of knowledge (Lomas, 2007).

The structure of the EXTRA program

In 2003, the Government of Canada provided CHSRF with an endowment of CDN\$25 million and a directive to train senior healthcare leaders in the application of research evidence in their work. Traditional approaches to management decision-making focus heavily on the construction, comparison and choice of competing options to address a given problem. Contrarily, the EXTRA approach recognizes that healthcare leaders work in very complex systems and make many decisions on any given day, affecting many patients who have unique circumstances and varying ability to benefit from a particular intervention (see e.g. Walshe and Rundall, 2001). As such, a "capacity-building" approach was pursued, which acknowledges the increasing supply of research and the corresponding need to nurture the practical skills of managers and their organizations to be able to conduct and use research on an ongoing basis in their work, as understood through a "4A" taxonomy: acquiring, assessing, adapting and applying the results of research (Thornhill et al., 2009), with the overall mission to develop capacity and leadership to optimize the use of research-based evidence in Canadian healthcare organizations (see Box 9.2).

Crucially, the program was funded by government at the urging of the healthcare professions themselves – the Canadian Medical Association, but also the Canadian Nurses Association and the Canadian College of Health Services Executives – all of whom (in addition to a consortium of partners representing the culturally distinct province of Quebec) serve on an Advisory Council (including leaders – managers, nurses and physicians – in healthcare management) that guides the program's direction. The niche of the program was seen to be a focus on managerial leaders rather than clinical leaders, a bridging of theory and practice in healthcare, the creation of a network across

Box 9.2 Vision and mission for the EXTRA program (adapted from CHSRF, 2003)

Vision

A health system where nurses, physicians and health service executives collaborate in teams of evidence-based decision-makers, taking care of the health of the Canadian population.

Mission

To develop capacity and leadership to optimize the use of research-based evidence in Canadian healthcare organizations.

Core principles

- commitment to innovation to ensure the program makes a genuine contribution toward both individual development and organizational performance;
- a focus on linking theory to practice, and providing tools and strategies for fellows and their organizations to optimize the use of research-based evidence in their decision-making practices;
- encouragement of a collaborative leadership approach toward evidence-based change;
- reflection of the diversity of the Canadian health system and the people who work within it;
- availability to fellows and faculty who will participate fully in all program activities using the official language of their choice;
- commitment to ongoing evaluation and refinement of the program in response to performance and needs.

the country, and a focus on "systemic, rather than piecemeal change" (CHSRF, 2003).

The program has been modified somewhat over time, informed by the results of a rigorous and continuous evaluation. For example, an early focus on single fellows from healthcare organizations was modified to allow for the inclusion of "teams" of up to three linked fellows, with at least one of these fellows intended to be a physician, in order to permit the bridging of professional silos. Nonetheless, the traditional 24-month EXTRA fellowship was designed with a number of key features: (1) four residency sessions where selected fellows participate in intensive educational sessions led by a high-quality faculty, using principles of adult learning; (2) a required intervention project, where fellows apply research to an area for improvement within their own organization; (3) a horizontal "information management" curriculum that runs across the program, including web-based technology; (4) a mentoring system to coach fellows in the development and implementation of their intervention projects, by pairing them up with both academic leaders and senior decision-makers experienced in change management. The six modules spread out over the 24 months of the program were designed to focus on: (1) promoting the use of research evidence in healthcare organizations; (2) demystifying the research world; (3) becoming a leader for the use of evidence; (4) using evidence to create and manage change; (5) sustaining change in an organizational context, and (6) synthesis and storytelling. In addition, the program focuses on experiential learning of fellows; fellows are expected to collect and use both scientific evidence and practical experience to structure and adapt IPs. In residency settings the experiences of fellows are shared and discussed. It should be noted that in a new call for applications issued in 2012, the EXTRA fellowships were shortened to 14 months.

To graduate, fellows/teams in the EXTRA program are required, with their CEO, to present the results of their intervention project to a panel of experts. Thus, the intervention projects may be seen as niche experiments to provide care in a better way, but at the same time the organizations are all conducting niche experiments to understand better how EIDM may be incorporated within their workings. In sum, the program aims to create a community of change agents, who could play a role in scaling up these experiments (whether specific interventions or broader organizational lessons with respect to EIDM) and capacities to induce system-wide change.

Objectives of the program

The expected causal linkages in the EXTRA program are outlined in the EXTRA Logic Model (Figure 9.1). The EXTRA model of learning is expected to lead to increased capacity in EIDM. These capacities are then used in the organization, in initial and subsequent intervention programs, and by explicit and implicit knowledge sharing between the fellow and his or her peers. It is expected that this will induce organizational change, which positively affects the performance of service delivery in the health organizations. The rationale is that fellows, their organizations and their success stories are the hub by which a culture of EIDM will diffuse through and between organizations, ultimately resulting in improved health services and health outcomes in Canada at large (Anderson and Lavoie-Tremblay, 2008; Anderson, 2011). As Sullivan and Denis (2011), the academic coordinators of the program, have noted, the EXTRA program objectives focus on three distinct but interrelated levels: professional development, organizational performance and ultimately health system benefits.

- *Professional development:* The EXTRA program focuses on building the capacity of healthcare leaders who are considered to be influential within their professions and organizations. In so doing, the program aims to build the capacity of these individuals to be able to use and contextualize evidence, and also enable collaboration across disciplines and to break down persistent professional silos.

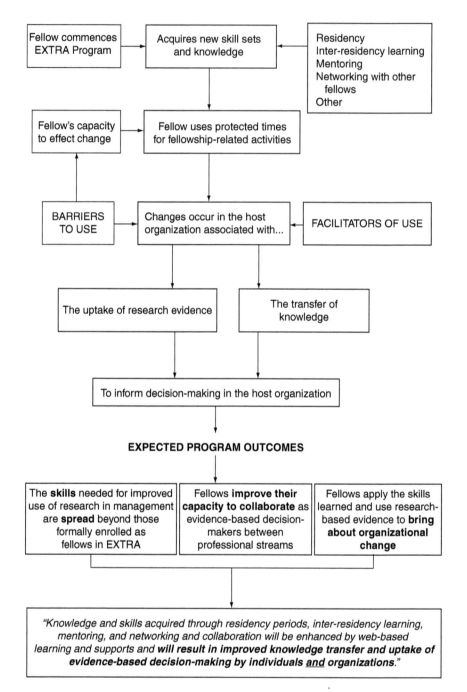

Figure 9.1 The EXTRA Logic model

- *Organizational performance:* The program focuses on both the application of evidence within the context of the EXTRA program fellows, as well as reinforcing the organization's own culture of EIDM.
- *Health system benefits:* The expectation is that, over time, the benefits to organizational performance will filter down to the level of the health system.

9.4 Results of the EXTRA program and bottlenecks encountered

The academic roots and early successes of the program have been captured comprehensively by its founders (Denis et al., 2008). In addition, the EXTRA program has been evaluated extensively since the early days of the program, with an external team of university-based researchers conducting a longitudinal evaluation of changes occurring with the fellows and their organizations over time, relying heavily on models for evaluating the effectiveness of training programs on learners (Kirkpatrick, 1994). As a result, the preponderance of data relates to the fellows' perceptions of the value of the program and changes resulting in their organizations. Nonetheless, these findings hold significant value as they have been replicated over time, and comprise the views of leaders within healthcare organizations, who are uniquely positioned to assess the changes occurring and their value (Anderson, 2011). In addition, these findings have been augmented by additional evaluations commissioned by CHSRF to assess the value of specific components of the program, such as the role and value of the mentoring function, the success factors for intervention projects, the return on investment of the program for fellows and organizations (Anderson and Lavoie-Tremblay, 2008; Denis et al., 2008; Anderson and Donaldson, 2010; Anderson, 2011; Sullivan and Denis, 2011), and three case studies of IPs (Flemons et al., 2008, Flemons, 2011; Roy et al., 2011; Postl, 2011). Finally, the first author's insights, based on participatory observation in the EXTRA program, contribute to the findings in this section.

We do not attempt to capture the full range of data regarding the impacts of the EXTRA program in this chapter, but rather to reflect more generally on some of the major contributions of the EXTRA experience to fellows and their organization, with respect to the objectives of the program in the areas of (1) professional development, (2) organizational performance, and (3) health system benefits. The third component covers parts of the second objective of the program, namely organizational performance, but then is specifically related to diffusion. In Box 9.3 at the end of this section we draw some conclusions on the basis of the EXTRA Program.

Professional development

The EXTRA program has trained more than 200 health system executives to date, of whom 40 percent are health service executives, 36 percent nurse executives and 24 percent physician executives. The geographical spread of the fellows reflects the population distribution in Canada.

Fellows in the EXTRA program report major improvements during the course of the program in their knowledge and skills in both using research in intervention projects and in their abilities for change management – the two key components in EIDM (see Table 9.1). A significant number of fellows report that they use research evidence "most or all of the time" in their own organizations, and in collaborating with other organizations. They also say that they have improved their knowledge of how to manage change, and have an enhanced ability to collaborate with their peers across the different professional streams represented in the program. Post-program, they express some concerns about their ability to sustain these collaborations, and some have called for the creation of structures to ensure ongoing collaboration, such as the establishment of a "College of Fellows" (Flemons, 2011: 192).

Competence-building came about largely through the training modules, which were overall rated as very good to excellent, with the exception of module 4 (*the use of evidence to create and manage change*). In addition, the inter-residency training allowed for learning in a network of peers. One of the most prominent results from an evaluation of the IPs was that this created the opportunity to translate the theoretical knowledge into practice; on average over 90 percent of fellows said that their intervention project built capacity for EIDM (finding, assessing adapting, creating and applying evidence) (Sullivan and Denis, 2011). This was further strengthened by the constant mentoring and desktop support, which was perceived as very useful in progressing in the learning on EIDM.

Table 9.1 Use of evidence in the EXRA program

Use of research evidence	Percent change over time (baseline to fourth residency)			
Fellows rate their own use of research evidence…	Cohort 1	Cohort 2	Cohort 3	Cohort 4
Fellows who state they use research evidence (most or all of the time)	29+	76+	23+	17+
Fellows use research evidence when collaborating with professionals in *host* organization (all of the time, most of the time)	38+	60+	28+	17+
Fellows use research evidence when collaborating with professionals in *other* organizations (all of the time, most of the time)	29+	44+	21+	17+

Source: Based on Anderson (2011). Evaluation survey data, various years.

Organizational performance

Each fellow conducted an IP (n = 200) related to EIDM within the scope of the fellowship. The fellows generally felt supported in the IP by the fellowship program and their host organizations. Approximately 70 percent of fellows said that their CEOs actively supported the IPs and were given enough resources to conduct the IPs. However, more than half of the fellows were restricted in the time they could spend on their IPs.

This resulted in a diverse range (e.g. hospital care, community-based care) and scope (e.g. organizational, multi-site) of IPs in the program. The program evaluation team has divided the IPs over three main categories. Of the 95 intervention projects reviewed in the paper on effectuating change through the IPs, 12 percent were considered conceptual IPs dedicated to generate knowledge that could be used as the foundation for future innovations; 46 percent of the intervention projects were more formative in nature as the fellows and their organizations moved toward developing a direct intervention; and 42 percent of IPs were direct interventions that focused predominantly on either improving the health outcomes of individuals or improving organizational efficiencies. Anderson (2011) used the same categorization for interventions, but reported a lower percentage of direct interventions. From our observations, most IPs were geared toward optimization of processes, where learning focused often on improving the efficiency of care. A major factor in this has likely been the fact that the IPs were endorsed by their sponsoring organizations and assessed on criteria that include the degree of organizational support (and therefore the likelihood of success). As a result, IPs that were rated successful rarely challenged dominant cultures, structures and practices within an organization and the health system.

Most fellows expected some change to occur on the basis of their IPs, but indicated that the time span of the fellowship (24 months) was often too short to demonstrate tangible results from the IP in terms of system-level outcomes. The two following comments, the first from a fellow and the second from a key researcher in the evaluation, demonstrate this:

> To date, several key foundational components have been accomplished that set the stage for longer term implementation and outcomes.... Full implementation of the wEb will extend beyond the 14 month EXTRA intervention project time frame. (Inta Bregzis, Cohort 3).
>
> (Sullivan and Denis, 2011: 30)

> In many cases our review was not able to easily identify the extent to which direct impact was achieved or not.
>
> (Anderson, 2011)

We recall from the EXTRA Logic Model that the program objective is less about the tangible result from the IPs, and more about increasing EIDM and, subsequently, health outcomes. Fellows did indicate that they expected the definite impact of the IPs was to contribute to a change in culture toward EIDM. This effect of the IP is put forward succinctly by a fellow from cohort 3:

> The IP is the beginning of the journey towards creating an EIDM nurturing environment. Baby steps were taken to put in place elements of an EIDM program using evidence-informed strategies that are respectful of the organizational strengths and culture. (Micheline St. Marie, Cohort 4).
>
> (Anderson, 2011: 12)

One message emerging from the EXTRA experience is that for the program to be successful in bringing about positive change, the organization as a whole must accept the need for change. A number of (successful) fellows clearly indicated that the success of an IP concerns more than the capacity of fellows and resources available. Future evaluation efforts may document the effects of the 2012 redesign to focus on shorter 14-month fellowships, but greater use of inter-professional teams in pursing health improvement projects. Quintessence for success is the extent to which shared norms and values are established within the organization, and strong networks are forged to structure and support the change process. As an example, the Chief Executive Officer of the Winnipeg Regional Health Authority, an organization that was an early and enthusiastic adopter of the EXTRA program, with six senior leaders enrolled in the program, has written that "Essentially, a shift in values and norms in the members of an organization must precede successful change" (Postl, 2011: 156). Postl suggests that for change to be lasting, organizations need to both accept the need for change and adopt a "sustainability model" to ensure that changes are consistent with the direction in which the organization is going (Postl, 2011: 162).

Health system benefits

The EXTRA program rationale is that through the competences of fellows and the impact of their IPs, EIDM will indirectly diffuse over and among organizations to have a positive impact on the health system. Thus the EXTRA program had quite a passive and indirect approach toward inducing diffusion, compared to other efforts. Nonetheless, there are some evident results. A significant number (75–100%) of fellows report some changes toward EIDM in their organizations, including cultural changes such as increased or even routine use of evidence, changes related to uptake of the findings of the fellow's intervention project (both within and beyond the organization), and the creation and application of tools and strategies for evidence-informed decision-making. As an example, in the Monteregie health and social services system of Quebec, leaders report that the program has been critical to implementing a number of significant improvements related to the development of integrated health and social services for citizens of the region, including improvements in public and population health. In fact, they report that without EXTRA, change would have been much more challenging, if not impossible (Roy et al., 2011: 172). Fellows also indicated that through the EXTRA program partnerships with the research community were created that had previously been non-existent, through the process of pairing each fellow with a university-based academic mentor, as well as the ongoing support of university-based regional mentoring centers across the country.

In Box 9.3 we have described formal and informal activities through which fellows aim to establish diffusion within their organizations. Most of these concerned informal transfer of knowledge among colleagues, such as leading by example. In some organizations formal protocols were established to guide the transfer of knowledge.

Fellows and researchers indicated that possibly the greatest success of the program is to create a determined group of change agents, namely the fellows, who share a feeling of togetherness, and have established lasting networks. The group of change agents share the belief in the need for EIDM to create ongoing loops of service improvements. Nevertheless, one evaluation clearly concludes that the group of change agents is far from sufficient to have a system impact: "No EXTRA site we studied came close to having any kind of critical mass" (Champagne et al., 2011: 68).

Not surprisingly, the fellows report significant challenges related to the use of evidence in their organizations and the wider health system. In their organization they face time pressures and competing priorities, which make it difficult to stay on top of emerging knowledge, progress in the IP and to

---

Box 9.3 Strategies for knowledge exchange by the EXTRA fellows (adapted from Anderson, 2011)

Informal tacit knowledge exchange

- Fellows leading by example with the use of research evidence in their own role and function.
- Increasing awareness by talking about "evidence" at all levels of meetings.
- Encouraging others to use evidence when presenting arguments.
- Encouraging trainees to use evidence.
- Asking questions, encouraging exploration of evidence to support ideas.
- Informally transferring knowledge among colleagues.

Formal knowledge exchange

- Modifying content of presentations and discussions in formal meetings with senior management.
- Modifying content of presentations and discussions in formal meetings with staff.
- Use in development and of Best Practice Guidelines.
- Incorporating into procedures for patient care.

carve out the time necessary for reflection. They also face challenges in getting their peers and subordinates to be open to using and contextualizing evidence in a more structured way. One fellow suggested that his organization never fully embraced the vision of the CHSRF as it relates to advancing evidence-informed decision-making, and this was a major factor that limited the success of his initiative, along with other factors including the lack of organizational stability (Flemons et al., 2008: 188). Taken as a whole, the experiences of fellows resulting from their IPs show how the (health) system and its turbulent environment hindered the diffusion of the culture of EIDM (at the same time hindering the diffusion of the IPs).

Box 9.4 Some conclusions/lessons from the EXTRA program

On the fellows

- EXTRA is capable of attracting leaders throughout the health system.
- The inter-residency training leads to improved knowledge and skills on EIDM.
- The combination of theory (modules) and practice (IPs) was key in activating competence for EIDM.
- The mentoring model proved to be successful in guiding the 14-month learning program.

On the IPs

- EXTRA is capable of igniting niche experimentation.
- The programs set up (conducting an IP which is scientifically supported) leads to a variety of evidence-informed experiments (IPs).
- The fellows and their IPs are generally well supported by their organization, and from our examples this support is crucial in the change process toward a culture of EIDM.
- At the same time, it appeared that some factors of success (establishing networks and shared norms and values) and failure (lack of frame reflection) clearly came forward through the program, without intentionally working on these issues.

On diffusion through the organization and the system

- The program has established some diffusion in organizations by creating a group of change agents.
- *Possibly the most important lesson* to learn is that the EXTRA program is not a silver bullet for successful diffusion; it has been successful in initiating a culture of EIDM, but lacks actual mechanisms to guide fellows and organizations in the active diffusion – scale-up – of EIDM in organizations and the health system.
- The efforts of the fellows have demonstrated organizational, regime and landscape barriers that hinder diffusion.

9.5 Transition management and the EXTRA program

The results of the EXTRA program clearly demonstrate that the system innovation process embarked upon is one with great potential. A growing number of change agents and power holders in the system have acquired competences for EIDM and have experimented with these in their organizations with some success. Nevertheless, the program is far from establishing a practice of public innovation through EIDM in the Canadian health system. In this section we will highlight what EXTRA can learn from Transition Management (TM) and vice versa.

What can TM learn from the EXTRA program?

The lessons that the EXTRA program offers those involved in TM are two-fold. First, we believe that the language and arguments of the EXTRA program enable better ways of regime shifts through adaptation. Second, the focus on competence for system innovation is an interesting addition to the toolbox of TM.

The EXTRA program does not use the same argument to justify the need for systemic change. TM focuses on the persistent problems that hinder change, resulting in rhetoric of "us" (the agents of change) against "them" (the regime) (see, e.g. Loorbach, 2007; Broerse and Bunders, 2010; Grin et al., 2010). The Canadian example shows us that similar problems, like EBM, can also be framed as building blocks of the systemic change process. In doing so they aim to address both the success factors of these building blocks and those elements that need change, which are often commonly understood by actors working in the health system. The Canadian government, via the CHSRF, stipulated a path of adaptation for system change (for pathways of change, see Chapter 3, this volume, and De Haan, 2010). This enabled them to focus on entrenched building blocks, rather than directly taking a role of opposing current regime features. Transition theorists could argue that the EXTRA program aims for optimization, rather than innovating the care system (e.g. optimizing EBM or optimizing public funding), and therefore they do not explicitly target persistent problems. Contrarily, we argue that this is indeed system innovation, or at least a constellation change. The EXTRA program aims for change in culture and practice: the introduction of EIDM and the need for contextualizing health procedures. The program sees that this requires new competences of agents, as well as a change in organizational culture and subsequent structures.

We consider the focus on competence (also referred to as capacity), comprising skills, attitudes and knowledge, a useful addition to the transition management toolbox. In TM, emphasis is placed on the competences of leaders, front runners, in transition processes, most notably those conducting niche experiments (Loorbach, 2007; Van den Bosch, 2010). In TM, the competences of leaders to induce change are observed through their practices, but they are not actively trained. In Chapter 7 of this volume, competences of those involved in transition experiments are distilled that show resemblance with competences trained in the EXTRA program. Both emphasize (1) communication – being a team worker and being able to translate theory into practice and vice versa; (2) networking – building bridges between communities of practice; (3) system thinking – understanding the big picture; (4) tenacity – being an ambitious leader and learning from failure, and (5) daring to take risks – which in TM is more related to entrepreneurship while in the EXTRA program this refers to stimulating innovation and organizational learning.

Thus, largely similar competences are needed, but whereas the EXTRA program only marginally addressed the guidance of the experiment through the competences of the fellows, TM, conversely, only marginally builds competences of the innovators through guiding the experiments. We stress that building competences should fulfill a more central role in TM besides niche experimentation. Competences bridge practical skills, knowledge and attitudes, and we found that this can change practices of actors, but also the thinking in the system. One of the most profound effects of the EXTRA program was the group of change agents who shared a vision of EIDM that was created over the course of the program. We argue that next to acknowledging the need for specific competences and describing them, TM can add the training of competences to its toolbox.

Lessons from Transition Management (TM) and system innovation literature

Transition Management offers a number of lessons to their Canadian system innovation counterparts. In this section we will address the challenges that EXTRA experiences and provide lessons from TM to deal with these challenges. These lessons may be divided among the focus on long-term change, the management of niche experimentation to stimulate learning on and scale-up of EIDM, and anticipating regime resistance.

The focus on long-term change

Possibly the most important lesson TM offers is to realize that transitions may take up to 15 to 50 years (Rotmans et al., 2004; Rotmans, 2005; Loorbach, 2007). Actors within the Canadian governments, the CHSRF, the EXTRA program and the fellows generally anticipated rapid results. Clearly the evaluations of the EXTRA program demonstrate that the IPs need more time to mature, and the diffusion of the IPs and the system-wide adoption of EIDM need even longer. Many of the fellows indicated that it is too early to demonstrate the effect of IPs, especially on the health outcomes. Moreover, the diffusion of EIDM through the system will take time, as the critical mass of change agents has as yet not been reached. The EXTRA program, in its design, hardly made the need for a long-term process explicit. As noted previously, in 2012 the managers redesigned the program and reduced the length of the fellowships to 14 months, with a greater focus on inter-professional teams. Alongside this change, the program has highlighted more focus on timely implementation of interventions and has focused less on culture change (Canadian Nurse, 2012). EXTRA now resides within a new organization, since the CHSRF has rebranded itself as the Canadian Foundation for Healthcare Improvement (henceforth CFHI) which is no longer a significant research funder and places a greater focus on healthcare improvement and change management.

The transition curve (Rotmans et al., 2001), a theoretical model which distinguishes phases in transitions (pre-development, development, takeoff, acceleration and stabilization), enables us to understand that the process embarked upon is just in its development phase; the new sets of cultures and structures have yet to take off and diffuse system-wide. The fellowship program led to niches of changes in which the fellows, with newly acquired competences, experimented with EIDM. These niches have been largely successful in increasing organizational capacity and may have even induced organizational change (Anderson, 2011), but the culture of EIDM and subsequent structures have as yet only marginally diffused to other settings. TM stresses that those involved in system innovation must have an attitude that anticipates this long-term process. We believe that this may curb dissatisfaction with the marginal changes achieved at a system level, and may prevent lock-in or backlash of the change process.

From the perspective of managing this long-term change process, TM tells us to more explicitly include holistic visions of desirable futures in our programs, and backcast (Drehborg, 1996; Loorbach, 2007) from that point onward. The backcasting refers to the selection of experiments/IPs (as discussed in the following section). We argue that the visions in the EXTRA program very much resemble a "short-term-objective," and therefore may lead to forecasting change: "A health system where nurses, physicians and health service executives collaborate in teams of evidence-based decision-makers, taking care of the health of the Canadian population" (CHSRF, 2003).

This vision may focus too much on establishing collaborative teams, rather than on a long-term vision of (sustainable) change. In doing so it appears that the approach resembles forecasting, the program focuses on an observed trend – lack of the use of scientific and contextualized evidence – and tries to stipple out a route to change the course of that trend. This may not justify the complexity and uncertain nature of the management of system innovation.

We thus believe that the EXTRA program could make the long-term process of the IPs, the organizational change and the diffusion of EIDM throughout the system more explicit. This may be further strengthened by placing more emphasis on the long-term vision of change (vision assessment) and approach the change process more from the perspective of backcasting.

The management of niche experimentation

The focus in the EXTRA program concerns the competences of fellows (which we address in a later phase as a lesson for TM), rather than the experiments (IPs) of the fellows. The IPs are primarily supported through the mentoring approach. TM, on the other hand, sees the experiments as central; we believe that the EXTRA program can learn from the experiences of TM with managing the experiments.

Work on the governance of transitions bears perhaps the most important lessons for healthcare planners looking to improve the health system, particularly through planning and the use of local experiments. Here the work of Charles Lindblom (1979) is clearly a strong influence on TM researchers, with his notions of incorporating incremental improvements within ideas of a long-term vision for change. Provided that efforts at incremental improvements involve policy-makers in both their design and conduct, local projects can indeed influence adaptations in some of the structures outside healthcare organizations which can so often limit their reach, impact and sustainability – but only if the barriers encountered in the projects can actually be traced back to the offending structures (Loorbach, 2007; Grin et al., 2010; Schuitmaker, 2010; Van den Bosch, 2010). Currently, the EXTRA program does little to trace back offending structures and make regime adaptations that may be needed to accelerate system change. It is largely expected that within organizations they deal with offending structures and advocate for change themselves; clearly this is a missed opportunity, since regime players (the Canadian government and the CFHI) are the founders/managers of the program. The CFHI is in an excellent position to serve as an intermediary to align niche and regime activities, as described by Grin et al., (2006; see also Grin, 2010). A more systematic collection and analysis of offending structures that arise from the experiments may be used by the EXTRA managers to inform policy-makers for necessary top-down restructuring. In addition, deliberative approaches may be conducted to structure the problems and their offending systemic structures (see e.g. Hisschemöller and Hoppe, 1995; Essink, 2012).

In addition, the selection of experiments (IPs) is largely determined by the selection of the fellows, who are chosen on the merit of their position in the organization (leaders) and the likelihood that their experiment will succeed. This resulted in experiments that were rather focused on optimization, had a short-term (one- to two-year) perspective, did not necessarily require the use and generation of contextualized evidence and did not per se focus on contributing to EIDM in the long term. We believe that the nature of the IPs could be more attuned toward contributing to the program's long-term vision: the shift to EIDM at an organizational and system level. When the EXTRA program more specifically backcasted from their vision, IPs could be selected that require the application and generation of evidence by a variety of stakeholders (see e.g. Loorbach, 2007; Van den Bosch, 2010; Chapter 7, this volume).

Transition Management researchers have developed three steering mechanisms to successfully guide transition experiments: deepening, broadening and scaling up (Van den Bosch and Rotmans, 2008; Chapter 7, this volume). We believe these mechanisms will be a useful addition to the mentoring model in the EXTRA Program to stimulate learning and diffusion/scale-up of the experiments and at the same time anticipate organizational and regime resistance. Below we will briefly highlight the steering mechanisms, to show how these can potentially curb observed limitations of the EXTRA program.

Deepening largely covers the innovation period, and is in many ways similar to applied research. In addition, it involves learning about societal challenges and their solutions, rather than working toward a predefined objective/solution. Thus it involves social learning and developing different perspectives (Röling, 2002; Grin, 2006; Van den Bosch, 2010), thereby shifting actors' thinking about cultures, structures and practices. TM researchers (see e.g. Loorbach, 2007; Van den Bosch, 2010; Grin et al., 2010) all stress the importance of framing, and frame reflection (Schön and Rein, 1994), and that the experiment should have a long-term approach. By frame reflection we mean that actors are capable of understanding how their frames of reference may inhibit successful change and contribute to maintaining the status quo. Subsequently change agents can adjust interpretive frames (e.g. values, assumptions) to contribute to problem-solving strategies required in system innovation (see e.g. Grin, 2010). This is even more pertinent, as this is not only required within the IP but also within the organization and the health system: "diffusing the culture of EIDM."

The two other steering mechanisms (broadening and scaling up) may aid in tackling bottlenecks in the EXTRA program. Broadening entails repeating the experiment in a variety of contexts and linking the experiment to other innovations and structures, and attracting more actors in the process of innovation. This phase increases the stability of the innovation, so that it can ultimately be rooted in the dominant system (Van den Bosch, 2010). Scaling up means embedding the innovation with its collection of cultures, structures and practices, in the dominant way of thinking, doing and organizing (ibid.). At the start of the experiment most activities address elements of deepening. Nevertheless, it is crucial that broadening and scaling-up activities are employed at the start of the experiment. Broadening and scaling up can be useful to the EXTRA program, as it concerns further learning on what EIDM "means and needs" to embed system-wide. Furthermore, actively engaging in these processes directly serves as actively engaging diffusion of EIDM. Here we only touched upon the added value of these experiments; it is not in the scope of this chapter to address the "how" of using these mechanisms. For further insight we refer to Chapter 7 of this volume.

Anticipating regime resistance

The work to date in transition management thus bears some important lessons for those working in healthcare improvement, particularly those who have been frustrated by the impact of outside forces upon attempts to make change within healthcare organizations – what transition researchers define as "regimes." As Mokyr (1990: 299) has put it, niche innovations are important, but "the environment into which these seeds are sown is, of course, the main determinant of whether they will sprout."

A very relevant issue, raised by various authors including Smith (2007) and Grin (2006, 2010), relates to this need to simultaneously influence both practices and institutional development. If we are to influence both change in local practices and also provide scrutiny of structural arrangements, there may be the need for a so-called "intermediary planning" process that prevents this from undergoing a process of "going back and forth between adapting structure and deliberative processes of reflexive design [that] may lead to experimentation without closure, unless some decision is taken at some place" (Grin, 2010: 274). For governments that might look to set up organizations to support experiments in healthcare, whether quality improvement or other processes of EIDM, this is an important lesson to bear in mind. At this stage in the evolution of EIDM, there is a very real risk that practitioners in healthcare environments continue with worthy experiments that continuously identify structural impediments to change, while policy-makers continue with grand plans for "system reform" that do not acknowledge the difficult businesses of changing even basic processes within healthcare organizations. Intermediary planning – and intermediary organizations that might be set up to facilitate such planning – must be constructed with this challenge in mind.

The EXTRA program, and/or its current host the CFHI, can act as catalyst for this sort of activity. The organization, or program, should set up communicative and learning networks with regime players, such as financers of care, policy-makers and patient organizations. By doing so, they can share lessons learned from the program and together embark upon pathways of change and incorporate views and priorities of other stakeholders in the design of the program.

9.6 Conclusions

The purpose of this chapter has been to describe and extract lessons from the EXTRA program from the perspective of system innovation and vice versa. In the EXTRA case, system innovation, the transition, implies a shift toward broader and contextualized use of "evidence" by healthcare professionals and leaders, which constantly in a reflexive manner contributes to improving the health system performance: "a culture of EIDM." Our analysis shows that the EXTRA program has been effective in improving the use of research evidence to bring about organizational change. Fellows reported that they and their organizations apply contextualized research more often and have adopted a culture more appreciative of EIDM. The EXTRA program provides a fresh perspective to the management of system innovation, but it is by no means a panacea to achieve it. Furthermore, there was a lack of attention for scaling up; it is unclear whether the EXTRA program had a positive effect on EIDM in the Canadian health system.

This Canadian example explicitly uses contested elements of its system, including professionalism, public funding and EBM, as part of the building blocks for change through adaptation. By doing so the program is appealing for actors in the system who have accepted the need for change. We hypothesize that in the health system, a more appreciative approach toward the current features of the regime may be beneficial in drawing many (powerful) actors into the change process. However, we understand that in doing so the reproduction of problems that are the result of regime structuration may be overlooked; therefore explicating the contested elements of these factors is imperative.

Moreover, the program also teaches those involved in the management of system innovation that we can train change agents. In most theory on system innovation the competences we need are well described: stimulate social learning, transdisciplinary knowledge production, frame reflection and "experimenting" (e.g. Loorbach, 2007; Broerse and Bunders, 2010; Grin, 2010; Van den Bosch, 2010). However, in system innovation and TM literature these are not used to "train" or "create" change agents. EXTRA aims precisely to do this, although some aspects are not yet well developed. A focus on the competences of actors in addition to niche experiments is an interesting tool in the management of system innovation. Through building competences the agency of actors in "hostile" regimes can be more directly influenced. Therefore we propose that the management of system innovation should put more emphasis on building competences in addition to the niche experiment. We do not presume that this is a panacea for success, but it can be a facilitator.

Another main lesson that may be extracted from our exploration is that the EXTRA program takes a rather passive attitude toward scaling up a culture and practice of EIDM. It is expected that through a group of change agents and their IPs this will occur, but we have learned that organizations and the systems are rather resistant to these change processes, and the competences and IPs for EIDM may end up as part of a patchwork of nuclei of change without having a system impact. CFHI and the EXTRA program may consider a more active role in scaling up the competences and cultures needed for EIDM, and use the lessons learned from the IPs on regime resistance and best practices toward EIDM. EXTRA and the CFHI can more actively communicate with actors in associated sectors of the regime. The CFHI should thus "broker" between the niche and regime to align the change processes. At the same time, we recognize that this more activist role could pose a very real threat to the relationships with the key actors in the system whose support has been so critical to the substantial successes of the program to date. CFHI and its partners will need to carefully consider whether this balance can be struck and maintained.

Above, we described differences between TM (system innovation paradigm in the Dutch context) and the EXTRA program, but let us also stress the remarkable similarities between the two. Both clearly work from the perspective that the *system* itself needs change rather than piecemeal change and acknowledge the need for a vision of change. In addition, in the EXTRA program as well as in TM the need for bottom–up experimentation is stressed. Through these experiments actors should learn about the changes needed and build learning networks through which experiences are disseminated so that a group of change agents emerges who can successfully challenge dominant regime practices.

Apart from the lack of attention for scaling up, another shortcoming is the uncritical approach of scientific knowledge. On the positive side, new partnerships were created between the fellows and a university-based mentor with support from a university-based regional mentoring center to increase access to scientific evidence. However, the way in which the scientific evidence had been produced was not reflected upon. The contextualization of scientific knowledge is viewed as an end-of-pipe process – only during the experimental use of the scientific knowledge is the context of application taken into account. Scholars increasingly criticize the process of scientific knowledge production for its reductionist, positivist character and decontextualization (e.g. Nowotny et al., 2001; see also Chapter 10, this volume).

As also put forward elsewhere (Broerse et al., 2010b), the management of system innovation is about (1) inducing change through agency via experimentation and by building competences of actors, and (2) by adapting overarching structures and building system-wide competences. While it cannot be denied that diffusion has been limited up until now, we take a more optimistic stand that change may occur in due time, and that it requires a timeframe much longer than the 14 months of the current EXTRA fellowship.

Note

1 In November 2012, CHSRF became the Canadian Foundation for Healthcare Improvement (CFHI), with a new focus and programming mandate.

10 Toward a needs-oriented health research system

Involving patients in health research

Janneke E. Elberse, Willem I. de Boer and Jacqueline E.W. Broerse

10.1 Introduction

In previous chapters, the health*care* part of the health system was mainly under scrutiny. In this chapter the focus will be on the *research* part of the health system and its innovation from a supply-driven toward a needs-oriented system by means of active patient involvement.

The function of the health research system is to generate knowledge through "scientific inquiry" focusing on improving the health of people (Pang et al., 2003). It spans the entire range from biomedical research, clinical research, public health research and epidemiological research to care research. The health research system is located at the intersection of the health system and the general research system. As such it contributes to the health system by generating knowledge and innovations (Hanney and Gonzalez Block, 2006). Research systems rely on particular research methods and techniques that are accepted as "scientifically" valid and reliable within the currently presiding paradigm. The health research system comprises a wide variety of actors that interact in a stabilized manner, following standard procedures and actions, and sharing scientific paradigms. The most important actors are researchers and research institutes, health professionals, national funding agencies, charity foundations, policy-makers, the pharmaceutical industry, patient organizations and individual patients (Caron-Flinterman et al., 2007). In the incumbent regime of health research, patients and patient organizations are not considered powerful actors playing an "active" role; rather, patients are "objects of study." The health research regime is basically supply-driven: the ideas and interests of the knowledge and innovation suppliers – researchers and the pharmaceutical industry – are driving the research process.

Although the knowledge generated by health research has led to considerable improvements in quality of life and a longer and healthier lifespan, the health research system is also criticized. Newly developed health innovations do not always address relevant problems in current health practices, nor do they effectively meet the needs of patients (Chalmers, 1995; Grant-Pearce et al., 1998; Tallon et al., 2000; Corner et al., 2007; Petit-Zeman et al., 2010). Mismatches have been identified between what is scientifically known and investigated and what patients would like to know about their disease or treatment, or would like to be treated for (Liberati, 1997). For example, people with rheumatoid arthritis indicate that fatigue is an important issue for them, but hardly any research has been done in addressing this issue (Kirwan et al., 2005). In another case, research in the area of dementia is very much focused on treatment and medication while little is known about how to live with dementia in dignity. In addition, most tests for dementia focus on developed limitations, such as no longer being able to write or read, instead of still existing possibilities. This is experienced as negative and burdensome by patients (Broerse et al., 2011). The methods used in health research are not always considered "patient-friendly" because they are too invasive or painful in relation to possible benefits. Moreover, innovations are developed for a "general population" rather than being focused on individuals. In randomized clinical trials, for example, interventions are often tested on a "homogeneous, standardized" group of patients. Interventions, prescriptions and other innovations are therefore not necessarily suitable for each individual (Schuitmaker, 2010). Questions such as how treatments will affect the elderly (Cherubini et al., 2011; Gurwitz and Goldberg, 2011), pregnant women or children (Burns, 2003; Pandolfini and Bonati, 2005) are often not addressed. These mismatches seem to be rooted in certain features of the health research system that have so far been the cornerstone of its success. These features have led to preferences for certain topics or domains and specific methodologies, while not taking into account patient perspectives, resulting in knowledge gaps. The focus of research does not always reflect the needs of patients or other stakeholder groups, such as care providers.

In the past three decades, patients have garnered more influence in the decision-making processes in the healthcare domain, and now this development is also becoming apparent in health research. Patients are demanding a stronger voice within health research (Caron-Flinterman, 2005; Elberse, 2012; Schipper, 2012), and there is growing support for the idea that the involvement of patients in health research could lead to a more needs-oriented focus, addressing their needs and wishes. Taking into account the mismatches in health research described above, it would be interesting to investigate if this more active role for patients could induce a system innovation toward a more needs-oriented health research system.

Patient involvement in health research may be defined as patients being actively involved in, and having an influence on, decision-making processes in health research (Elberse et al., 2011). Usually, various levels of patient involvement are distinguished, ranging from providing information to researchers about their disease or experiences to being an influential counterpart (Oliver et al., 2008; Abma et al., 2009). Patients' experiential knowledge acquired by living and coping with an illness, sickness and/or disease can complement scientific knowledge, resulting in better-informed decisions (e.g. Popay et al., 1998; Nordin, 2000; Telford et al., 2002; Caron-Flinterman et al., 2005a). Patient involvement may increase the levels of social support for and acceptance of research, and enhance legitimacy (Whitstock, 2003). It is also argued that patients have the right to be consulted in decisions that directly affect their lives. In principle, patients could be involved in all phases of the research process, from agenda setting to implementation and utilization of the results (Abma et al., 2009). Various scholars emphasize that involvement throughout the research process will have the highest impact (Hanley et al., 2004; Hewlett et al., 2006; Wyatt et al., 2008). Patient involvement will lead to a redefinition of power relations among patients, researchers and other important players in the field (Beresford, 2007; Lindenmeyer et al., 2007; Ward et al., 2010).

There are different societal trends supportive of a more needs-oriented health research system: first, the changing role of patients in healthcare. Patients have become increasingly outspoken and empowered over the past three decades (Traulsen and Noerreslet, 2004; Barbot, 2006; Epstein, 2008; Williamson, 2008). Various patient organizations advocate their active involvement in care, research and policy (Williamson, 2010), and this involvement is increasingly recognized as important by other actors (Baggott and Forster, 2008). In particular with regard to healthcare services, patients have become more actively involved through client advisory boards and client satisfaction surveys on the quality of care facilities as well as shared decision-making on individual treatment (Blume and Catshoek, 2003; Elwyn et al., 2010; Brown et al., 2011). Second, trends like "democratization of science," "increasing societal demand for utilization of knowledge" and "public accountability" (Frodeman, 2000; Fuller, 2000; Nowotny et al., 2001; Chopyak and Levesque, 2002; Collins and Evans, 2002) may put pressure on the health research system to become more needs-oriented.

In numerous countries, patients are increasingly involved in health research. The UK in particular seems to be a front-runner; developments started there already in the mid-1990s. In 1996, INVOLVE was established with funding from the National Institute for Health Research (NIHR). This national advisory group stimulates and supports active patient and citizen involvement in care, public health and research (Hanley et al., 2004). The involvement of patients and the public is institutionalized in the UK, where the idea of patient involvement is already more accepted than elsewhere. However, initiatives may also be seen in other countries, including Canada, Sweden (Keizer and Bless, 2010; Kjeken et al., 2010), Italy (Mosconi et al., 2007), France (Vololona, 2003; Barbot, 2006) and especially Australia (Saunders and Girgis, 2010; Payne et al., 2011). The same applies to the Netherlands, as evidenced by many experiments with various approaches. In this chapter we will focus on the Dutch situation. Different actors in the Netherlands have taken up the challenge of realizing patient involvement in health research. The various experiments conducted in this country provide the opportunity to learn about effective methods for patient involvement in health research and possible future directions for a system innovation.

This chapter presents the activities of one of the pioneers in patient involvement in health research in the Netherlands: the Netherlands Lung Foundation (Teunissen et al., 2013). We also introduce another important pioneer in this area: ZonMw. This is followed by a discussion of the various other activities involving patient involvement in health research in the Netherlands as a manifestation of niche-level initiatives that may lead to a system innovation. Furthermore, the most important features of the health research system are described based on literature study, document analysis, interviews, informal conversations and observation. Many niche-level initiatives encounter the regime features that subsequently act as barriers to the structural involvement of patients in health research. Various strategies based on insights from transition management studies will be discussed that may provide a way forward, including processes of "deepening," "broadening" and "scaling up."

10.2 Patient involvement in health research in the Netherlands

The Netherlands Lung Foundation as pioneer of patient involvement

The Netherlands Lung Foundation (NLF), founded in 1960, is considered one of the pioneers of patient involvement in health research in the Netherlands. It is a research-funding agency as well as a patient organization. The NLF promotes the interests of people with asthma and chronic obstructive pulmonary diseases (COPD) by stimulating research and improvement of care for patients. Recently, they extended their focus to lung conditions in general, including "orphan lung diseases." They are financed by donations, and on average 25 percent of their income is spent on health research, which is around four million euros per year. The NLF is one of the biggest health-funding agencies in the Netherlands. Its patient section promotes patients' rights, providing information on lung diseases to patients and citizens and trying to stimulate awareness of lung problems. There is a strong relationship between the NLF's funding and advocacy sections. Because of the combination of funding agency and patient organization, the NLF has an extensive network including both researchers and patients.

The research agenda of the NLF had previously been set by the scientific advisory board in consultation with leading researchers and health professionals (Caron-Flinterman et al., 2005b). However, in 2003 the program managers for research and patient involvement thought it could be important to involve patients in agenda-setting for three reasons. First, it was assumed that patient involvement could result in a broader perspective on lung research due to their experiential knowledge; it could provide insight into their needs and ideas, leading to a more needs-oriented focus. Second, the NLF wanted to investigate to what extent they had spent research funding in line with patients' needs. Furthermore, involving patients in research agenda-setting could strengthen the connection between the patient organization and funding agency. At the same time not much was known about how to realize patient involvement in health research decision-making. For its 2005 to 2008 research agenda, the NLF wanted to include the perspectives of patients as well as those of health professionals and researchers.

Since no methodology was available, the NLF contacted the Athena Institute of the VU University Amsterdam, where experience was available on involving resource-poor farmers in research agenda-setting through the so-called Interactive Learning and Action (ILA) approach (Broerse and Bunders, 2000; Roelofsen et al., 2008; Swaans et al., 2009). Researchers from the VU adapted the previously developed methodology to the context of patient involvement in research agenda-setting. Specifically, the project, which was considered an experiment by all partners, involved testing of the adapted methodology.

The agenda-setting project took place from July 2003 to June 2004. In the ILA approach, research topics are identified and priorities set in interaction with various stakeholders. Each of the different stakeholders is assumed to have its own perspective, and all these perspectives are relevant for addressing the issues at hand. Enhancing a dialogue about relevant topics among and between stakeholders will lead to personal and mutual understanding of the different contextual perspectives and experiences. This will result in a better-informed and more needs-oriented research agenda. The approach comprises six phases (Abma and Broerse, 2010), of which the first four phases were mainly executed by VU University and the last two phases by the NLF:

1   *Initiation and preparation.* A project team is established. A first assessment is made of the problems, ideas, opinions and wishes of patients and other stakeholders, and a start is made in creating conducive social conditions.

2   *Consultation.* Due to asymmetry in power, the various stakeholder groups are initially consulted separately, using interviews and focus groups to develop a list of issues that are relevant from the perspective of each stakeholder group.

3   *Prioritization.* Stakeholder groups cluster the different research topics and rank them in order of importance, resulting in a list of research topics per stakeholder group.

4   *Integration.* In a carefully structured dialogue meeting, participants exchange information, address conflicts and integrate research agendas, resulting in one joint research agenda.

5   *Programming.* The joint research agenda is translated into a coherent program or action plan.

6   *Implementation.* Participants determine and take action, monitor progress and evaluate the results.

This approach follows different principles to create an appropriate setting to include patients. These principles are described in Box 10.1.

Box 10.1 Principles of the model for patient participation in health research

- *Active engagement of patients:* Extra attention is paid to the wishes and needs of patients and their inclusion in the various phases.
- *Good social conditions:* Realization of a genuine dialogue between stakeholders requires the creation of conducive social conditions, including openness, trust and respect.
- *Respect for experiential knowledge:* The research methods used need to enable patients to articulate their problems and needs, and their needs and concerns are visibly incorporated into the process.
- *Dialogue:* A genuine dialogue needs to ensure that participants listen to each other during the process and learn about their own and each other's perspectives and experiences, which may eventually result in an adjustment of their opinions.
- *Emergent and flexible design:* Since the issues of stakeholders cannot be known in advance, the design cannot be predetermined. The design emerges gradually in conversation with all parties, although the basic ground pattern and separate phases of the methodology are preset.

The execution of this experiment in research agenda-setting is extensively described by Caron-Flinterman et al. (2005b, 2006). This experiment showed that patients are able to articulate their main problems and needs, and to prioritize research topics in a facilitated process. Patients also suggested new research topics which were not mentioned by the other stakeholders, such as co-morbidity and interaction between medications. They did not just prioritize care research, social research or focus only on their own problems as was expected by some researchers; they prioritized biomedical research topics and considered future generations.

The programming phase was initially delayed due to some controversy over the implications of the research agenda for the structure of the NLF research program. The research agenda was used from 2005 until 2009. However, it seems that the topics indicated as important by patients, such as co-morbidity and drug interaction, were not taken up by the research community; no project proposals on these topics were submitted.

Despite the problems encountered in the programming and implementation phases, the NLF considered patient involvement important and beneficial. In 2008 it was decided that the research agenda be updated and extended (Elberse et al., 2012a). Besides asthma and COPD, the NLF wanted to include rare chronic lung diseases (pulmonary fibrosis, pulmonary arterial hypertension and the respiratory aspects of cystic fibrosis and sarcodiosis). Since the first agenda-setting project took considerable time and effort, it was deemed necessary to develop a less time-consuming and less expensive version of the methodology. The aims for this new version according to the NLF were to include the perspectives of patients, researchers and health professionals, and to realize a justifiable level of patient involvement.

The different steps as described in the ILA approach were followed in the new version as well. During the initiation phase (2009), a project team was established comprising three staff members of the NLF (including a patient), a researcher and a research advisor of VU University. To speed up the process, some decisions were taken by the project team after receiving feedback from the stakeholders. This implies that the level of participation of stakeholders was mainly advisory.

In the consultation/prioritization phase, a questionnaire was sent to members of the scientific advisory board (20 researchers/health professionals and two patients), in which they could indicate which topics of the former agenda should be kept, changed or removed, or which new ones should be added. The priorities on rare lung diseases were obtained through semi-structured interviews with the researchers and health professionals. This input was discussed together with the questionnaire in a plenary session with the scientific advisory board. During this meeting, the former research agenda was scanned, updated, validated and prioritized.

To assess the problems, needs and perspectives of patients, focus groups were organized. After documenting their problems and needs in the first exercise, the topics were prioritized to gain insight into the arguments and rationale behind the priority-setting. Next, research topics were clustered thematically by the project team. Subsequently, a web-based questionnaire was developed for the patient stakeholder group to validate and prioritize the research topics. The results showed that patients suffering from different lung diseases indicated topics specifically relevant for their lung disease along with more general topics, such as disease causes and development. For example, people suffering from lung fibrosis assigned high priority to the reduction of the side effects of Prednisone, while those suffering from pulmonary hypertension indicated improving the method of administering medication as important.

In the integration phase, the project team evaluated and compared the perspectives from the different stakeholders. Two separate agendas were formulated: one for asthma/COPD research and one for research on the rare chronic lung diseases. The two agendas were sent to the people involved to check for completeness. Finally, the scientific advisory board of the NLF examined the agendas for feasibility from a scientific perspective.

The development and execution of this adapted process were realized in a time span of only five months. Patients were satisfied with this approach and considered focus groups a useful method to gain insight into their experiential knowledge, and to provide the opportunity to meet and share personal stories (peer support). Within the two agendas, the overlap between research themes was substantial with respect to basic, translational and applied research. In the details, the priorities of patients and professionals differed (Elberse et al. 2012a). Interestingly, also during this second experiment, differences were observed with respect to the topics of co-morbidity and drug interactions, which were given high priority by patients, while again researchers did not prioritize these topics. The topics of side effects of drugs, unpleasant administration techniques and specific drugs for children were introduced by patients. This may be explained by differences in the frameworks of patients and professionals. While professionals are often highly specialized, focusing on part of the respiratory condition, patients have a more contextualized focus and consider "co-morbidity" as part of their condition. However, the NLF has indicated that funding research in relation to drug development does not fall within their mandate; it is considered the domain of pharmaceutical companies. Other differences were observed with respect to the topics of "smoking" and "stop smoking." These topics were prioritized by health professionals (because great benefits can be obtained for respiratory conditions if people stop smoking), while patients and researchers indicated that they did not consider these topics relevant. Patients felt that it was not necessary to fund more research on "smoking and stop smoking" because they already know that smoking is bad for them. Some had decided to quit smoking already, while others decided not to stop despite the known risks. They believed that more research and knowledge would not convince those who still smoked to quit.

The NLF has also developed initiatives in other areas of patient involvement. First, the NLF has changed its guidelines for proposal writing. When researchers now apply for funding, they need to submit a "lay summary" so that patients are capable of judging the proposals for themselves. Different patients judge the summaries for relevance, burden versus benefits, possible impact on quality of life, intelligibility of information, and the level of involvement of patients. The judgment of the patients is taken into account when funding decisions are made.

Second, a pool of about 20 patients has been established by the NLF. Patients receive a two-day training course on patient involvement to prepare them to engage in research and gain insight into how researchers work and think. They receive basic knowledge of evidence-based medicine, ethics and research methodologies, as well as training in communication skills to collaborate with researchers in a constructive manner. They are also exposed to methodologies for consulting other patients to generate a more broadly shared or intersubjective "patient perspective." Furthermore, the NLF provides follow-up training sessions focusing on specific competences also needed to engage in healthcare and research policy. These patients are being asked to act as advisors or evaluators on scientific or research advisory boards developing guidelines in respiratory care, project-related ethics boards, and advisory boards for the improvement of care, or as patient representatives during conferences. By training patients, the NLF establishes a group of "professional patients" who are empowered and competent to become an accepted voice in decision-making processes, advocating the needs of patients. It is assumed that professional patients who are capable of integrating individual patient stories into a more broadly shared patient perspective will be more easily accepted as an equal partner in the field.

Third, the NLF participates in various international projects in which patient involvement plays a role. Examples include PROactive and U–BIOPRED of the Innovative Medicines Initiative (IMI). The main aim of PROactive is to develop Patient Reported Outcomes (PROs) measuring how people with COPD experience physical activities. PROs may be used in clinical trials as outcome measures. In order to develop PROs, patients are involved on the level of active consultation to provide insight into essential elements regarding physical activities. U–BIOPRED focuses on different types of severe asthma and aims to find biomarkers for this disease with the hope that this understanding will consider individual characteristics and be used for further therapy-related investigations leading to personalized medicine. The role of patients as active partners is similar to those in PROactive. In both projects, patients provide advice on communication and dissemination aspects.

Fourth, the NLF tries to make patient involvement visible for the research community by presenting its patient involvement initiatives at scientific conferences and via publications (Elberse et al., 2012a). During its annual scientific symposium, the NLF strongly promotes active patient involvement in scientific lung research. Examples are presented to show researchers the benefits of active patient involvement (AstmaFonds, 2008, 2009). It lobbies for more patient involvement nationally as well as internationally.

The vision of the NLF with respect to patient involvement is that it should become "normal practice." As described above, the NLF has undertaken various experiments, learning and improving along the way. It developed forms of patient involvement when no appropriate methodologies were available. It assumed a leading role among health-funding agencies in the Netherlands. Several funding agencies have copied these initiatives.

ZonMw, another pioneer

The Organization for Health Research and Development (ZonMw) is also an important player in the field of patient involvement in health research in the Netherlands. ZonMw finances health research, varying from basic research to prevention or care research. It is mainly supported by the Dutch Ministry of Health, Welfare and Sports (VWS). ZonMw applies different approaches for enhancing patient involvement in research.

Involvement of patients is not a general policy within ZonMw; whether or not it is pursued is left to the program secretaries. Patient involvement is realized in about a quarter of the 80 programs. Improvements could be made especially in the more biomedical oriented programs (Van Bijsterveldt and Van Mechelen, 2011). Recently, ZonMw organized seminars for program coordinators and secretaries to provide more insight into patient involvement and create more enthusiasm. In addition, workshops are held to develop more know-how and to stimulate employees to involve patients in their programs.

Several program secretaries have decided to involve patients in the agenda-setting procedure for their program, such as mental disabilities (Nierse et al., 2006; Nierse and Abma, 2011), Health technology assessment and spinal cord injuries (Abma, 2005, 2006). Although the input of patients was not always clearly visible in the programs, the initiatives contributed to the understanding of how to involve patients.

ZonMw is also experimenting with an adapted procedure for the "call for proposals," whereby applicants are obliged to indicate how patients are involved in the research project, and this is even a condition for obtaining funding in some programs. Although patient involvement is not a strict criterion for funding, it does force researchers to think about this issue. Researchers indicate that they are indeed stimulated to consider patient involvement, but at the same time they do not feel pressured to involve patients in their research given the absence of additional budgets for it.

In some programs, patients help appraise the project proposals. ZonMw established a patient advisory board, which may be asked to review proposals. Initially, patients were asked to review complete proposals – often in English and containing much scientific terminology – in a short amount of time. This was unrealistic, and patient reviewers indicated that they could not form a good judgment on the basis of the material provided and at such short notice. Nowadays, applicants are requested to write a summary in layman's terms, including only essential elements of the proposal. In addition, the number of proposals per person has been reduced. The process is regularly evaluated and improved.

In 2009 ZonMw started the special program "Patient involvement in care, research and policy" with the aim of stimulating research on patient involvement to gain insights into its methods, effects, impact and criteria. In so doing, ZonMw seeks to stimulate evaluation of the different initiatives, foster structural implementation of patient involvement in these three areas, and create awareness of the importance of patient involvement by the different actors (ZonMw and VSBfonds, 2009). In total, a budget of 2.7 million euros was available for the program.

Besides the different approaches toward realizing patient involvement in health research, ZonMw tries to connect people with experiences with, or interest in, patient involvement in health research and to stimulate mutual learning by organizing annual symposia on patient involvement in research. This facilitates the creation of alignment between different stakeholders and contributes to the development of shared visions and goals. Since its start in 2003, the number of participants at this annual symposium has grown steadily, indicating that an increasing number of people are interested in patient involvement in health research. It should be noted, however, that the symposia are rarely attended by biomedical and health scientists.

Other initiatives in the Netherlands

Besides the NLF and ZonMw, there are other important players in the field. Several other funding agencies are also experimenting with patient involvement in their practices, albeit on a smaller scale. Different funding agencies have involved patients in establishing their research agenda, for example, the Burns Foundation (Broerse et al., 2010c), the Diabetes Foundation (Broerse et al., 2006), the Kidney Foundation (Abma et al., 2007), the Heart Foundation (Elberse et al., 2007, 2011) and the Dutch Alzheimer Society (Broerse et al., 2011), or have included patients in their scientific advisory boards (e.g. the Diabetes Foundation, the Kidney Foundation, and the Dutch Arthritis and Rheumatism Foundation).

Among patient organizations, the Dutch Arthritis Patients' League (RPB) plays a leading role in patient involvement. It set up the "network patient research partner" in 2008, financed by the Dutch Arthritis and Rheumatism Foundation, through which patients are being trained to become a "patient research partner" in research projects (Hewlett et al., 2006; De Wit et al., 2014).

Activities concerning patient involvement may also be witnessed in the area of clinical trial research and pharmaceutical companies' practices, for example, Duchene Parents' Projects and PatientPartner. PatientPartner[1] is a partnership between different European organizations funded by the European Commission, which focuses on "promoting the role of patients in the clinical trial context" (Smit, 2009). The KWF, the Breast Cancer Patient Organization (Borstkankervereniging Nederland, BVN) and BOOG Study Center (Borstkanker onderzoeksgroep, BOOG) are experimenting with the active involvement of patients in the set-up and execution of clinical trials (Pittens et al., 2012), and the Dutch Cancer Society is including patients in their project appraisal procedures through a patient advisory committee.

Looking at the various activities undertaken by funding agencies, patient organizations and others, it becomes evident that most concern patient involvement in research agenda-setting (although it should be noted that the majority of funding agencies still do not include patients in their agenda-setting procedures). It is not surprising that this approach is often employed to realize more patient involvement by different actors (Abma and Broerse, 2010). First, there is a thoroughly evaluated methodology for agenda-setting available. Second, the different charity foundations, organized in the Collaborative Health Foundations, regularly meet and inspire each other. Third, setting a research agenda seems to be an isolated, clearly defined step in the research process. The process has a clear span of control and leads to a tangible end product for a research-funding agency. Last but not least, the involvement of patients in setting a research agenda does not demand major changes in procedures.

However, various scholars have raised concerns whether, after participatory agenda-setting, it will not be "business as usual," i.e. professionals once again dominate decision-making processes on what topics are researched in health research (Caron-Flinterman, 2005; Broerse et al., 2010a). Articles that focus on patient involvement in the phases after agendas have been set (i.e. programming and implementation) are very scarce. According to Stewart et al. (2011), setting priorities with different stakeholders does not have much impact on healthcare and health policies. Recently a study on the evaluation of the programming and implementation phases of eight Dutch agenda-setting projects was conducted by Metamedica (VUmc) and the Athena Institute (VU University). This study, funded by ZonMw/VSBfonds, shows that the role of patients was generally marginal after priorities were set (Pittens et al., 2014). Funding agencies as well as researchers have their own procedures, culture and structures. Not all see the benefits of continued involvement of patients and often there is a lack of knowledge how to involve patients more structurally. Other important findings are that although patients have a surplus value as they add new topics to the agenda and prioritize different topics compared to professionals, these "new" topics are not always implemented by funding agencies or picked up by researchers. In case of burns, itching was highly prioritized by patients and included in the research program, but for some years no proposals for research were received on the topic. Extra incentives were needed to stimulate researchers to write a proposal on itching.

Another concern is that collaborations among patients, funding agencies and researchers are often not sustained. Initiatives are usually one-off events, with no continuity, feedback or future planning (see also Jordan et al., 1998; Stevens et al., 2003).

Moreover, there is a lack of thoroughly evaluated initiatives which is also extensively mentioned in the literature (Beresford, 2007; Staniszewska et al., 2008; Broerse et al., 2010a). The methodologies employed and lessons learned are rarely evaluated, and feedback from experiments is restricted. Consequently, there are as yet few "proven" effective methodologies or "best practice" models to guide those individuals and organizations that would like to experiment with patient involvement in health research.

Yet another concern is that health researchers rarely take up the role of initiator or advocate of patient involvement. They rarely participate in organized debates on patient involvement in research (Moens, 2010). Besides, researchers, policy-makers and health professionals are rarely supporting the required changes for the effective involvement of patients in research.

10.3 Regime features as barriers to patient involvement

Although the number of initiatives for realizing patient involvement is increasing, involvement of patients in research is still far from being common practice within the health research system, and barriers are encountered. Based on case studies, interviews with a broad range of stakeholders and the literature study we conducted, it becomes apparent that the encountered barriers are related to certain features of the health research system. Realizing structural patient involvement seems to require a radical change in organizing, thinking and doing from the different actors involved. However, the current structure, culture and practice of the health research system developed over time, resulting in a dominant, stabilized way of organizing itself, as well as thinking and acting (Van Raak, 2010). The features that form a barrier for patient involvement are identified below.

Academic research community

Decision-making dominated by experts in research

Traditionally, decisions on health research are made by experts. While the NLF, ZonMw and a number of other funding agencies are slowly changing their procedures for funding by including patients in the decision-making processes, many funding agencies still do not consider this an improvement and prefer to retain a more academic structure. Including patients in decision-making processes means that the autonomy of researchers is challenged and that the focus on scientific quality may shift toward a focus on societal relevance. It means that the current procedures will need to be adapted to include new criteria, such as societal relevance, more attention for benefits versus burden, and providing a lay summary, but also room for new topics. Since there are few experiences to build upon, this process of adaptation is one of experimentation. For example, the first time patients appraised project proposals for ZonMw, they had major difficulties coping with the procedures: there were too many proposals with too little time to read them, they were mostly in English with much jargon, and no guidance was given on how to judge them. By "trial and error," the procedure for patient involvement is being adapted and improved.

The negative opinion on patient involvement held by some members of scientific advisory boards and the uncertainty about the additional value of their input make many charity funds reluctant to adapt structures and procedures to realize the involvement of patients (Caron-Flinterman et al., 2007; Broerse et al., 2010a). An often-heard argument is that patients are biased and subjective, will only focus on research projects that can lead to a personal benefit and lack the right knowledge. As one researcher put it: "Patients lack the knowledge and experience. They are not used to work with biomedical information so I think it is really difficult." Furthermore, some researchers are convinced that they already know what patients need and want, and therefore involvement is not needed: "I do not see the added value of involving patients in research ... a good clinical researcher knows the patients and knows the things that are relevant" (researcher).

Specialization

The health research system is highly specialized, and categorized into a range of scientific disciplines (Pang et al., 2003). Researchers often specialize in a certain type of research (e.g. genetics, tissue engineering) and focus on a specific disease (e.g. cancer, asthma, depression) or organ (e.g. heart, lung, kidney) instead of the patient. The strong specialization within the health research system complicates the interaction among researchers and health professionals, policy-makers and patients. The problems which patients with chronic diseases face are often interdisciplinary and integral by nature, such as co-morbidity, psychosocial issues related to a somatic condition, pain or fatigue. Such problems rarely fit specializations. This leads to under-researched areas; interdisciplinary problems brought in by patients are often not addressed by researchers. The aforementioned topic of "itching" of burns survivors is a good example. Another example is the topic of co-morbidity, which was mentioned by patients as an important topic in the research agendas of the NLF. It was considered a difficult topic by the scientific advisory board, however, because of the question of who should fund research on co-morbidity, as the NLF only provides funding for research on respiratory conditions. Moreover, it is hard to find researchers who are able to do research across different disciplines. Conducting interdisciplinary research is often less attractive to many researchers, since there are few interdisciplinary approaches (Wilson, 2000), and this type of research leads to outcomes that tend to be less appreciated or understood by peers.

The value of scientific knowledge

Researchers define "true" knowledge as data generated through the use of robust scientific research methodologies (Caron-Flinterman et al., 2005; Bijker et al., 2009). Non-scientific knowledge, such as the experiential knowledge of patients, is judged to lie much lower in the knowledge hierarchy (Blume, 2005). Experiential knowledge is regarded as "a personal story," as subjective and, thus, "difficult to generalize," instead of being considered usable knowledge; patients are emotionally attached and therefore endanger objectivity. "Patients have too many personal issues to give their opinions at the level of decision-making" (Researcher). Furthermore, researchers often do not know how to integrate experiential knowledge into their research; they focus on scientific excellence and theoretical purity, and the input of patients does not correlate with that. Patients are usually considered lay-people, without the required knowledge to contribute anything relevant to the scientific research endeavor (Caron-Flinterman, 2005). The idea of patients becoming co-authors of an article, after being involved in research, is not considered beneficial.

> There are going to be problems with publications. Reviewers are going to say: that is a patient, not a researcher, we are not going to accept this. Yes, I think many researchers will be skeptical, it will not be accepted easily.
>
> (Researcher)

The strong focus on validated scientific methodologies in health research does not leave room to integrate experiential knowledge and thus forms a barrier to patient involvement in health research. For example, researchers use validated questionnaires. In different case studies patients have pointed out that the questions were unclear, irrelevant or not well described. However, researchers are reluctant to change validated questionnaires. "About some question in a questionnaire patients say: that is a weird question. But if they fill it in and you don't ask what they think about the question, in the end the results seems to have a good predictive value" (Researcher).

Changing opinions toward acknowledging patients' experiential knowledge as a valuable input requires a fundamental change in the scientific paradigm, incorporating a broader, non-hierarchical view on knowledge, and an acknowledgment of the uncertainty and fallibility of scientific knowledge.

Scientific excellence

Within research, there is a strong focus on scientific excellence, generating scientific knowledge that can be published (see also Hessels, 2010). Spending time with patients to discuss a research project is often considered a distraction from research instead of a possible improvement of work. Researchers are more inclined to pick up research topics that lead to publishable results in disciplinary, internationally renowned journals. "People do the things that give them profit, if you get profit for multiple publications you're going to write many publications. In that case it is not profitable to increase the length of your research process by patient involvement since patient involvement will take more time" (Researcher). Research with mainly a societal impact rarely improves career perspectives. High-tech research is preferred over research on more common symptoms, such as low back pain or ear infections, while high-tech research does not always lead to innovations which address the needs of patients or users. Frenk (1992) stated that scientific excellence and practical relevance are difficult to combine because they are measured in totally different ways. Little attention is paid to communicating results to a non-scientific audience and implementing generated knowledge in practice (Lavis et al., 2003; Jacobson et al., 2004). Although growing attention for the societal relevance and practicality of research is being witnessed among funding agencies, career advancement and appreciation of researchers are still primarily related to publication rates and citation scores as part of the required benchmarking by governments and university boards (Aksnes and Rip, 2009; Hessels, 2010).

These features of the research community – decision-making by experts in research, strong specialization, the high value of scientific knowledge and relevance – do not allow the system to operate optimally in contributing to improvement of the quality of life of patients. Despite the positive impact of health research, the health research system favors certain research, methodologies and topics over others, resulting in a gap between what is researched and what patients experience as problematic or functional.

Pharmaceutical industry community

Much health research is initiated and conducted by pharmaceutical companies, which focus on medicine and treatment development. Most are big multinationals, striving to make a profit. In most pharmaceutical companies, patient involvement is a rare phenomenon. Many barriers to realizing more patient involvement seem to be in place in pharmaceutical companies. First, as in the academic research community, most companies mainly consider patients as "subjects of study." They are satisfied with the current situation and do not see a need for change. Second, there is a lack of awareness of the potential benefits of patient involvement and how patients may become more actively involved (how to do it). At the same time, there is a lack of best practice examples. Third, rules and regulations prohibit many forms of contact between pharmaceutical companies and patients, and it is unclear which forms of patient involvement are allowed. Fourth, local companies are usually not independent but affiliated to a multinational. These local companies have little influence on the policies of the central board of the multinational (Fransen, 2009; Broerse and Elberse, 2010). Despite the many barriers, there are visible developments (O'Connell and Mosconi, 2006). Some initiatives, like the Patient-Industry and PatientPartner, lobby for a more active role of patients within private research.

Although R&D companies currently do not involve patients actively in their research, these companies nevertheless engage with patient organizations; various patient organizations receive a substantial part of their funding from pharmaceutical companies. Several scholars have raised concerns that authentic involvement of patients in research agenda-setting may be jeopardized by pharmaceutical companies because of these donations (Coulter, 2004; Abelson et al., 2007). In previous agenda-setting processes in which we were involved, the focus was on the identification of unmet needs – needs that are by definition not yet developed/marketed by the private sector. We have no indication that patients, participating in the focus groups, interviews and dialogue meetings, were directly influenced by pharmaceutical companies (see e.g. Elberse et al., 2012b). However, we cannot rule out that there is an indirect influence, given the highly contextualized and diffuse character of the process of needs articulation, as well as the internalization of medical rationality by patients. Moreover, around the time of the market introduction of pharmaceutical products for unmet patient needs, policy coalitions between pharmaceutical companies and patient organizations to realize accelerated (conditional) market approval have been regularly observed; at this point pharmaceutical companies and patients share a common interest in bringing new technologies and therapies more quickly from the bench to the bedside (e.g. Kukk et al., 2016).

Patient community

The patient community also has features that may not be conducive to their involvement in research. Patient organizations and communities are not always effectively organized to make a strong demand of the research community and are easily ignored. Traditionally, patient organizations focus on peer support, providing information and advocating for good care. To be actively involved in health research has been considered a possibility only in the past decade. Due to the growing attention paid to the patient community by different actors, ranging from governmental organizations to care organizations, the workload of the patient community is also increasing. Therefore, patient organizations need to choose between different activities, and often the priority for becoming involved in health research is low. They prefer to invest time in care-related issues and peer-support activities.

The patient community usually lacks resources – money, manpower and time (because many people in the patient community work voluntarily). Although the Dutch government is trying to address this problem by investing money in the professionalization of patient organizations, it is a slow process. It is complicated by the ambiguous term "professionalization." Some consider a patient organization professional if they employ "professionally" educated staff or when the organization is well structured, while others believe that being professional entails the ability to represent the "general patient population" or being able to represent the voice of the patients during discussions and decision-making.

Researchers wishing to involve individual patients in research sometimes complain about the limited interest patients have in participating in health research. There are various reasons for this. First, patients feel they lack knowledge about scientific research and, thus, have little to contribute (Broerse et al., 2010a; Caron-Flinterman et al., 2005a). They often do not value their experiential knowledge and lack self-confidence. The general thought is that decision-making on health research should be left to experts. Second, the jargon used by many researchers discourages patients from becoming involved. Third, most patients consider themselves ignorant regarding the implications and benefits of health research for their personal lives. The effects of care are often directly evident for patients while the effects of health research are "distant" and "complex." As a result, there has been little direct interaction between researchers and patients in the past.

10.4 Deepening, broadening and scaling up

Although the number of initiatives at the niche level is increasing and supporting landscape developments are putting pressure on the health research system, there is still little sense of urgency to change the incumbent regime among different actors, particularly academic researchers and pharmaceutical companies. According to many actors, the health research system is functioning satisfactorily. It facilitates the development of high-quality medical innovations that improve the quality of life for millions of people. Dominant players consider the gap between generated knowledge and patients' needs relatively small and therefore feel there is no need to involve patients. This idea is strengthened by the limited proof of the benefits and effectiveness of patient involvement in research. Although there is a growing body of literature on patient involvement in research, not much has been published on the effectiveness and impact on health research. As long as people are not convinced of the benefits, they will not take the time or effort to be part of these initiatives (see also Rogers, 1995). Combined with the fear of delays and complications of decision-making processes, stakeholders believe that the benefits – if any – do not outweigh the disadvantages.

System innovations only occur when changes transcend from the niche level to the regime level (Kemp and Rotmans, 2005). The next question is: How could a shift toward a more need-oriented health research system be enhanced? A system innovation requires knowledge, best practices and methodologies, resources like money and time, a shared vision, and a growing network of actors willing to invest time and take risks. Furthermore, the creation of supporting structures and regulatory frameworks is important. In the transition literature, three central mechanisms are described through which experiments contribute to a system innovation or transition: (1) deepening, by learning as much as possible in a specific context, (2) broadening, by linking and repeating the experiment in different contexts, and (3) scaling up, by embedding the experiment in the incumbent regime, changing the dominant way of organizing, thinking and acting (Rotmans and Loorbach, 2006; Van den Bosch and Rotmans, 2008; Raven et al., 2010). These "steering" notions focus on the importance of creating space for learning processes at different levels, while at the same time stimulating interaction between experiments and the broader context and actively working on embedding the new practices to increase the impact of the experiment at a higher scale level (Van den Bosch and Rotmans, 2008; Van den Bosch, 2010). In a transition process, all three steering notions need to be attended to simultaneously. In the current developments, some steering mechanisms are already being applied, mostly deepening and broadening. Momentarily, not many actions can be seen for scaling up patient involvement in health research. In this section we will briefly introduce the notions "deepening," "broadening" and "scaling up," and provide indications based on these notions of how to continue to enhance a system innovation toward more needs-oriented health research.

Deepening

Deepening involves social learning processes in a specific context, implying shifts in thinking about culture, structure and practice, their relationship with other actors and the broader context (Röling, 2002; Van den Bosch and

Rotmans, 2008). Experimenting with and learning from transition experiments could lead to the enhancement of a shift in structure, culture and practice (Schot and Geels, 2007). Learning may be considered as an interactive process to develop or obtain knowledge, competences, norms and values. Attention should be paid to experiment-based learning of the possibilities and constraints of patient involvement. It is also relevant to gain insight into the expectations and attitudes of the actors involved (Raven, 2005). It is important to shape the different expectations to ensure that they are realistic and to identify which aspects vary. New, innovative experiments demand open-minded people willing to experiment with new practices (Van den Bosch and Rotmans, 2008; Van den Bosch, 2010). In addition, change agents with a strong drive are essential for a system innovation.

As described above, different experiments are taking place, and change agents with a strong drive to change are present. ZonMw is stimulating learning in the field of patient involvement in research by providing subsidies for the execution and evaluation of experiments to gain insight into experienced barriers, solutions, enabling factors, effective methods and evidence of impact and benefits (ZonMw and VSBfonds, 2009). When transition experiments are evaluated, experiments can be improved and adapted, leading to best practices. Gaining insight into the impact and benefits of patient involvement in health research can remove an important barrier for researchers. It may lead to convincing proof-of-principle concerning the added value of patient involvement in research. In addition, there is a strong need for developing new approaches for patient involvement in health research, because currently there is a lack of knowledge on how to put patient involvement into practice throughout the research cycle. Effective approaches have been developed for only some steps in the research cycle (e.g. agenda-setting).

Second, not all research projects are suitable for patient involvement, and a balance needs to be found between the involvement of patients and the benefits for the research project. However, clear criteria are lacking to identify suitable research projects (De Wit et al., 2014). In addition, there are various forms of participation, and some are more suitable than others in certain research projects. The intrinsic and potentially utilitarian value of basic health research should not be underestimated, and therefore the question of whether all types and phases of health research should be subjected to the influence of patients is legitimate. Experiments are needed to clarify this issue. The involvement of patients in health research is not a plea for putting a patient next to every researcher. It addresses the question of how patients can be effectively involved, leading to a more needs-oriented system.

Third, it is important to focus on the experiences and expectations of researchers and other actors. Researchers have barely had a say in how experiments were shaped or executed. This was mostly decided upon by funding agencies, and to some extent by patients and their representatives. It is also important to keep track of how attitudes and expectations change over time and how the expectations of the different actors involved may be aligned.

Fourth, the sustainability of collaboration among the different actors warrants attention. If active involvement stops after a project is finished – as is now often the case – interaction and learning between researchers and patients barely evolves. Patients will develop more confidence over time and will be able to provide more useful input and become more accustomed to the practices within health research (Shea et al., 2005; Kirwan et al., 2009). Researchers need more time to become familiar with the involvement of patients and how to handle their input based on experiential knowledge. Collaboration often only continues if the different actors involved have an intrinsic motivation (Jansen et al., 2008). Therefore, it is important to understand why people want to become involved in an experiment. Actors need to be motivated to continue collaboration in order to create new routines.

Broadening

Broadening entails the notions of repeating experiments in different contexts (Raven, 2005; Geels and Raven, 2006; Rotmans and Loorbach, 2006) and linking experiments to other functions. Experiments which are considered successful can be repeated in a different setting while applying the lessons learned and adapting the experiment to the new context. Guiding principles can be established based on previous experiments to provide direction and support for new experiments (Raven et al., 2010).

Most initiatives with patient involvement are ad hoc and single events (Jordan et al., 1998; Stevens et al., 2003; Caron-Flinterman et al., 2005). However, repetition of experiments in different settings is essential in the development toward a needs-oriented health research system. For example, the involvement of patients in research agenda-setting was repeated by different actors, including funding agencies and the Health Council of the Netherlands (RGO, 2006, 2007; Gezondheidsraad, 2010; Elberse et al., 2012b). This led to a "best practice" and guiding principles which actors can follow (Abma and Broerse, 2010).

Initiatives with patient involvement in healthcare, health policy and education are also taking place and may stimulate involvement of patients in research. Most actors are involved in all the different domains. For example, the NLF is also experimenting with patient involvement in healthcare and care improvement. Some researchers are care providers, for example, clinicians. This may lead to synergy.

The involvement of more actors in current niche developments will help create momentum in order to influence the regime. Therefore, the approach used by ZonMw, namely focusing on connecting people, is essential. Networking is also beneficial for creating awareness and connecting different experiments; actors from different experiments can stimulate and learn from each other. It is important to gain insight into the different approaches, underlying visions, methodological steps, effects and impacts on society and patients as well as science and health research. When these insights are well documented, interested stakeholders can experiment and reflect upon the approach and make possible adaptations. In addition, discussions can lead to new ideas and visions, which are important in stimulating the system innovation even further. The national and international lobbying for more patient involvement by several front runners is important to make people aware of possibilities and create a larger network.

To generate interest in different actors to become involved in activities, they need to be motivated to take risks. Intrinsic motivation can be enhanced by making the benefits of involving patients clearly visible. In order to change the dominant way of acting and thinking in research, researchers should first become aware of the effectiveness and usefulness of involving patients. Currently, experiments are often not published, nor shared in other ways (Crawford et al., 2011). For example, many scientific journals are not interested in articles on patient involvement. As a result, knowledge obtained during experiments with patient involvement is not easily accessible, and researchers rarely encounter examples of patient involvement within "their" international scientific literature. Visibility can be created by publishing the results of patient involvement in research in journals read by biomedical and health scientists, or by presenting work at conferences in their field.

Scaling up

Scaling up refers to activities to embed the new culture, structure and practices at the regime level, leading to fundamental changes in the dominant regime (Van den Bosch and Rotmans, 2008). This steering notion is the most challenging one. Considerable resistance may be encountered, and institutional barriers have to be overcome. It is of major importance to involve key figures who are willing to change as well as to have access to resources and support (Van den Bosch, 2010). It is also important that landscape developments support this shift. In the case of patient involvement in health research, landscape developments such as increasing patient empowerment, democratization of science and public accountability may be considered supportive for a shift toward a more needs-oriented research system.

Although more supportive structures seem to be coming into existence (e.g. funding agencies requesting lay summaries or statements about how researchers will realize patient involvement in their research), most funding agencies are hesitant to reject research proposals because they insufficiently address this criterion. Care should also be taken that such incentives do not lead to tokenism. Tokenism is the involvement of patients without giving them real influence, creating a false appearance of the involvement of patients in health research (Beresford, 2003; Pronk, 2007). Researchers indicate that the risk of tokenism will be present when they are obliged by financers to realize patient involvement without receiving further support, additional money or guidance (Moens, 2010). In other words, it is not sufficient to change the conditions for funding research; it should be accompanied by a support package including making additional funds available for patient involvement, providing training opportunities to increase competences and developing more appropriate accountability systems.

10.5 Concluding remarks

Allocating an active role to patients within health research seems to be quite a radical change. To realize such a change, a system innovation would be needed affecting institutional and funding structures, and established ways of working change. It is expected that such a drastic change will take time and effort, and will need to overcome various barriers, given the resistance of regimes to change. However, considering the current developments, a system innovation from a supply-driven health research system toward a needs-oriented health research system by means of patient involvement may be possible. Currently, there seems to be commitment from a growing number of organizations in the system to effect a change toward a more needs-oriented health research system. Front runners like the Netherlands Asthma Foundation and ZonMw can be identified. They stimulate different "followers" in these developments, who have also started to experiment with different approaches of patient involvement. The current initiatives are still fragile, however.

The current change agents with respect to patient involvement have expressed a particular need for more appropriate methods and increased competences at the niche level and adjusted procedures at the regime level. In order to enhance this shift, the effectiveness and usefulness of the different experiments should be analyzed more thoroughly and made more visible to the different potential change agents, so people can learn from each other. More importantly, the impact of patient involvement on health research, patients and other actors should be made more visible. Specific attention should be paid to the interaction between the niche and regime level.

Despite the obstacles of enhancing a system innovation toward a more needs-oriented health research system, different initiatives show that the involvement of patients could induce this shift. The contribution of the experiential knowledge of patients to health research processes may lead to closing the gap between needs and what is researched. However, to become truly needs oriented it will also be necessary to include yet other stakeholders who have had little voice in health research thus far (e.g. citizens (or the public), incidental care users and informal caregivers). When only patients are involved, we have regularly observed that public health needs or the burden of caregiving are underrated or even overlooked (e.g. Broerse et al., 2010). Indeed, in the few instances in the Netherlands where citizens were involved in research agenda-setting (e.g. in the case of dementia (Broerse et al., 2011)), topics related to prevention and healthy living received more attention.

Related to the different phases described in transition theory, there are indications that the system innovation toward a more needs-oriented health research system is in the take-off phase. During this phase, the development of change gains momentum, resulting in structural changes. The current health research regime is losing support for its practices and structures on some fronts. Niches are gaining support, and more approaches are emerging. There is a growing interest in patient involvement in health research from different actors, such as patient organizations, government-related organizations like ZonMw and RGO, and charity foundations. Funding agencies are involved in different approaches, and are taking actions and setting up different experiments. Since many charity foundations have close relations with both a patient community and a research community, they may be able to influence the parties and bridge cultural and structural gaps effectively. The concept of patient involvement is also slowly becoming visible in scientific papers and conferences within the system and in formal policy documents. These points indicate that this may be the beginning of a shift toward a more needs-oriented health research system in the Netherlands.

Note

1 www.patientpartner-europe.eu/en/home.

Part III

Reflections

11 The future of health systems

Beyond the persistence of contemporary challenges

Jacqueline E. W. Broerse and John Grin

11.1 Introduction

In the Introduction to this volume, we stressed the increasing discrepancy between the central, persistent problems in the health domain and its incumbent regime (structures, cultures and practices). We argued that this regime was shaped by the typically modern, conventional biomedical paradigm, in which health and disease are (virtually exclusively) located in the (universal) body, and may be controlled by professional intervention with little room for patient agency. From that modernization theoretical perspective (Grin, 2010: 228–231; 2012) the persistence of three major contemporary challenges to health systems may be understood in different ways: problems with affordability, quality, acceptability and accessibility result from following this paradigmatic orientation too long and too exclusively; the difficulties of dealing with non-communicable diseases arise as they have more complex pathologies, located not merely in the body but in (interactions among) bodily processes, life practices, life conditions and patient agency; and the increasing care demand, associated with aging, which often involves non-communicable diseases (NCDs), is difficult to meet until this is taken into account. Meeting these challenges requires appreciation of the limits of the classical paradigm, moving to a more integral orientation on health and disease. Current attempts to reach what we called a "sustainable" health system – transcending existing shortcomings regarding, and tensions between, affordability, quality, acceptability and accessibility of care – often fail because they largely neglect these elements, as explicitly demonstrated by Van Raak and De Haan (Chapter 3). In this final chapter, we seek to articulate what we have learned from the preceding chapters on the "why and how" of the persistence of contemporary challenges, as well as on opportunities and problems implied by contemporary experimental practices that might contribute to a more sustainable healthcare.

The preceding chapters, each in its own way, have shown what we may see if we adopt a transition perspective on modern health systems. Importantly, there is more to say on these issues. While "high modernism" has shaped many different societies, with different ideological bases and associate structures (Scott, 1998: 88ff.), the precise nature of the structures of the health system have obviously also been shaped by the historical development of that system, and the wider society in which it is embedded (e.g. Pierson, 2004; Skocpol, 2008; Marsh, 2010). This historical development, shaped by deeper structures of the health regime and other regimes, affects the precise distribution of inequalities in access, disease prevalence and mortality rates (e.g. Wilkinson and Picket, 2006; Picket and Wilkinson, 2015). It is also about how the supply-oriented nature of health systems has come with high private profits for pharmaceutical industries, unequal access for patients, legal protection of intellectual property and funding from public resources (e.g. Perehudof et al., 2010). It is, for that matter, about understanding how such conditions may change, as is now starting to happen through the WHO's Prequalification of Medicines Programme ('t Hoen et al., 2014). The integration of such factors into transition thinking has been taken up in fairly recent studies on the politics of transitions (Grin, 2012b; Hoffman, 2013; Pel et al., 2016; Avelino and Wittmayer, 2016; Castán Broto, 2016; Swilling et al., 2016; Avelino et al., 2016). Whereas the preceding chapters have occasionally referred to changes on that level through the impact of, for instance, nineteenth-century state formation, economic globalization and the emergence of neoliberalism, they largely leave this level out of consideration, as we will do here.

Within this scope, we will synthesize the upshot from these chapters by discussing the following questions:

- How did system innovations and transitions emerge in the health domain in the past, and how do the insights presented here shed light on the origin of persistent problems currently encountered?
- What visions on sustainable healthcare are, implicitly or explicitly, articulated in the contemporary innovations discussed in this book?
- What may we learn from the successes and, especially, failures of these contemporary innovations on the nature of these problems and the features in health systems on which the development to sustainable healthcare critically depends?
- What do the answers to these questions, as well as earlier insights from transition studies, suggest about strategies for remedying persistent problems through structural change in health systems?

As the above qualifications imply, when developing these lessons further in a particular health system and society, it is obviously important to situate them historically in the development of that system and society.

11.2 Evolution and key properties of modern healthcare

Since the Enlightenment, the guiding orientation of healthcare has been that quality of life and quality of care could be improved through scientific and technical advances. As Chapter 2 by Berkers extensively demonstrates, due to this orientation, a transition toward centralization, specialization and use of technology took place. Professionals became central, while patient agency was underemphasized. These structural characteristics co-evolved with developments in care, research and policy practices. Other co-evolving regime features included the central place of the hospital, the differentiation between care and cure, and the dominance of the supply side characterized by conventional medical rationality, which locates health and diseases in the body, neglecting the interaction between health, body, life practices and life conditions. The health system vastly improved and became accessible to all segments of the population by the establishment of compulsory health insurance. Increasingly, citizens were socialized in a rudimentary version of this particular understanding of health, both implicitly, through practices of healthcare, and explicitly, through education. Together with this "proto-professionalization" (De Swaan, 1996), particular relationships between professionals and patients crystallized, whereby professional interventions were mutually recognized as a key determinant of health and patient agency was being de-emphasized, if not outright neglected.

In order to understand this historical transition, in Chapter 3 Van Raak and De Haan distinguish constellations in the evolving health system. Some of them centered around particular practitioners (such as surgeons and doctors until 1865 and, more recently, specialists and general practitioners after 1930), while others centered around institutional arrangements (hospital and nursing homes for the entire period, and also, as of the early twentieth century, funding, Cross Work and public health). Three transition patterns appear helpful to map and explain transition dynamics in the health system: *re-constellation* or top-down regime change through landscape developments; *adaptation* of the incumbent regime to landscape pressures; and *empowerment* of novel practices through the creation of an associate niche regime.

Most of the dynamics initially emerged from a pattern of re-constellation, in which incumbent practices, structures and cultures underwent landscape pressures that all tended to push toward societal and scientific modernization: Napoleonic changes in society and government, and subsequent state and nation formation. Thus, conventional medical rationality was central, and over time its elaboration in research and treatment practices led to the emergence of other patterns. While the physician, and later the general practitioner, largely evolved from adaptations in the professions of surgeons, who resisted too much change, specialists went through an empowerment pattern enabled by a successful program of scientific advance that neatly divided human health into different categories of bodily (dys-)functioning. The weight of the specialists' constellation also increased due to its dynamic interaction with other constellations. The hospital constellation gradually adapted to the process of specialization. Over time, following the introduction of specialist reimbursement and compulsory health insurance in the 1930s and 1940s, the funding constellation empowered and shaped the specialist constellation. Thus specialists eventually out-competed general practitioners who, since the 1970s as an ultimate confirmation of the specialization-oriented system, have been formally made gatekeepers to specialist care. The role of Cross Work, after it had first grown through empowerment (due to provisions established to resolve nineteenth-century social problems), gradually grew weaker on account of individualization.

This, admittedly very rough, summary of Van Raak and De Haan's account indicates how the dynamics of constellations and their mutual inter-action help to understand developments that have prompted, for instance, compartmentalization, medicalization and less attention for patient agency.

While this modernization transition has indeed led to very significant improvements in individual and population health, over time drawbacks of modern healthcare have become clear as well. Affordability became a real issue from the early 1970s onward, when economic globalization gave rise to a debate on the sustainability of advanced welfare states. Starting more or less simultaneously, other features became objects of debate, such as the (underestimated) side-effects of interventions and the dominance of professionals. As Berkers vividly shows in Chapter 2, critique was often framed in unprecedentedly strong terms, such as the "dehumanization" of patients and profit-seeking behavior of medical specialists and the pharmaceutical industry. Frequently, critical views were associated with new social movements, gaining momentum on the waves of landscape developments such as secularization, individualization and emancipation. In this sense, modern healthcare shared the fate of many other "expert" systems (cf. Beck et al., 1994); Berkers shows how this led to a variety of interesting experimental practices.

At the same time, however, the health system appeared relatively immune to these pressures. While, for example, the agricultural regime started to destabilize by the mid-1980s due to the pressure from new social movements and critical intellectuals emerging as of around 1970 (Grin, 2010: 249–264), and the food consumption and retail system started to gradually transform since around 2000 (Spaargaren et al., 2012), the health system maintained many of its structural features, as well as the aforementioned orientation on conventional medical rationality (see Chapter 2 by Berkers and Chapter 3 by Van Raak and De Haan). This lack of fundamental change is especially clear from the nature of most health system reforms that occurred in later decades, inspired by concerns about balancing core values such as quality, affordability, acceptability and accessibility. To be sure, it would be wrong to conceive of these reforms as homogeneous attempts. As the historical chapters in Part I indicate, it is more accurate to say that, for a long time, there have been several parallel strands of concern linked to the following issues: cost control and efficiency improvement, closely tied to the more general debate on neoliberal welfare state reforms and much less shared by main players in the health system (Martineau and Buchan, 2000); quality, such as the allegedly reductionist conventional medical rationality, medicalization and lack of attention to diversity (Wieringa et al., 2005); accessibility or distributional issues (partly related to the affordability debate, as noted above); and finally, the limited degree of patient and professional autonomy (Mol, 2008), which ironically resulted from the succession of professional patronizing by government regulation in the 1970s, and increased market conform accountability and control mechanisms with the introduction of New Public Management in the 1980s (Tonkens et al., 2008; Newman and Tonkens, 2011; Tonkens, 2013).

Importantly, major tensions between these concerns have revealed themselves in contemporary debates and policies. The most salient tensions are linked to cost containment (for which there are strong political drives) on the one hand, and various other concerns (often emphasized by other actors, namely professionals and patients) on the other. While costs are increasing (due to more expensive treatments as a result of technological innovation from a structurally privileged supply system, and an increased demand as the result of an aging population combined with unhealthy lifestyles, partly shaped by other social systems, like food and labor), quality, acceptability and accessibility concerns do not seem to improve. At the same time, there has been widespread doubt as to how reducing costs could be done without further jeopardizing quality, acceptability and accessibility. Van Raak and De Haan argue that this tension between different goals is rooted, at least partly, in two key factors behind the system's success – compulsory sick funds and specialist reimbursement – that together undermined earlier mechanisms of cost control. Referring to the chapter by Berkers, we may add that the simultaneous medicalization, intra-muralization and reduced attention to patient agency have further contributed to the tension between the goals of costs, quality and accessibility.

Earlier strands of reform had in common that they barely, if at all, addressed these elements – least of all the adverse effects of the strong dominance of conventional medical rationality (privileging the development of expensive equipment and drugs over prevention and patient care) at the expense of other rationalities. As argued above, this rationality shaped incumbent practices and structures into a self-reproducing, persistent system that thus resisted earlier reforms.

Some of the innovative practices that emerged in recent years reflect, to a greater or lesser extent, a different orientation: a more integral view of health and illness and a focus on the patient and patient agency (see Chapter 2), yielding different meanings and priorities to the various goals for reforms. In Section 11.4 we will discuss how, ironically, such practices as discussed in this volume in particular, disturbingly often encounter barriers that upon closer inspection appear to be expressions of these structural features. But let us first discuss the normative orientations implied in these practices.

11.3 Different elaborations of sustainable healthcare

The innovative practices, discussed in Part II of this volume, each reflect, and are shaped by, a desire to reorient healthcare practice toward some optimal balance between quality, affordability, acceptability and accessibility: what in our introductory chapter we called a "sustainable" health system. This is an essentially contestable notion because each of these criteria may be interpreted in different ways, as is true of the way they are weighed vis-à-vis each other, reflecting differences between contexts as well as the outcome of interactions in the networks involved (Essink et al., 2010; cf. Grin, 2006). The innovative practices discussed arose from the initiators' sense that some key values of the health system are not properly met through current health practices. In rebalancing values these various sustainability visions share, in some way or another, what we wish to call a "human–integrative" orientation on the issues mentioned above. That is, they integrally consider body and mind, the patient and his or her context, health and other social systems, as a basis for tailor-made provisions and to foster patient agency. This contrasts with conventional medical rationality, with its strong focus on the body and professional intervention. In the different cases, the sustainability vision provided a sense of direction for change and aligned the different actors.

One example has been elaborated upon in Chapter 6 by Ródenas and Garcés on the Sustainable Socio-Health Model that ties together concerns about "quality of life and death," recent "explosions of investments in healthcare" and "accessibility also for future generations." This proposed model requires the reorganization of health and social systems into a more integrated, individual client-oriented system in long-term care. On the shop floor, case management teams operationalized this idea, defining personal care pathways based on a careful study of the needs and possibilities of each client and shared decision-making among the team, the client and the main informal caregiver.

Another, more radically deviating, orientation was articulated in the Dutch Transition Program in Long-term Care, set up as a response to concerns of those most directly involved: professionals in primary healthcare and their clients. This effort emphasizes how human needs and values are under pressure in a highly fragmented system, focusing on diseases that may be remedied by specialized health professionals (rather than on integral health and patient agency), and in which many connections have been broken (between management and shop floor, between funding schemes and the substance of care, and between care professionals and care receivers). As such this program's focus is more radical, since care is defined as tailor-made, yielding much more responsibility and agency to clients and professionals. It emphasizes empowering people in self-management while supporting societal participation, so-called "Together Care" or "Community Care." Professionals need to respond to clients, providing tailor-made, flexible care. As in the Spanish case, care professionals were to be supported by broader societal organizations providing a range of services and integrating health and social care. The Dutch program, however, was geared toward a different set of key problems: "lack of diversity in care," "not being able to remain living at home comfortably" and "lack of human contact."

The vision emerged from, and then started to shape, ten existing, and, later, 16, new experiments, demonstrating what sustainable future care *could* look like. Most of these projects involved more responsiveness to the patient's varying needs, offering much less standardized care and more room for professional judgment. Cases in point were projects involving Assertive Community Treatment (or ACT-Youth, on tailor-made, individual care for youngsters) and telecare (whereby patients may even co-determine if, when and how care is needed), projects discussed by ter Haar-van Twillert and Van den Bosch in Chapter 8. As was reported elsewhere on telecare, nearly all clients and professionals, after initially being rather skeptical (fearing "technicalization"), became really positive very soon after embarking on a pilot. About two-thirds of the clients felt more secure due to telecare and thought they could remain living at home much longer, while about one-third felt more autonomous in their daily lives. Moreover, increased contact with care professionals was widely mentioned as an additional benefit. Of the care professionals, a large majority felt better able to appreciate their clients' situation, and the amount and nature of needed care; nearly all believed that telecare enabled continuous "proximity" where necessary, and indicated that video connection, much more than by telephone, implied real contact with their clients (Peeters et al., 2013).

A vision of sustainable long-term healthcare, promoting patient agency, is also at the core of Workplace Health Promotion (WHP); in Chapter 5, Vaandrager et al. explain the underlying novel understanding of health. The conventional pathogenic model is used in conjunction with the salutogenic model, which includes work and life practices and agency of employees in understanding how they may maintain and improve their health. Both employees and employers thus appear to have many opportunities to turn work into a health-promoting endeavor rather than a health-threatening one.

A human-integrative orientation may be found in practices discussed elsewhere, such as community-based recovery and rehabilitation approaches in mental health and disability care (e.g. Corrigan et al., 2007; Amering and Schmolke, 2009; Thornicroft et al., 2010; WHO, 2011) and integrated, user-centered approaches in long-term care (e.g. Leichsenring et al., 2013). Such approaches typically focus on clients' active involvement by providing (1) a multi-sectoral strategy that empowers them to gain access to integrated services in education, employment, health and social welfare, while (2) taking their capacities and aspirations (instead of their *disability* and impairments) as a starting point, and (3) decisions on care and services are jointly made by professionals, clients, family members and informal caregivers. Inspired by such initiatives, the WHO (2011: 65) has emphasized the opportunities to simultaneously address accessibility, affordability, availability and quality by stressing clients' needs, possibilities and agency.

Evaluation studies, however, show that the implementation of these approaches is rarely supported by the incumbent regime. Community-based rehabilitation, for instance, is reported to require the scaling up of new "thinking" on disability care and mental healthcare, implying a need for cultural change as well as new competences and infrastructures (WHO, 2011). The experiments in this book clearly show that sustainable development involves an open-ended orientation; in practice it is shaped through mutual learning processes, as is further elaborated in the next section.

11.4 Where incumbent regimes do not help promote sustainability: learning from innovative practices

The above finding is not unique for community-based rehabilitation. The chapters in Part II have shown that setting up innovative practices with a different orientation is far from simple, and is bound to run into – and is often constrained by – a range of obstacles. These obstacles often appear to be expressions of the structural and cultural dimensions of the incumbent regime, in line with the basic claim from transition theory that problems are so persistent because even serious attempts to resolve them eventually tend to reproduce the incumbent regime (Rotmans, 2005; Grin et al., 2010: 2–3; on healthcare see Moret-Hartman et al., 2007). Schuitmaker and ter Haar-van Twillert (Chapter 4, this volume, p. 87) extend this claim, promoting the insight that such obstacles are caused by the embedment of practices in a system which "actively creates barriers for innovations that are not compatible with the existing regime in that system." Emphasizing this self-reproduction of the incumbent health system in innovative practices, they propose to understand the persistent problem as the substantive health problem at stake *plus* the mechanisms of self-reproduction. As a corollary, carefully analyzing difficulties emerging from innovative practices may not only inform the further development of these practices but also provide guidance to strategies for regime transformation, facilitating broadening and scaling up. We will elaborate on this point further in Section 11.5.

Below, we will draw upon previous chapters' analyses of specific innovative practices to identify which features of incumbent health regimes, as discussed in Section 11.1, appear most important in producing barriers against experiments that introduce more sustainable healthcare practices. Such factors include specialization and compartmentalization within healthcare and between health and other domains, the supply-driven character of the health system, the medical rationale including evidence-based medicine, and the role of regime players in innovative care practices. Interestingly these factors are remarkably consistent in different practices discussed in Part II, whether involving prevention, cure, care or health research.

Specialization and compartmentalization

The incumbent health regime is characterized by divisions within healthcare (e.g. different health professions, primary/secondary/tertiary care) and between health and other domains (e.g. social welfare). As we have seen, the historical analyses in Chapters 2 and 3 show how specialization within the health system, as reflected in particular in specialized departments within a growing number of hospitals following World War Two, enabled the development of routine, standardized procedures and a continuous monitoring of patients, and thereby contributed to a radically modernized medical practice with successful health outcomes. However, as Van Raak and De Haan argue, the downside of this specialization is the consequent fragmentation and discontinuity in healthcare. Paradoxically, then, it yields a reduction in the quality of care and increasing costs (e.g. when patients with co-morbidities or unclear disease manifestations go through a range of referrals from one medical specialist to another, neither of whom can adequately remedy the patient's complaints). From the early 1970s this gave rise to concerns about the sustainability of the modern health system, as well as critique on the nature of the care provided.

At the same time, specialization complicates transformative efforts toward more integrated approaches. This may be seen especially from the case studies on the Sustainable Socio-Health model in Spain – where case management teams encountered resistance from specialists with a distaste for being managed – and on telecare in long-term care – where primary care professionals were challenged to invest, in their local contexts, in organizing an integral care network (with primary and secondary professional caregivers, as well as informal caregivers), while, moreover, many professionals were not keen to participate in multidisciplinary teams. In addition, the health research system shows divisions among different scientific disciplines. Specialized scientists focus on a specific disease or organ, and even specific types of research, largely ignoring the problems patients experience as a person (body and mind) within a certain context. Chronic disease patients, for instance, tend to experience very complex problems (with physical, psychological, social and economic dimensions) and often include co-morbidities. Such complex problems require interdisciplinary and integral research approaches, as argued by Elberse et al. (Chapter 10, this volume). The specialist focus on a particular bodily function or organ also tends to reinforce the dominance of the reductionist conventional medical rationality (11.1) and to de-emphasize the role of the mind, life practices and life conditions.

The consequent *compartmentalization* between care and other domains, such as welfare, seems to be another recurring problem. In the Valencia case management experiments, differences emerged between the social welfare and health systems regarding organization and available resources, impeding the management of a unique portfolio of resources to realize tailor-made care. Moreover, inter-system structures on which to build were lacking, restricting the coordination of resources and services. Plausibly, such difficulties, rather than being limited to Spain, are as widespread elsewhere as the institutional separation between care and welfare.

In fact, the case of the Dutch telecare project (Chapter 8), which also involved trans-sector collaboration, encountered similar barriers. The video screen forming the heart of the telecare arrangement provided clients with a gateway to a range of services from other sectors than health (e.g. welfare, leisure and retail), and with a chance to co-decide on how to draw upon and combine them, so as to optimally fit with their life practices. Yet, implementation was frequently hampered by the division between domains such as care and well-being, and between primary and secondary care institutions. Apart from problems of cooperation between professionals and community members and between professionals, funding was complicated due to financial regulations and reimbursement rules that reflect institutional divisions.

Compartmentalization between care and other domains appeared to be a particular problem in the case study on Workplace Health Promotion (WHP). At the basis of WHP is the recognition that employees are, in principle, able to maintain their health, provided that they have proper resources (including incentive structure, team spirit, collegial atmosphere) and some real agency (e.g. to manage their workload). Thus, the workplace becomes essentially part of the "health-producing system." In one WHP experiment (KPN), compartmentalization appeared to strongly dominate thinking of in particular the firm's occupational health specialists and managers, who each in their own specific ways understood WHP to mean that employees would take more responsibility for their own health. Compartmentalization was significantly overcome in another participating organization, a hospital: after explicit discussion on the need for and nature of a balance between employer and employee responsibility, management developed an organizational strategy to make the hospital a more health-promoting workplace.

The supply-driven character of health systems

The contemporary quality debate also points to another, not entirely unrelated issue: historically, the development of healthcare has been dominated by medical rationality and a linear "innovation-diffusion" pattern (Rogers, 1995), making the health system strongly supply-driven. Thus treatment is based on the following:

1   products developed and produced by pharmaceutical companies, often closely collaborating with publicly funded research institutes;
2   products admitted to the market by governments;
3   treatments reimbursed by insurance companies;
4   treatments selected by care professionals.

Patients are downstream this linear process and therefore situated primarily as receivers of care with very limited input in decision-making processes upstream. In addition, deeply embedded in the healthcare regime and reinforcing this supply orientation is patients' inclination to put the responsibility of good care in the hands of care professionals (Schuitmaker and ter Haar-van Twillert, Chapter 4). In sum, while this supply-driven health system has led to considerable improvements in quality of life and life spans through developing new technologies, provisions and protocols, there are also crucial flaws. As we have seen (11.3), many of the innovative practices discussed here propose a patient- or client-centered approach (reflecting a human-integrative orientation), which presumes new roles of and relations among all those involved and interrelated institutional provisions. Hence, actors will easily encounter inertia and resistance.

For instance, patient organizations frequently believe that newly developed health innovations do not always address relevant problems in current health practices, nor do they effectively meet the needs of *all* patients. Mismatches occur between scientific knowledge produced and what patients would like to know or would like to be treated for and in what way. In Chapter 10, Elberse et al. discuss experiments seeking to address these flaws through involving patients in decision-making on health research. These experiments encountered discursively as well as institutionally rooted resistance. A range of researchers and health professionals argued that patients, acting on the basis of narrow self-interest and lacking sufficient scientific knowledge, should leave these issues to the professionals. In addition, patients were reluctant to take up this new role and deploy agency, and often felt they lacked competencies.

More downstream, experimental care practices implementing patient- or client-oriented approaches are likely to run into the incumbent, supply-driven regime. One illustrative case is that of the Sustainable Socio-health Model. Its shift to a tailor-made type of care, and shared decision-making between the case management team, client and informal caregivers requires different routines and attitudes from all involved. In Chapter 6, Ródenas and Garcés describe the reluctance among some professionals to work in a more client-oriented way, as it challenges their autonomy and status.

Another case in point is that of medically unexplained symptoms, discussed by Schuitmaker and ter Haar-van Twillert in Chapter 4. Here, patients appeared sometimes disinclined to accept the active role presupposed in the experimental practice based on the recognition that doctors are not always capable of being "custodians" of people's health because of their specialized backgrounds, the standardized treatments at their disposal, and the compartmentalized institutions of which they are a part. Hence patients and clients are attributed agency; they are seen as unique individuals with relevant knowledge, specific needs and preferences, and who bear co-responsibility for their own health. Yet, making patients take up that agency required some persuasiveness and trust-building – they were accustomed to patient–doctor relationships that historically emerged in supply-oriented health systems. This particular, dominant definition of relationships is closely related to the nature of conventional medical rationality.

Conventional medical rationality

Earlier in this chapter we characterized conventional medical rationality as one with a focus on (1) diseases, (2) located in the body, and (3) to be remedied by an outside, medical intervention. Body and mind are considered (4) separate entities, while (5) the body is conceived of as universal. Disease is understood in a reductionist way, as a matter of malfunctioning of some of its parts. Complaints are thus translated in these terms that serve to identify proper treatment through highly standardized interventions designed to remedy bodily deficiencies.

This orientation has yielded knowledge development and care practices that are extremely successful in dealing with the types of health problems (infectious diseases, etc.) which until recently dominated the healthcare agenda. The epidemiological shift discussed in our introduction chapter, however, has yielded novel types of health problems centered around NCDs. Conventional medical rationality underemphasizes some factors that are more often than not part of NCDs' more complex pathologies: lifestyles, life conditions and psychological well-being. A related matter is that conventional rationality offers little scope for patient agency as a contribution to health. Even more strongly, closely associated with this particular rationality on the supply side is the "proto-professionalization" of patients: the internalization of an elementary form of conventional medical rationality by patients (cf. Section 11.1). To be sure, proto-professionalization is part of the success story of modern healthcare – think, for instance, of hygienic behavior and a basic insight into self-help and timely recognition of particular symptoms. Yet, the other side of the coin is that conventional medical rationality also pervades patients' responses (which, we note in passing, also explains the limited success of market-driven health system reforms in which patients are viewed as well-informed, price-conscious, critical consumers of care). This presupposed critical role of the "demand side" is only applicable to some small subgroups of patients, while most patients need support to be able to exercise agency (e.g. Naiditch et al., 2013).

Similarly, conventional medical rationality, proto-professionalization and associate relationships may imply barriers to novel practices. We have already noted that it was a key challenge for doctors involved in innovative treatments for MUPS to convince patients to take up more agency.

Conventional medical rationality's historical success and deficiencies to address current problems come together in several other case studies, producing major barriers in innovative projects that appear to be structural features shaped by conventional medical rationality: *funding* procedures and a range of underlying procedures, especially the complaint-diagnosis-treatment sequence and the notion of evidence-based medicine. The cases of medically unexplained physical symptoms (MUPS) and ACT-Youth both illustrate how defining a diagnosis and, subsequently, an associate treatment was a quintessential requirement for reimbursement. However, by their nature, MUPS do not allow for a clear diagnosis – it is about *medically unexplained* physical symptoms (see Chapter 4). The core of its success is to lead the patient away from a focus on some bodily defect, and stimulate her or his agency in exploring ways to deal with their own health. The idea is that such agency is partly a success in its own right, and partly may induce changes in complex pathologies. ACT-Youth focuses on youngsters suffering from multiple, interacting problems. It offers a balanced set of care provisions, tailor-made to a youngster's needs. A diagnosis of their mental health problem(s) is deliberately discarded, pre-empting fixations on a given set of problems and opening up routes that include and stimulate the youngster's agency (see Chapter 8). However, insurance companies appeared unwilling to reimburse a treatment absent a proper diagnosis, with due consequences for the continuity of the activities of the ACT teams.

Another key expression of medical rationality is the current reliance on one particular mode of evidence-based medicine (EBM). The concept was originally proposed by the Evidence-Based Medicine Working Group led by Canadian physician Gordon Guyatt (Guyatt et al., 1992). The rationale is that clinical practice guidelines should only include effective diagnosis and treatment options of which effectiveness is proven by scientific research. Detailed guidelines have been elaborated for care professionals on how to incorporate EBM in their practices (e.g. Guyatt et al., 2008). EBM has become the core of a powerful discourse on responsible care, institutionalized in formal and informal rules governing policy, care and funding practices.

The "evidence" in EBM is supposed to be based on meta-analyses of randomized clinical trials (RCTs) – the "gold standard" within the EBM approach (Timmermans and Berg, 2003). As Pawson (2002a) has pointed out, such studies focus on particular categories of interventions, asking what effect interventions from a specific category have and answering that question through aggregation of a set of earlier evaluations (a "meta-analysis"). EBM is thus essentially based on some key assumptions of dominant medical rationality: a focus on bodily defects, a generic understanding of the body, interventions as the sole factor restoring health, a neglect of contextual factors and patient agency, and bodily effects as outcome measures.

RCT-based EBM is thus theoretically and methodologically appropriate toward measuring linear causal relations between a singular intervention and short-term effects. RCT-based EBM may fall short, however, in analyzing the effectiveness of novel practices that essentially recognize the more complex, often non-linear pathologies that characterize NCDs. Effectiveness may then be expected to rely on non-linear mechanisms, context and individual agency. In the clinic for unexplained diseases, in order to ensure the continued support of the clinic by the hospital, the initiators had to demonstrate the cost-effectiveness of their innovative treatment. Based on both the hospital's rules and the specialists' own convictions, an RCT was the "self-evident" way to do so. However, the intended outcome – improved quality of life – is hard to measure in RCTs; and it is co-dependent on the context and agency of the patient.

Similar problems have been encountered in a case study of interventions in irritable bowel syndrome (Moret-Hartman et al., 2007). Here, medicinal intervention is seen as crucial, not because of the effect of the drugs per se, which is high (50–70%) but no higher than that of a placebo, suggesting that factors like stress are crucial (co-)determinants of irritable bowel syndrome. Doctors prescribe a drug nevertheless because they feel doing so is crucial to ensuring the trustful relationship needed to persuade patients to adopt agency.

Regime players as change agents?

The innovative practices to address persistent problems, described in this volume, are usually initiated by players from the incumbent regime. For instance, the new clinic for treating patients with MUPS was set up by two medical specialists in an academic hospital who were dissatisfied with the health system's inability to organize adequate care for these patients (Chapter 4). Key players in the Transition Program in Long-term Care were established care organizations and the Ministry of Health (Chapters 7 and 8). The Canadian EXTRA program was initiated and funded by the Canadian Health Services Research, and higher level health professionals were central in its realization (Chapter 9). Pioneers for a more needs-oriented health research system in the Netherlands were two large research-funding organizations (Chapter 10). Our findings resonate with those of a recent volume investigating innovative practices in long-term care in Europe, in which, typically, as Nies et al. (2013: 330) note, health professionals are the pioneers.

That mainly regime players initiate niche experiments seems typical for the health system. In the car mobility sector (Geels et al., 2012), outsiders (start-up companies) often acted as front runners and pioneers, although regime actors appeared crucial for a sustainability transition because of regime assets needed to scale up innovations. The front runners in transition processes in food practices – as discussed in Spaargaren et al. (2012) – were highly diverse, including both insiders (e.g. farmers and retailers) and outsiders (mainly environmental NGOs and consumer organizations, but also (activist) consumers) to the food system. In the case of the energy domain (Verbong and Loorbach, 2012: 321), change agents were often outsiders to the system (niche actors), although "the examples of the major changes in the electricity and gas regimes during the last decade demonstrate that regime actors have been actively involved in those changes."

The specific role of regime players as change agents in the health sector may be the result of the fact that conventional medical rationality is so highly valued and deeply embedded in the health system. This has been a cornerstone of our modern health system, and the way to ensure effective and safe care. However, as a consequence, the health system has become rather "closed." Treatments not backed by scientific evidence as to their effectiveness are considered as "alternative practices" and thereby positioned in the social system of "alternative or complementary medicine" (e.g. Angell and

Kassirer, 1998; Zollman and Vickers, 1999) – if not as "quackery" and "pseudoscience." In addition, as Van Raak and De Haan (Chapter 3, pp. 52–53) mention, throughout the history of healthcare, alternative medicine practices have had "no major material or cultural magnitude within or impact on the health system." Relative "outsiders" to the regime are therefore exceptionally constrained in initiating niche experiments.

However, most innovative practices, even when initiated close to the regime, will encounter major difficulties. This is partly due to the fact that the agency of regime players tends to be influenced relatively strongly by the culture, structure and practice of the incumbent regime (cf. Grin, 2003; Roep et al., 2003; cf. Grin et al. (2004) on agricultural transitions). For example, the neurologist who initiated the clinic for unexplained diseases was strongly convinced that healthcare interventions should be evidence-based (based on RCTs) and also knew he would be held accountable in these terms by his peers. Thus, setting up an RCT was a self-evident step, in spite of the fact that – as Schuitmaker and ter Haar-van Twillert (Chapter 4) argued – this was methodologically not an appropriate approach. In addition, in the Transition Program in Long-term Care many of the innovating care organizations tended to revert to incremental change instead of the envisioned radical change in structure, culture and practice. Moreover, government, as provider of the funds for the transition experiments, relied on conventional financial procedures and required "SMART" project plans – which both constrain the flexible learning processes that need to take place in transition experiments. Significantly, in the experiments with patient-centered health research practices (Chapter 10), the research funding organizations that actively involved patients in the research agenda-setting process usually returned to business-as-usual when it came to implementing the agendas.

All this should not come as a surprise. The historical chapters have shown the crucial role of conventional medical rationality, both directly and indirectly, through shaping the institutional rules and regulations. Although this has been important for developing and practicing effective and safe interventions, a more human-integrative orientation is needed to meet current challenges, and this requires a much broader rationality.

So how to proceed?

It is crucial to address the various obstacles discussed above if we are to realize more sustainable healthcare. Further evidence for their relevance is found in health studies literature of innovative care practices with a human-integrative orientation. For example, initiatives in the field of community-based rehabilitation, such as discussed by Thornicroft et al. (2010) and WHO (2011), often suffer from a lack of relevant knowledge or skills among health professionals because current training curricula are geared to preparing students for conventional care practices. In addition, the care infrastructure does not support community-based, integrated and people-centered medical care and rehabilitation services because it relies almost exclusively on centralized, specialized facilities. Last but not least, current policies and financial schemes usually reflect the current fragmentation of services.

Similarly, Nies et al. (2013), in reviewing recent literature on innovations in long-term care in Europe, identify five obstacles encountered in novel care practices for client-centered integrated care: the traditionally highly fragmented silos of health and social care systems, the "Taylorist" division of work ("with distinct tasks for home helps, geriatric aides, registered nurses, therapists and a range of other specialized job profiles" (p. 32)), home care restricted to meeting physical needs, a supply-driven tradition and a shared understanding of the patient as a passive recipient of care. In addition, in the same volume Billings (2013) points at the difficulty of establishing evidence on innovative practices in the complex, multifaceted context of long-term care mainly as a result of the strong focus on evidence-based medicine among policy-makers and stakeholders.

As a final example, Van der Ham et al. (2013) in their analysis of various innovative mental healthcare practices in tertiary care (non-ambulant specialist care), ambulant crisis care and clinical guideline development (focusing in particular on facilitating client agency and integrated care), explicitly point to the discrepancy between the incumbent regime (with its strong emphasis on the hospital as the center stage of medical action), and the practice, structure and culture required for effective implementation of these novel rehabilitation approaches. It is hardly surprising that precisely in fields within the health system where patients' care needs are most complex – multifactorial, multifaceted, requiring behavioral change and patient agency, such as care for chronic patients, long-term care, mental healthcare and disability care – the negative side-effects of the dominance of the rational–reductionist paradigm are felt most urgently.

Thus, the barriers identified in this book and other literature are strongly congruent. What a transition perspective may add is (1) the insight that these barriers are rooted in the incumbent regime, and (2) insights and strategies on how such problems may be overcome. To this we now turn.

11.5 Toward transition strategy for sustainable healthcare: key requirements and opportunities

Key requirements

What do the above findings imply for strategies to address the challenges now facing modern health systems? A *first* key requirement is to move away from an exclusive reliance on conventional medical rationality – focusing on professional intervention in bodily effects – toward a wider, human-integrative orientation – with attention to body, mind, life practices and life conditions and their interactions – thus giving patient agency a place next to professional intervention. As we have seen, the strong cultural embedding (proto-professionalization) and structural embedding (e.g. funding routines relying on EBM; relations between R&D, professionals and patients) of conventional medical rationality may imply key challenges in meeting this requirement.

A *second* key requirement is the careful scrutiny of institutional features that have co-evolved with conventional medical rationality, especially those that appear to hamper innovative practices following this orientation: features which hinder cooperation among different specialisms within the care system and among healthcare actors and actors from other domains; and institutionalized relations that – often unintentionally – privilege the supply side, including the interrelated rationality, and discourage patient agency. Scrutinizing them is important in solving two problems. The first is to maintain such practices running and "on course" in spite of these barriers. The second, as emphasized in the preceding chapters, is the need to spend some real effort on "scaling up" experimental practices. Both problems imply a need for identifying and overcoming institutional barriers.

Against this background, a *third* key requirement for any transition strategy is to promote institutional changes. We know from transition studies (e.g. Geels and Schot, 2007; Grin, 2010, 2012a) that this may involve strategically drawing upon exogenous trends (the "landscape" in MLP terminology), given the pressure they may imply for incumbent structures and practices. Such agency may help shape transition pathways (Grin et al., 2011). More specifically, we may learn from the car mobility domain that drawing upon exogenous trends becomes even more crucial when innovations tend to come from the incumbent regime (Wells et al., 2012) and when a system is characterized by culturally deeply embedded assumptions (Dudley and Chatterjee, 2012). As Geels and colleagues (2012: 363) argue, this leads to two problems for policy-makers, which the preceding analyses of the health domain also underscore: many citizens may be more supportive of the incumbent regime than of novel practices, and policy-makers depend on key actors from the incumbent regime, *including* for the definition and realization of experiments. Geels et al. (2012: 361–366) conclude that in such cases transition strategies should ideally, in addition to niche experiments, pay attention (1) to cracks in the incumbent regime and incremental changes in that regime; (2) to assisting and promoting transformative change at the demand side; and (3) to cultural trends (Sheller, 2012: 187–192) and other exogenous trends that may yield appeal and dynamics to novel practices and structural change (Dudley and Chatterjee, 2012), including changes in the relationships among state, science, market and civil society ("the institutional rectangle," as Grin (2012b) has demonstrated for the transition of modernizing food production and consumption, 1945 to 1970).

But what are relevant trends, *how* do they yield "regime cracks" and *how* may they contribute to the success and scaling up of transition experiments?

Exogenous trends, regime cracks and opportunities for transition practices

One trend challenging the incumbent regime is demographic change. As discussed in the Introduction, aging occurs in many modern countries (partly as an effect of the success of modern health systems). Other challenges – and opportunities for change – come from a second long-term trend: individualization, which has yielded a new generation of elderly – more independent, active and with less passive trust in (Giddens, 1991) and respect for the authority of caregivers – and contributed to a more diverse population. Taken together, these developments put pressure on the incumbent regime: they tend to give rise to a larger and more complex care demand; they undermine the legitimacy of standardized care practices, without much consideration of lifestyles and other individual circumstances and characteristics. In addition, in principle, they provide a basis for legitimizing practices with more patient agency and autonomy.

Yet, as we have seen, the virtually uncontested conventional medical rationality and the aforementioned institutional features have hitherto largely pre-empted a transition toward a sustainable health system. Earlier, many governmental system reforms – such as recent welfare state reforms toward "responsibilization" of citizens as patients or informal caregivers, and earlier reforms aimed at transforming the system through introducing a strong "demand side" in the "care market" – failed because the limits of conventional medical rationality were not considered, and pioneers and patients were hardly empowered to transcend institutional constraints. Similarly, as we have seen, these factors also inhibit the transformative potential of experimental practices that seek to elaborate a more human-integrative orientation to care.

We wish to emphasize here that the potential of individualization has been under-exploited. Explicit elaboration, and presentation, of human-integrative practices as strengthening autonomy among patients and care professionals, and as accounting for more diversity in life practices and lifestyles, may help give these practices both legitimacy and momentum. Workplace Health Promotion, ACT-Youth and telecare, for instance, could thus be promoted. Another example is "Buurtzorg" (Neighborhood Care; cf. Nies et al., 2013: 32; Hotta, 2014), one of the other projects from the Dutch Transition Program in Long-term Care (see Box 11.1 and also Box 7.2). Such innovations also benefit from another sociological trend: the emergence of network society, constituted by contemporary communications infrastructures (Van Dijk, 1999; Castells, 1996). This too offers perspectives for transition strategies.

The crucial point to recognize when linking novel practices to these trends is the following. It has been demonstrated that improved patient and professional satisfaction, better labor productivity and accessibility of care in these projects are essentially associated with the implied increased patient and caregiver agency and tailor-made care. Plausibly, the hitherto limited success of many governmental healthcare reforms in modern societies is partly due to precisely a lack of attention to these factors. This so-called "reconstellation" pathway (Van Raak and De Haan, Chapter 3, this volume) thus tends to fail

Box 11.1 "Buurtzorg"

In the context of the Dutch project on "Buurtzorg", which has meanwhile taken root in other countries as well, such as Sweden, the USA and Japan (Monsen and De Blok, 2013), evaluations have shown that families appreciate help tailored to their needs and situation. These families experience improved accessibility, and personal contact, while care workers appreciate integral care and cooperation between professionals from different organizations. Furthermore, professionals, informal caretakers and families appreciate mutual cooperation, as well as more specific referrals to specialists (Hoeven-Mulder et al., 2014). Data on care demand reduction are not yet available, but the researchers argue that such reduction is plausible. Another evaluation (Schouten, 2013) reports that 80 to 90 percent of both clients and professionals claim to be content or very content with "Buurtzorg" on a variety of criteria. Over the first six months, productivity, defined as the percentage of hours actually spent on care, increased for these teams from 64 up to 71 percent; this must be compared with a 62 percent target and 56 percent reality for the organization as a whole.

to realize the intended effects: quality is not being improved, nor is equity reduced; if costs are curbed, this often occurs at the expense of quality and equity. One way of understanding this finding from health studies (e.g. Gwatkin, 2001; Whitehead et al., 2001; Stambolovic, 2003; Pollock, 2005; De Savigny and Adam, 2009; Mills and Ranson, 2012) is by realizing that such reforms may only succeed to the extent that they manage to shape the agency of professionals, patients, policy-makers and other actors involved in care, funding and life practices. If the latter is difficult to achieve even for grassroots initiatives aiming to do so, it could hardly be expected that initiatives launched with limited knowledge of practice would be more successful.

While the 2008 financial crisis has yielded additional fuel to governmental reforms, it is salient to recognize that the undertones have remained rather constant: less governmental expenditure, more efficiency, new modes of management focused on cost control, and a shift of responsibility from government to insurance companies, citizens and their employers. Citizens are primarily seen as healthcare "consumers" and health professionals as spenders, who should be persuaded (through rhetorical and financial measures) to better take into account the collective interest. These reforms largely miss the point that many of these people *wish* to have more autonomy but precisely find it hard to gain that autonomy in the incumbent regime. There is ample reason to think that, where patients and caregivers do get more agency – in spite of the barriers implied by that system but helped by the sociological trends mentioned above – this yields much better prospects for sustainable healthcare on all dimensions: quality, accessibility, acceptability *and* affordability (see also Box 11.1). Let us now explore transition strategies that may help to draw upon such opportunities.

11.6 Novel solutions to current challenges: outline of potential transition strategies

In this section we outline the most crucial elements of transition strategies in healthcare, embodying the key requirement of moving away from an exclusive reliance on conventional medical rationality, carefully scrutinizing the institutional features that have co-evolved with that rationality, and promoting changes in those institutional features that hamper innovation, by strategically drawing upon regime cracks and long-term trends to generate legitimacy and momentum.

Visions shaping distributed agency and concerted action

Visioning – the development of a long-term vision or normative orientation toward change – is a crucial activity in transition management (e.g. Rotmans et al., 2001). Through a joint process of articulating expectations among a range of stakeholders, visions of a sustainable future are developed. Importantly, these visions should not be understood as blueprints for action, but rather as "horizons of expectation" (Grin, 2000). Expectations inform human action and are normally rooted in past experiences; they are therefore bounded by the horizons of these experiences – in our case the horizons implied by conventional medical rationality. Visioning must be elaborated as finding novel horizons of expectation (Grin, 2010: 269–271), as a contribution to replacing the dominance of the past over the future (Beck et al., 2003; Lissandrello and Grin, 2011).

As part of a transition strategy in healthcare, visioning could help articulate a rationality beyond conventional medical thinking and interrelated practices and institutional features. That would help mitigate the above-mentioned drawback of the fact that insiders to the health system are often the ones to undertake innovative practices. Visioning could help to maintain the benefits of their involvement while maintaining a human-integrative orientation in experiments.

However, there is a certain risk that visions can become footloose. Although the value of visioning has been shown in innovative practices, for example, in the energy system, hype–disappointment cycles may occur when expectations were not met by initiated experiments (Raven, 2012). The question we posed in the Introduction to this volume is to what extent guiding sustainability visions are fruitful in conducting experiments for health system innovation. Clearly, many experiments discussed in Part II were guided by a sustainability vision, which usually took a human-integrative perspective (see Section 11.2). In the cases of workplace health development (Vaandrager et al., Chapter 5), long-term care in Spain (Ródenas and Garcés, Chapter 6) and the EXTRA program (Clements and Essink, Chapter 9), a vision provided the inspiration and guidance for setting up the experiment.

In the Transition Program in Long-term Care (Van den Bosch and Neuteboom, Chapter 7), a shared sustainability vision was initially lacking and was developed in the course of the program. This case showed that, apparently, it is not a prerequisite to develop a full-fledged, articulated shared sustainability vision right from the start, as is usually done in transition management (Loorbach, 2007; Rotmans and Loorbach, 2010). Initially, a shared drive to change the dominant structure, culture and practice of the regime can also provide a strong binding force. Yet a vision was crucial to define a balanced portfolio of experiments; to maintain projects on transition course against regime inertia and resistance notwithstanding; and to strategically connect them to landscape trends and "regime cracks," thereby supporting their scaling up.

Doing experiments and linking them to dynamics at the niche, regime and landscape levels

As we have argued above, experiments to deal with a specific health problem on the basis of a human-integrative orientation are also crucial. In performing experiments, timely recognizing and overcoming institutional barriers that may hamper or derail such experiments and inhibit their scaling up are of key importance. The *method of reflexive design*, as described by Schuitmaker and ter Haar-van Twillert (Chapter 4, this volume), may provide a way forward in supporting such an endeavor by providing in-depth insight into the mechanisms by which resistance to change is effected in specific experiments. The method entails a historically informed system analysis and an actor-guided system analysis focusing on a specific innovative practice.

In a historically informed system analysis the embedding of the persistent problem at stake is unraveled by looking for the features that are part of the *success* of the system, as well as by reviewing earlier critiques. Frequently, according to reflexive modernization theory (Beck, 1997), the factors underlying success also generate the objects of critique, since they underlie the side-effects and blind spots of the system as well.

An actor-guided analysis is done iteratively around a transition experiment. The reproduction of structural features is analyzed from the perspective of the experimenting actor(s). It is investigated (1) how the new care practice organizes itself, (2) what premises and expectations underlie the practice, (3) what kind of support or impediment the practice experiences, and (4) what the possible link is between the success factors (with negative side-effects), the way the practice seeks to address these factors and how the practice is supported or impeded. This method is very promising, and could be operationally elaborated, drawing upon experiences with reflexively designing sustainable livestock systems (Bos et al., 2009, 2012).

With regard to particular experiments, it may thus be possible to identify the institutional features that appear at odds with the experiment at hand. In order to translate this into a strategy for institutional changes, it is advisable to link up with "regime cracks" and ongoing efforts for regime adaptation, as well as with "landscape" trends. As an illustration, telecare, with more agency and autonomy for patients and nurses as core elements, could be (and, in fact, has been) related to regime cracks, in particular the discrepancy between demands for, and the availability of, nursing capacity in case of continued regime practices. Institutional changes were given legitimacy by demonstrating that telecare could reduce demand, lead to higher labor productivity as well as improved labor satisfaction *if, and only if,* telecare practices would be elaborated such that autonomy for patients and nurses alike would be improved. Initiators also argued that such autonomy would become increasingly appropriate, given long-term trends associated with individualization. Appeals for adapting funding rules became more convincing when it was argued that more tailor-made practices, with increased autonomy for patients and caregivers, were obviously ill-served by rules focusing on reimbursing generically allocated provisions.

Running transition programs

Various chapters have discussed conscious attempts to influence the direction and speed of system innovations. One notable example is the Transition Program in Long-term Care (see Chapter 7 by Van den Bosch and Neuteboom), which was largely set up according to the Transition Management (TM) approach (see Introduction to this volume). In this program, TM notions, developed in the energy domain and other domains, were applied to the health domain. The Program Team established a transition arena – a setting in which actors jointly analyze problems, design and implement solutions and develop new insights through learning processes and apply strategies related to deepening, broadening and scaling up. Deviating from earlier TM, the program's efforts did not start from a strategic problem analysis and visioning but rather built on existing experiments, which were subsequently "transitionized" (Avelino, 2009; Van den Bosch, 2010) and served as stepping stones for developing a diagnosis of the incumbent regime and a vision of a sustainable health system. More than commonly in TM, therefore, the Program Team already ran into system barriers right at the start of the initiative, inducing changes to the TM "guidelines," which led to interesting insights. For example, since a shared vision and transition agenda was not developed before selecting innovations, the Program Team instead established so-called *TM selection criteria* to choose radical innovations with transition, learning and growth potential, and addressing a persistent problem in long-term care. Another lesson was that with the number of projects growing, it is important explicitly to define and maintain a *"balanced" portfolio* that adequately covers the various dimensions of transition to practices reflecting a more human-integrative orientation. While this was attempted in order to explore the full scope of the care sector, Van Raak and De Haan's spaghetti metaphor for transition dynamics also suggests that this is crucial to making various innovations add up to an overall transition.

The program also emphasized *learning about funding*. Cost-effectiveness is obviously crucial for the experiments involved, as well as for their broadening and scaling up. More importantly, funding rules may have to change: from a supply-side, standardized focus on reimbursing health interventions toward a mode of funding that promotes, and draws upon, patient agency and tailor-made care.

Another important lesson was that the explicit *formulation of scaling up object-ives and strategies* is highly conducive in maintaining focus and structuring experiments. In addition, as Elberse et al. underscore in Chapter 10, it is important to *develop and present "best practices" as showcases* to make the benefits and the "how to" visible. This will inspire and motivate others to take the risk of experimenting beyond the regime in their own context (cf. Geels and Schot, 2010: 84–85), eventually causing mutual reinforcement among the "spaghetti" of innovation strands.

Moreover, Van den Bosch and Neuteboom emphasize the need to *coach project leaders* and support them in reflexively analyzing and addressing regime barriers. Clements and Essink, in their discussion of the EXTRA program (which they label as an example of TM *"avant la lettre"*), show that project leaders may not only benefit from coaching but also from *training* to enhance their competences to set up and manage transition experiments. While the importance of competences is frequently mentioned (e.g. Loorbach, 2007; Van den Bosch, 2010), it would be important to extend the TM toolbox with methods for building TM competences through well-targeted training programs.

Interestingly, Van den Bosch and Neuteboom emphasized *patient/client agency also as a contribution to TM*. Whereas in healthcare regime players are usually the ones to initiate innovative care practices (Section 11.4), Van den Bosch and Neuteboom found that the involvement of relatively new actors, such as patients, was a crucial aid in maintaining a transition orientation in experiments. This resonates with accounts of "consumer" agency in food transitions (see e.g. the chapters by Grin, Van Otterloo, Klintman and Bostrom, Oosterveer and Spaargaren in Spaargaren et al., 2012), and it is cer-tainly an issue that warrants further investigation. In doing so, due attention must be paid to the reluctance of many patients/clients to take up their agency in bringing about system change (see the chapters by Schuitmaker and ter Haar-van Twillert, ter Haar-van Twillert and Van den Bosch, and Elberse et al. in this volume). This reluctance is an expression of the incumbent regime features, such as the proto-professionalization of patients (internaliza-tion of conventional medical rationality) and the subordinate and passive role implied in incumbent patient–doctor relationships. We therefore support Verbong and Loorbach's (2012) appeal – in the context of energy transition – to gain more insight into how the agency of users affects regimes, either in sustaining or destabilizing these regimes. In addition, we suggest that more research be done on how users may (be empowered to) take up an active role in transition processes (see e.g. Oldenziel and Hård, 2013).

11.7 Implications for future research in health studies

On establishing reliable, valid evidence

However well elaborated, transition strategies may fail unless the practices they help promote are evaluated in a way that does *not* reproduce conventional medical rationality. As we have seen (Section 11.3), this may easily happen when experiments are assessed on the basis of the unreflected application of standard evidence-based medicine.

To be sure, sustainable healthcare must be evidence-based – quality and cost-effectiveness of novel care practices must be established in reliable and valid ways. The issue at stake here, however, is: *What*, exactly, is reliable and valid evidence? Clearly, "gold standard" EBM comes with important a priori theoretical and methodological limits in evaluating human-integrative-oriented practices that seek to deal with health problems characterized by complex, non-linear pathologies. Such EBM relies on the meta-analysis of randomized controlled trials (RCTs). Methodologically, RCTs seek to establish the relationship between a particular intervention and its health effect. Theoretically, they embody conventional medical rationality, in which an intervention targets a bodily defect with a relatively direct causal connection to the health problem. In case of more complex pathologies, however, a health problem will involve complex interactions among intervention, body, mind, life practices, life conditions and patient agency. In such cases it is far from self-evident that, methodologically, working with RCTs represents the best approach to EBM in establishing the effectiveness of interventions.

Increasingly, proponents of EBM also view "evidence" as the combination of scientific evidence with knowledge derived from clinical experience of health professionals and the experiences of patients (Sackett et al., 1996; Rycroft-Malone et al., 2004). We also see moves toward new approaches to evidence for certain types of interventions. Pawson (2002a) argues that in cases where the effects of an intervention depend on (1) the context, and (2) the agency deployed in response to the intervention, a "realist synthesis" (Pawson, 2002b) is a much more appropriate form of evaluation. Realist synthesis focuses not on answering the question "What works?" but on the question "What works, for who, in what context, why and how?" (Pawson, 2006: 74). It is thus not about establishing an inventory of effective interventions but rather one of mechanisms (M), which, in interaction with the context (C), affect actors and thus yield certain outcomes (O). Interestingly, realist synthesis is increasingly applied in the evaluation of innovative health practices (e.g. Shepperd et al., 2009; Robert et al., 2012; Lodenstein et al., 2013).

In order to make sense of C–M–O relations identified from analyses, some basic knowledge is needed of the underlying "program theory." Pawson proposed to construct such a model in a "realist" meta-analysis essentially using a grounded theory approach (Glaser and Strauss, 1967). In addition, we argue, some rudimentary understanding is available in the form of informal knowledge from the patient and caregivers in primary care. This informal understanding may help develop a heuristic model that provides guidance to practice, being tested, enriched and further developed over time. Interestingly, by using such a rudimentary model for evaluating different types of innovative practices, it may be tested through, and enriched by, an increasingly comprehensive set of S–M relations. This may in and of itself lead to a better theory; and it may suggest questions for foundational research which may lead to further and deeper theory development (Grin, forthcoming). That way, evaluation of innovative practices may become the core of a novel knowledge infrastructure which in turn may contribute to interconnecting different strands of the spaghetti of innovation and thus become a catalyst for a wider transition (cf. Van Raak and De Haan, Chapter 3, this volume). We elaborate upon this in the following section.

Consolidating and scaling up interventions

Until recently, it was generally assumed that health interventions would diffuse and scale up once proven effective through RCTs. Health research shows surprisingly little attention to how such scaling up would occur, and the strong reliance on RCTs as the "gold standard" was left virtually unquestioned. However, over the past three decades numerous studies (often under the heading of translational, dissemination or sustainability research) have outlined a sobering picture; many "effective" interventions in a wide variety of care practices were not sustained after funding dried up, or failed to transfer to larger populations or different cultural settings (Simmons et al., 2007; Scheirer and Dearing, 2011; Stirman et al., 2012; Billings, 2013). Simultaneously, such studies usually leave readers puzzled about the reason for this limited sustainability and scaling up. What transpires from these studies is that innovations are often implemented and tested through small-scale, isolated, time-limited projects with a limited focus on the future. "While providing some inspirational ideas for practice improvement, they have neglected a range of other relevant issues not least their own sustainability and how they can be scaled up" (Nies et al., 2013: 332).

This has led to a new strand in health research focusing on the consolidation and scaling up of health interventions. Initially the main focus was on identifying enabling and constraining factors to diffuse health interventions (e.g. Glaser et al., 1983; Stirman et al., 2012; Billings, 2013). These include: (1) characteristics of the intervention (e.g. flexible, adaptable, inexpensive, simple interventions with evidence of effectiveness); (2) factors in the organization setting (e.g. good fit between the intervention and organization's mission and routines, an internal champion, capacity and leadership, and committed staff), and (3) factors in the community environment of each intervention site (e.g. supportive partnerships and continued funding), while emphasizing the interrelations and interactions among these factors (e.g. Scheirer and Dearing, 2011; Stirman et al., 2012). Thus it has become increasingly acknowledged that most health service interventions involve complex innovations requiring participatory, interdisciplinary approaches to implementation and that scaling up amounts to a non-linear process, whereby the various strategies aimed at implementation, consolidation and scaling up need to be multifaceted and adapted to the specific context (Medlin et al., 2006; Simmons et al., 2007). This is why research increasingly pursues the development of *heuristics* for improving scaling-up processes (e.g. Mangham and Hanson, 2010; Nies et al., 2013). Based on an analysis of experiments that successfully scaled up, Nies et al. (2013) list the following strategies: setting clear priorities, establishing agreed objectives, developing a social business case (stakeholder analysis and impact map), experimenting, training, strong leadership, partnerships, and long-standing commitments and investments by governments and other actors. In addition, it has been noted that aligning organizational procedures with particular interventions may help (Scheirer and Dearing, 2011; Stirman et al., 2012).

Although these heuristics share some notions with system innovation and transition theory, they are limited to integrating new interventions in mainstream healthcare, rather than explicitly viewing the obstacles as being of a systemic nature. But health research will learn most from transition studies – in ways discussed in this chapter – precisely by recognizing that in many cases it is ultimately the incumbent regime that has to change.

The studies presented in this book focus on pioneers in the application of transition studies to the health system, and much of the work has been based on the Dutch health system. This is why more historical, evaluative and action research is needed to deepen and generalize the findings to other contexts, including the following:

- comparative (historical) studies in different countries;
- studies on the relevance of sustainability as a guiding vision;
- experiments assessing strategies for deepening, broadening and, especially, scaling up;
- research on how users may (be empowered to) take up an active role in transition processes;
- comparative studies between transitions in health systems in welfare states and such systems in developing countries.

The various insights provided in this volume will hopefully inspire researchers to take up this challenge. We also hope that in a co-creation process between research and practice, stakeholders will set up and analyze transition experiments – building on the findings presented here – in order to contribute to the development of a more robust body of knowledge on system innovation and transition theory in the context of health systems. In time, this may lead to an increased capacity to deal effectively with the persistent problems in our health systems, bringing the increasingly widely shared vision of a sustainable health system closer to becoming a reality.

References

Abelson, J., Giacomini, M., Lehoux, P., and Gauvin, F.P. (2007) "Bringing 'the public' into health technology assessment and coverage policy decisions: From principles to practice." *Health Policy*, 82(1): 37–50.

Abma, T.A. (2005) "Responsive evaluation: Its meaning and special contribution to health promotion." *Evaluation and Program Planning*, 28(3): 279–289.

Abma, T.A. (2006) "Patients as partners in a health research agenda setting – The feasibility of a participatory methodology." *Evaluation and the Health Professions*, 29(4): 424–439.

Abma, T.A., and Broerse, J.E.W. (2010) "Patient participation as dialogue: Setting research agendas." *Health Expectations*, 13(2): 160–173.

Abma, T.A., Nierse, C., Van de Griendt, J., Schipper, K., and Van Zadelhoff, E. (2007) *Leren over lijf en leden. Een agenda voor sociaal-Cwetenschappelijk onderzoek door nierpatienten. Eindrapportage ten behoeve van Nierstichting en Nierpatienten Vereniging Nederland*, Maastricht: Universiteit Maastricht.

Abma, T.A., Nierse, C.J., and Widdershoven, G.A. (2009) "Patients as partners in responsive research: Methodological notions for collaborations in mixed research teams." *Qualitative Health Research*, 19(3): 401–415.

Abraham, R. (1970) *Analyse van de geneesmiddelenreclame door middel van advertenties in medische vakbladen*, Haarlem: der Toorts.

Achterhuis, H. (1983) *De markt van welzijn en geluk*, Baarn: Ambo Uitgevers.

Achterhuis, H. (1988) *Het rijk van de schaarste. Van Hobbes tot Foucault*, Utrecht: Ambo Uitgevers.

ACT-Youth (2005) *Business Plan ACT-Youth*, Rotterdam: GGZ Groep Europoort.

ACT-Youth (2008) *Annual Report, Transition Programme in the Care*, January.

Actiz (2007) *Zorg op afstand, Dichterbij "Meer van hetzelfde werkt niet meer. Het moet echt anders,"* Utrecht: Actiz.

Ahgren, B., and Axelson, R. (2007) "Determinants of integrated health management: Chains of care in Sweden." *The Internal Journal of Health and Planning Management*, 22(2): 145–157.

Aksnes, D.W., and Rip, A. (2009) "Researchers' perceptions of citations." *Research Policy*, 38(6): 895–905.

Amering, M., and Schmolke, M. (2009) *Recovery in Mental Health: Reshaping scientific and clinical responsibility*, World Psychiatric Association, Chichester: John Wiley & Sons.

Anderson, M. (2011) "Evaluating the first years of the EXTRA Program." In T. Sullivan and J. Denis, *Building Better Healthcare for Canada: Implementing Evidence*, Montreal: McGill-Queen's University Press, pp. 122–150.

Anderson, M., and Donaldson, S. (2010) *Effecting Change through the Intervention Projects, Making an Impact: Draft Final Report Prepared for the Canadian Health Services Research Foundation*, Ottawa: Canadian Health Services Research Foundation.

Anderson, M., and Lovoie-Tremblay, M. (2008) "Evaluation of the Executive Training for Research Application (EXTRA) Program: Design and early findings." *Health Policy*, 4(2): 136–148.

Angell, M. (2004) *The Truth about the Drug Companies. How they deceive us and what to do about it*, New York: Random House.

Angell, M., and Kassirer, J.P. (1998) "Alternative medicine – The risks of untested and unregulated remedies." *New England Journal of Medicine*, 339(12): 839–841.

Antonovsky, A. (1993) "The structure and properties of the sense of coherence scale." *Social Science and Medicine*, 36(6): 725–733.

Applebaum, R., Straker, J., Mehdizadeh, S., Warshaw, G., and Gothelf, E. (2002) "Using high-intensity care management to integrate acute and long-term care services: Substitute for large scale system reform?" *Case Management Journal*, 3: 113–119.

Arts, B., and Van Tatenhove, J. (2004) "Policy and power: A conceptual framework between the 'old' and 'new' policy idioms." *Policy Sciences*, 37(3/4): 339–356.

Astmafonds (2008) *Verslag Wetenschappelijk Jaarsymposium 2008.*

Astmafonds (2009) *Verslag Wetenschappelijk Jaarsymposium 2009.*

Avelino, F. (2009) "Empowerment and the challenge of applying transition management to on-going projects." *Policy Sciences*, 42(4): 369–390.

Avelino, F., Grin, J., Jhagroe, S., and Pel, B. (eds) (2016) Special Issue on the Politics of Transitions. *Journal of Environmental Policy and Planning*, 18(5): 557–672.

Avelino, F., and Rotmans, J. (2009) "Power in transition. An interdisciplinary framework to study power in relation to structural change." *European Journal of Social Theory*, 12(4): 543–569.

Avelino, F., and Wittmayer, J.M. (2016) "Shifting power relations in sustainability transitions: A multi-actor perspective." In J. Grin, S. Jhagroe, and B. Pel, Special Issue on the Politics of Transitions. *Journal of Environmental Policy and Planning*, 18(5): 628–649.

Baart, P., Van Capelleveen, C., Iedema, P., Raaijmakers, T., Vaandrager, L., and Der Weduwe, K. (2003) *Workplace Health Promotion*, Woerden: NIGZ.

Bacon, F. (1626) *Nova Atlantis.*

Baggott, R., and Forster, R. (2008) "Health consumer and patients' organizations in Europe: Towards a comparative analysis." *Health Expectations*, 11(1): 85–94.

Bains, M. (2003) "Projecting future needs: Long-term projections of public expenditure on health and long-term care for EU Member States." In OECD, *A Disease-based Comparison of Health Systems: What is best and at what cost?* Paris: OECD, pp. 145–162.

Balbus, J.M., Barouki, R., Birnbaum, L.S., Etzel, R.A., and Gluckman, P.D. (2013) "Early-life prevention of non-communicable diseases." *The Lancet*, 381(9860): 3–5.

Baranski, B., Vaandrager, L., Martimo, K., and Baart, P. (2003) *Workplace Health in the Public Health Perspective: Policy requirements and performance indicators for Good Practice in Health, Environment, Safety and Social Management in Enterprises (GP HESME)*, Copenhagen: World Health Organization.

Barbot, J. (2006) "How to build an 'active' patient? The work of AIDS associations in France." *Social Science and Medicine*, 62(3): 538–551.

Batalden, P., and Davidoff, F. (2007) "What is 'quality improvement' and how can it transform healthcare?" *Quality and Safety in Health Care*, 16: 2–3.

Bauer, G., Davies, J.K., and Pelikan, J. (2006) "The EUHPID Health Development Model for the classification of public health indicators." *Health Promotion International*, 21(2): 153–159.

Beck, U. (1992) *Risk Society: Towards a New Modernity*, New Delhi: Sage.

Beck, U. (1997) *The Reinvention of Politics. Rethinking modernity in the global social order*, Cambridge: Polity Press.

Beck, U., and Beck-Gernsheim, E. (2002) *Individualization: Institutionalized individualism and its social and political consequences*, London: Sage.

Beck, U., Bonss, W., and Lau, C. (2003) "The Theory of Reflexive Modernization Problematic, Hypotheses and Research Programme." *Theory, Culture and Society*, 20(2): 1–33.

Beck, U., Giddens, A., and Lash, S. (1994) *Reflexive Modernization: Politics, tradition and aesthetics in the modern social order*, Stanford, CA: Stanford University Press.

Beddington, J., Cooper, C.L., Field, J., Goswami, U., Huppert, F.A., Jenkins, R., Jones, H.S., Kirkwood, T.B.L., Sahakian, B.J., and Thomas, S.M. (2008) "The mental wealth of nations." *Nature*, 455: 1057–1060.

Belleman, S. (1977) "Ontwikkelingen in de vraag naar specialistische hulp." *Medisch Contact*, 32: 13.

Bensing, J.M. (2000) "Bridging the gap. The separate worlds of evidence-based medicine and patient-centered medicine." *Patient Education and Counseling*, 39: 17–25.

Beresford, P. (2003) "User involvement in research: Exploring the challenges." *Nursing Times Research*, 8(1): 36–46.

Beresford, P. (2007) "User involvement, research and health inequalities: Developing new directions." *Health and Social Care in the Community*, 15(4): 306–312.

Berkhout, F., Angel, D., and Wieczorek, A. (2009) "Asian development pathways and sustainable socio-technical regimes." *Technological Forecasting and Social Change*, 76(2): 218–228.

Berman, P. (1995) "Health sector reform: Making health development sustainable." *Health Policy*, 32: 13–28.

Bernabei, R., Landi, F., Onder, G., Liperoti, R., and Gambassi, G. (2008) "Second and third generation assessment instruments: The birth of standardization in geriatric care." *Journal of Gerontology Series A Biological Sciences Medical Sciences*, 63(3): 8–13.

Beswick, A.D., Rees, K., Dieppe, P., Ayis, S., Gooberman-Hill, R., Horwood, J., and Ebrahim, S. (2008) "Complex interventions to improve physical function and maintain independent living in elderly people: A systematic review and meta-analysis." *The Lancet*, 371: 725–735.

Bijker, W.E., Bal, R., and Hendriks, R. (2009) *The Paradox of Scientific Authority*, Cambridge, MA, and London: The MIT Press.

Billings, J. (2013) "Improving the evidence base." In K. Leichsenring, J. Billings, and H. Nies (eds), *Long-term Care in Europe: Improving policy and practice*, Basingstoke and New York: Palgrave Macmillan, pp. 299–324.

Billings, J., and Leichsenring, K. (2005) *Integrating Health and Social Care Services for Older Persons. Evidence from nine European countries*, Aldershot: Ashgate.

Bindman, A.B., Grumbach, K., Osmond, D., Vranizan, K., and Stewart, A.L. (1996) "Primary care and receipt of preventive services." *Journal of General Internal Medicine*, 11: 269–276.

Binnenkade, C. (1973) *Honderd jaar opleiding tot verpleegkundige in Nederland*, Amsterdam: Faculty of Medicine, VU University Amsterdam.

Blech, J. (2003) *Die Kranheitserfinder: wie wir zu Patienten gemacht werden,* Frankfurt am Main: Fischer.

Blok, G. (2004) *Baas in eigen brein, Antipsychiatrie in Nederland, 1965–1985,* Amsterdam: University of Amsterdam.

Blume, S.S. (1992) *Insight and Industry: On the dynamics of technological change in medicine,* Cambridge, MA, and London: The MIT Press.

Blume, S.S. (2005) "Wetenschapper in dovencultuur." In H. Haaster and Y. Koster-Deese, *Ervaren en Weten, essays over de relatie tussen ervaringskennis en onderzoek,* Utrecht: Uitgeverij Jan Van Arkel, pp. 147–152.

Blume, S.S., and Catshoek, G. (2003) "De patiënt als medeonderzoeker. Van vraaggestuurde zorg naar vraaggestuurde onderzoek." *Medische Antropologie,* 15(1): 183–204.

Boer, A. (1999) "Assessment and regulation of healthcare technology. The Dutch experience." *International Journal of Technology Assessment in Healthcare,* 15(4): 638–648.

Boot, J.M., and Knapen, M. (2005) *De Nederlandse Gezondheidszorg,* Houten: Bohn Stafleu van Loghum.

Bos, B., and Grin, J. (2008) "Doing reflexive modernisation in pig husbandry: The hard work of changing the course of a river." *Science, Technology and Human Values,* 33(4): 480–507.

Bos, B., Koerkamp, G., Gosselink, P.W.G., Jules, M.J., and Bokma, S.J. (2009) "Reflexive interactive design and its application in a project on sustainable dairy husbandry systems." *Outlook on Agriculture,* 38(2): 137–145.

Bos, B., Spoelstra, S.F., Groot Koerkamp, P.W.G., De Greef, K.H., and Van Eijk, O.N.M. (2012) "Reflexive design for sustainable animal husbandry: Mediating between Niche and regime." In G. Spaargaren, P. Oosterveer, and A. Loeber (eds), *Food Practices in Transition: Changing food consumption, retail and production in the age of reflexive modernity,* London: Routledge, pp. 229–256.

Bos, J.T., and Francke, A.L. (2006) *Tussentijds verslag experiment screen to screen,* Utrecht: Nivel.

Bos, J.T., de Jongh, J.D.M., and Franke, A.L. (2005) *Monitoring invoering videonetwerken in de thuiszorg,* Utrecht: Nivel.

Bosch, M. (2002) "Women and science in the Netherlands: A Dutch case?" *Science in Context,* 15(4): 483–527.

Bouma, J. (2006) *Slikken. Hoe ziek is de farmaceutische industrie?,* Amsterdam: Veen.

Bourdieu, P. (1990) *In Other Words Essays towards a Reflexive Sociology,* Stanford, CA: Stanford University Press.

Brandt, E. (2005a) "Kliniek voor onbegrepen ziektes; Behandelcentrum voor onverklaarde aandoeningen is kostenbesparend." *Trouw,* May 28.

Brandt, E. (2005b) "Lichamelijk onverklaarbare klachten poli." *Trouw,* July 19.

Braudel, F. (1976) *The Mediterranean and the Mediterranean World in the Age of Philip II,* New York: Harper & Row.

Bremer, G.J. (2006) *Huisarts zijn in het interbellum,* Rotterdam: Erasmus Publishing.

Broerse, J.E.W., and Bunders, J.F.G. (2000) "Requirements for biotechnology development: The necessity of an interactive and participatory innovative development." *International Journal of Biotechnology,* 2: 275–296.

Broerse, J.E.W., and Bunders, J.F.G. (eds) (2010) *Transitions in Health Systems: Dealing with persistent problems,* Amsterdam: VU University Press.

Broerse, J.E.W., and Elberse, J.E. (2010) *Patient Participation in the Practices of the Pharmaceutical Industry*, Annual Meeting of the Society for Social Studies of Science (4S), Tokyo, Japan.

Broerse, J.E.W., Essink, D., and Bunders, J. (2010b) "Reflections on persistent problems and strategies for health system innovation." In J.E.W. Broerse and J.F.G. Bunders (eds), *Transitions in Health Systems: Dealing with persistent problems*, Amsterdam: VU University Press, pp. 209–230.

Broerse, J.E.W., Elberse, J.E., Caron-Flinterman, J.F., and Zweekhorst, M.B.M. (2010a) "Enhancing a transition towards a needs-oriented health research system through patient participation." In J.E.W. Broerse and J.F.G. Bunders (eds), *Transitions in Health Systems: Dealing with persistent problems*, Amsterdam: VU University Press, pp. 181–206.

Broerse, J.E.W., Konijn, W., Elberse, J.E., and Pittens, C.A.C.M. (2011) *Onderzoeksagenda Dementie. Behoeften van mensen met dementie, mantelzorgers, burgers en onderzoekers*, Amsterdam: Athena Institute, VU University Amsterdam.

Broerse, J.E.W., Zweekhorst, M.B.M., De Groot, J., and Oud, A.M.M. (2006) *Patientenraadpleging Diabetes Fonds Amsterdam*, Amsterdam: Athena Institute, VU University Amsterdam.

Broerse, J.E.W., Zweekhorst, M.B.M., Van Rensen, A.J., and De Haan, M.J. (2010c) "Involving burn survivors in agenda setting on burn research: An added value?" *Burns*, 36(2): 217–231.

Brown, L., Tucker, C., and Domokos, T. (2003) "Evaluating the impact of integrated health and social care teams on older people living in the community." *Health and Social Care in the Community*, 11(2): 85–94.

Brown, M.M., Brown, G.C., and Sharma, S. (2005) *Evidence-based to Value-based Medicine*, Chicago, IL: AMA Press.

Brown, R.F., Butow, P.N., Juraskova, I., Ribi, K., Gerber, D., Bernhard, J., and Tattersall, M.H. (2011) "Sharing decisions in breast cancer care: Development of the Decision Analysis System for Oncology (DAS-O) to identify shared decision making during treatment consultations." *Health Expectations*, 14(1): 29–37.

Bruinsma, J. (2009) "Persoonlijk budget zorg leidt tot fraude." *De Volkskrant*, April 1.

Burns, J.P. (2003) "Research in children." *Critical Care Medicine*, 31(3): S131–S136.

Buse, K., Mays, N., and Walt, G.N. (2008) "Interest groups and the policy process." In K. Buse, N. Mays, and G. Walt (2012), *Making Health Policy*, London: Open University Press, pp. 101–121.

Buurtzorg (2008) *Annual Report District Care 2007*, Transition Programme in Long-term Care.

Callahan, D. (1973) "The WHO definition of 'health'." *The Hastings Center Studies*, 1(3): 77–87.

Callon, M. (1991) "Techno-economic networks and irreversibility." In J. Law (ed.), *A Sociology of Monsters: Essays on power, technology and domination*, London: Routledge, pp. 132–161.

Canadian Nurse (2012) "EXTRA Program revamped for 2012." *Canadian Nurse*, 108(1).

Caron-Flinterman, F. (2005) *A New Voice in Science. Patient participation in decision-making on biomedical research*, Zutphen: Wohrmann Print Service.

Caron-Flinterman, F., Broerse, J.E.W., and Bunders, J.F.G. (2005a) "The experiential knowledge of patients: A new resource for biomedical research?" *Social Science and Medicine*, 60(11): 2575–2584.

Caron-Flinterman, F., Broerse J.E.W., and Bunders, J.F.G. (2007) "Patient partnership in decision-making on biomedical research – Changing the network." *Science Technology and Human Values*, 32(3): 339–368.

Caron-Flinterman, F., Broerse, J.E.W., Teerling, J., and Bunders, J.F.G. (2005b) "Patients' priorities concerning health research: The case of asthma and COPD research in the Netherlands." *Health Expectations*, 8(3): 253–263.

Caron-Flinterman, F., Broerse, J.E.W., Teerling, J., Van Alst, M.L., Klaasen, S., Swart, L.E., and Bunders, J.F. (2006) "Stakeholder participation in health research agenda setting: The case of asthma and COPD research in the Netherlands." *Science and Public Policy*, 33: 291–304.

Carpenter, I., Challis, D., and Hirdes, J.P. (1999) *Care of Older People: A comparison of systems in North America, Europe and Japan*, London: Farrand Press.

Carretero, S., Garcés, J., and Ródenas, F. (2007) "Evaluation of the home help service and its impact on the informal caregiver's burden of dependent elders." *International Journal Geriatric Psychiatry*, 22: 738–749.

Casanova, C., and Starfield, B. (1995) "Hospitalizations of children and access to primary care: A cross-national comparison." *International Journal of Health Services*, 25: 283–294.

Castán Broto, V. (2016) "Innovation territories and energy transitions: Energy, water and modernity in Spain, 1939–1975." In J. Grin, S. Jhagroe, and B. Pel, Special Issue on the Politics of Transitions. *Journal of Environmental Policy and Planning*, 18(5): 712–729.

Castells, M. (1996) *The Rise of the Network Society (The Information Age: Economy, Society and Culture), Volume I*, Oxford: Blackwell.

CBS (n.d.) *Statline*.

Challis, D. (1993) "Programas alternativos en las prestaciones a la tercera edad: prestaciones domiciliarias y gestión individualizada por casos." In L. Moreno (ed.), *Intercambio social y desarrollo del bienestar*, Madrid: Consejo Superior de Investigaciones Científicas, pp. 365–397.

Challis, D., Darton, R., Hughes, J., Stewart, K., and Weiner, K. (2001) "Intensive care-management at home: An alternative to institutional care?" *Age Ageing*, 30: 409–413.

Chalmers, I. (1995) "What do I want from health research and researchers when I am a patient?" *British Medical Journal*, 310: 1315–1318.

Chalmers, I., and Altman, D.G. (1995) *Systematic Reviews*, London: BMJ Publications.

Champagne, F., Lemieux-Charles, L., MacKean, G., Reay, T., Duranceau, M., and Suàrez Herrera, J.C. (2011) *Knowledge Creation in Healthcare Organizations as a Result of Individuals' Participation in the EXTRA and SEARCH Programs*, Toronto: CHSRF.

Cherubini, A., Oristrell, J., Pla, X., Ruggiero, C., Ferretti, R., Diestre, G., Clarfield, A.M., Crome, P., Hertogh, C., Lesauskaite, V., Prada, G., Szczerbinska, K., Topinkova, E., Sinclair-Cohen, J., Edbrooke, D., and Mills, G.H. (2011) "The persistent exclusion of older patients from ongoing clinical trials regarding heart failure." *Archives of Internal Medicine*, 171(6): 550–556.

Chopyak, J., and Levesque, P. (2002) "Public participation in science and technology decision making: Trends for the future." *Technology in Society*, 24(1–2): 155–166.

Christensen, C.M., Grossman, J.H., and Hwang, J. (2009) *The Innovator's Prescription*, Europe: Mc Graw-Hill Education.

CHSRF (2003) *Proposed Program Design and Development*, Final Report of the Design Working Group, Canadian Health Services Research Foundation.

Chu, C., Driscoll, T., and Dwyer, S. (1997) "The health-promoting workplace: An integrative perspective." *Australian and New Zealand Journal of Public Health*, 21(4): 377–385.

CIHI (2011a) *Health Care Cost Drivers: The facts*, Toronto: Canadian Institute for Health Information.

CIHI (2011b) *National Health Expenditure Trends, 1975 to 2011*, Toronto: Canadian Institute for Health Information.

Clements, D. (2004) *What Counts? Interpreting evidence-based decision-making for management and policy*, Ottawa: Canadian Health Services Research Foundation.

Cohen, M.J. (2010) "Pursuing sustainable mobility in the face of rival societal aspirations." *Research Policy*, 39(4): 459–470.

Colin-Thomé, D., and Belfield, G. (2004) "Improving chronic disease management." *Department of Health*, 1–6.

Collins, H.M., and Evans R. (2002) "The third wave of science studies: Studies of expertise and experience." *Social Studies of Science*, 32(2): 235–296.

Comas, A., Wittenberg, R., Costa-Font, J., Gori, C., Di Maio, A., Patxot, C., Pickard, L., Pozzi, A., and Rothgang, H. (2006) "Future long-term care expenditure in Germany, Spain, Italy and the United Kingdom." *Ageing Society*, 26(2): 285–302.

Cooper, C.L., Quick, J.C., and Schabracq, M.J. (2009) *International Handbook of Work and Health Psychology*, Chichester: John Wiley & Sons.

Corner, J., Wright, D., Hopkinson, J., Gunaratnam, Y., McDonald, J.W., and Foster, C. (2007) "The research priorities of patients attending UK cancer treatment centres: Findings from a modified nominal group study." *British Journal of Cancer*, 96(6): 875–881.

Corrigan, P.W., Mueser, K.T., Bond, G.R., Drake, R.E., and Solomon, P. (2007) *The Principles and Practice of Psychiatric Rehabilitation: An empirical approach*, New York: Guilford Press.

Coulter, A. (2004) "Perspectives on health technology assessment: Response from the patient's perspective." *International Journal of Technology Assessment in Health Care*, 20(1): 92–96.

Crawford, M.J., Robotham, D., Thana, L., Patterson, S., Weaver, T., Barber, R., Wykes, T., and Rose, D. (2011) "Selecting outcome measures in mental health: The views of service users." *Journal of Mental Health*, 20(4): 336–346.

Culyer, A., and Lomas, J. (2006) "Deliberative processes and evidence-informed decision making in health care: Do they work and how might we know?" *Evidence and Policy*, 2: 357–371.

Dane, C. (1980) *Geschiedenis van de ziekenverpleging*, Utrecht: Lemma.

Dankers, J., and van der Linden, J. (1996) *Van regenten en patiënten: de geschiedenis van de willem arntsz stichting: Huis en hoeve, van der hoevenkliniek en dennendal*, Amsterdam: Boom.

Davidoff, F., Haynes, B., Sackett, D., and Smith, R. (1995) "Priority setting and the NHS: purchasing. First report sessions 1994–95." *House of Commons Papers*: 134–141.

Davies, B. (1992) *Care Management, Equity and Efficiency: The international experience*, Canterbury: University of Kent.

Davies, B. (1994) "Improving the case management process." In OECD (ed.), *Caring for Frail Elderly People: New directions in care*, Social Policy Studies No. 14, Paris: OECD.

Deber, R.B. (2003) "Health care reform: Lessons from Canada." *American Journal of Public Health*, 93(1): 3–24.

De Brantes, F., Rosenthal, M.B., and Painter, M. (2009) "Building a bridge from fragmentation to accountability: The Prometheus Payment Model." *New England Journal of Medicine*, 361: 1033–1036.

De Haan, J. (2006) "How emergence arises." *Ecological Complexity*, 3(4): 293–301.

De Haan, J. (2010) *Theory, Computational and Mathematical Approaches to Societal Transitions*, Rotterdam: Erasmus University Rotterdam.

De Haan, J., and Rotmans, J. (2011) "Patterns in transitions: Understanding complex chains of change." *Technological Forecasting and Social Change*, 78(1): 90–102.

Delnoij, D., Van Merode, G., Paulus, A., and Groenewegen, P. (2000) "Does general practitioner gatekeeping curb health care expenditure?" *Journal of Health Services Research and Policy*, 5(1): 22–26.

De Nationale Denktank (2006) *Recept voor morgen. Een frisse blik op betere zorg voor chronisch zieken*, Amsterdam.

Demoulin, L., and Felius, P. (2007) *ACT-Youth Experiment Scan and Process Advice, Transition Programme in the Care*. No publisher.

Denis, J.L., Lomas, J., and Stipich, N. (2008) "Creating receptor capacity for research in the health system: The Executive Training for Research Application (EXTRA) program in Canada." *Journal of Health Services Research Policy*, 13: 1–7.

Department of Health (1998) *Modernising Social Services: Promoting independence, improving protection, raising standards*, London: Her Majesty's Stationery Office.

De Rooy, M., and Steers, T. (1971) *Hoe mis het is. Een studie over maatschappij en inrichting*. Thesis.

De Savigny, D., and Adam, T. (2009) *Systems Thinking for Health Systems Strengthening*, Geneva: World Health Organization.

De Swaan, A. (1982) *De mens is de mens een zorg: opstellen 1971–1981*, Amsterdam: Meulenhoff.

De Swaan, A. (1996) *Zorg en de staat. Welzijn, onderwijs en gezondheidszorg in Europa en de Verenigde Staten in de nieuwe tijd*, Amsterdam: Bakker.

De Wit, M., Elberse, J.E., Broerse, J.E., and Abma, T.A. (2014) "Don't forget the professional – The value of the FIRST model for guiding the structural involvement of patients in rheumatology research." *Health Expectations*, DOI 10.1111/hex.12048.

Dick, B. (2004) "Action research literature: Themes and trends." *Action Research*, 2(4): 425–444.

Directorate-General for Economic and Financial Affairs (2002a) "Incorporating the sustainability of public finances into the Stability and Growth Pact." *European Economy*, 3: 62–74.

Directorate-General for Economic and Financial Affairs (2002b) "The long-term sustainability of public finances." *European Economy*, 3: 32–36.

Dirkzwager, A.J.E., and Verhaak, P.F.M. (2007) "Patients with persistent medically unexplained symptoms in general practice: Characteristics and quality of care." *BMC Family Practice*, 8(1): 33–43.

Dirven, J., Rotmans, J., and Verkaik, A. (2002) *Samenleving in transitie: Een vernieuwend gezichtspunt*, Den Haag: Innovatie Netwerk Groene Ruimte en Agrocluster.

Dixon, A., and Mossialos, E. (eds) (2002) *Health Care Systems in Eight Countries: Trends and challenges*, London: The London School of Economics and Political Science.

Djellal, F., and Gallouj, F. (2007) "Innovation in hospitals: A survey of the literature." *European Journal of Health Economics*, 8: 181–193.

Docteur, E. (2001) "Measuring the quality of care in different setting." *Health Care Financing Review*, 22(3): 59–70.

Drehborg, K.H. (1996) "Essence of backcasting." *Futures*, 28(9): 813–828.

Dudley, G., and Chatterjee, K. (2012) "The dynamics of regime strength and instability: Policy challenges to the dominance of the private care in the United Kingdom." In F.W. Geels, R. Kemp, G. Dudley, and G. Lyons (eds), *Automobility in Transition? A socio-technical analysis of sustainable transport*, New York: Routledge, pp. 83–103.

Elberse, J.E. (2012) *Changing the Health Research System: Patient participation in health research*, 's-Hertogenbosch: Uitgeverij BOXPress.

Elberse, J.E., Caron-Flinterman, J.F., and Broerse, J.E.W (2011) "Patient–expert partnerships in research: How to stimulate inclusion of patient perspectives." *Health Expectations*, 14(3): 225–239.

Elberse, J.E., Caron-Flinterman, J.F., and De Cock-Buning, T. (2007) *Naar een gezamenlijke visie op onderzoek bij kinderen met een aangeboren hartafwijking*, Amsterdam: Athena Institute, VU University.

Elberse, J.E., Pittens, C.A.C.M., De Cock-Buning, T., and Broerse, J.E.W. (2012b) "Patient involvement in a scientific advisory process: Setting the research agenda for medical products." *Health Policy*, 107(2): 231–242.

Elberse, J.E., Laan, D., De Cock-Buning, T., Teunissen, T., Broerse, J., and De Boer, W. (2012a) "Patient involvement in research agenda setting for respiratory research in the Netherlands." *European Respiratory Journal*, 40(2): 508–510.

Elwyn, G., Frosch, D., Volandes, A.E., Edwards, A., and Montori, V.M. (2010) "Investing in deliberation: A definition and classification of decision support interventions for people facing difficult health decisions." *Medical Decision Making*, 30(6): 701–711.

Elzen, B., Geels, F.W., and Green, K. (2004) *System Innovation and the Transition to Sustainability: Theory, evidence and policy*, Cheltenham and Camberley: Edward Elgar.

Emanuel, E.J. (1996) "Cost savings at the end of life: What do the data show?" *JAMA*, 275(24): 1907–1914.

Emirbayer, M., and Johnson, V. (2008) "Bourdieu and organizational analysis." *Theory and Society*, 37(1): 1–44.

Emirbayer, M., and Mische, A. (1998) "What is agency?" *American Journal of Sociology*, 103(4): 962–1023.

Engel, H., and Engels, D. (2000) *Case Management in Various National Elderly Assistance Systems*, Koln: Kohlhammer.

ENWHP (1997) "The Luxembourg declaration on workplace health promotion in the European Union." Paper presented at European Network for Workplace Health Promotion Meeting, November 27–28, Luxembourg.

Epstein, S. (2008) "Patients groups and health movements." In O.A.E.J. Hackett, M. Lynch, and J. Wajcman, *The Handbook of Science and Technologies Studies*, Boston, MA: The MIT Press, pp. 499–539.

Erasmus, D. (1518) *De lof der geneeskunde*.

Eriksson, M., and Lindström, B. (2008) "A salutogenic interpretation of the Ottawa Charter." *Health Promotion International*, 23(2): 190–199.

Essink, D.R. (2012) *Sustainable Health Systems: The role of change agents in health system innovation*, 's-Hertogenbosch: Uitgeverij BoxPress.

Essink, D.R., Spanjers, R., Broerse, J.E.W., and De Cock-Buning, T.J. (2010) "Sustainable health systems: The role of change agents in health system innovation." In J.E.W. Broerse and J.F.G. Bunders (eds), *Transitions in Health Systems: Dealing with persistent problems*, Amsterdam: VU University press, pp. 87–112.

European Commission (2006) "The impact of ageing on public expenditure: Projections for the EU25 Member States on pensions, health care, long-term care, education and unemployment transfers (2004–2050)." Economic Policy Committee, *European Economy*, No.1/2006.

Family Caregiver Alliance (2001) *Fact Sheet: Selected caregiver statistics*, San Francisco, CA: Family Caregiver Alliance.

Field, J., and Peck, E. (2003) "Mergers and acquisitions in the private sector: What are the lessons for health and social services?" *Social Policy Administration*, 37: 742–755.

Figueras, J. (2003) "Health system reforms and post-modernism." *European Journal of Public Health*, 13: 79–82.

Fine, M., and Glendinning, C. (2005) "Dependence, independence or interdependence? Revisiting the concepts of 'care' and 'dependency'." *Ageing Society*, 25: 601–621.

Fisher, E., Wennberg, D.E., Stukel, T.A., Gottlieb, D., Lucas, F.L., and Pinder, E. (2003a) "The health implications of regional variations in Medicare spending. Part 1: Utilization of services and quality of care." *Annual Journal of Internal Medicine*, 138(4): 273–287.

Fisher, E., Wennberg, D.E., Stukel, T.A., Gottlieb, D., Lucas, F.L., and Pinder, E. (2003b) "The health implications of regional variations in Medicare spending. Part 2: Health outcomes and satisfaction with care." *A Journal of Internal Medicine*, 138(4): 288–298.

Fitzpatrick, T. (1996) "Postmodernism, welfare and radical politics." *Journal of Social Policy*, 25: 303–320.

Flemons, W. (2011) "Conclusion: Supporting the individual as change agent and the organization as responsive to change." In T. Sullivan and J. Denis (2011), *Building Better Healthcare for Canada*, Montreal: McGill-Queen's University Press.

Flemons, W., Conly, J., and Eagle, C. (2008) *Emergency Department Overcrowding: Effecting system level change to improve patient flow through tertiary care emergency departments*, Final Intervention Project Report, Ottawa: Canadian Health Services Research Foundation.

Foucault, M. (2003) *The Birth of the Clinic: An archaeology of medical perception*, London: Routledge.

Fransen, C. (2009) *More than Research Subjects? The perspective of pharmaceutical companies on the active involvement of patient organisations in clinical trials in Europe*, Amsterdam: Athena Institute, VU University.

Freidson, E. (2001) *Professionalism, the Third Logic. On the practice of knowledge*, Chicago, IL: University of Chicago Press.

Frenk, J. (1992) "Balancing relevance and excellence: Organizational responses to link research with decision making." *Social Science and Medicine*, 35(11): 1397–1404.

Frodeman, R. (2000) "Science and the public self." *Technology in Society*, 22(3): 341–352.

Fuller, S. (2000) *The Governance of Science: Ideology and the future of the open society*, Buckingham: Open University Press.

Gallud, J., Guirao-Goris, J.A., Ruiz Hontangas, A., and Muñoz León, M. (2004) *Plan para la Mejora de Atención Domiciliaria de la Comunidad Valenciana 2004–2007*, Valencia: Generalitat Valenciana, Conselleria de Sanitat.

Garcés, J. (2000) *La nueva sostenibilidad social*, Barcelona: Ariel.

Garcés, J., Carretero, S., and Ródenas, F. (2011) *Readings of the Social Sustainability Theory: Applications to long-term care field*, Valencia: Tirant lo Blanch.

Garcés, J., Carretero, S., Ródenas, F., and Alemán, C. (2010a) "A review of programs to alleviate the burden of informal caregivers of dependent persons." *Archives of Gerontology and Geriatrics*, 50(3): 254–259.

Garcés, J., Carretero, S., Ródenas, F., and Sanjosé, V. (2008) "Variables related to the informal caregivers' burden of dependent senior citizens in Spain." *Archives of Gerontology and Geriatrics*, 48(3): 372–378.

Garcés, J., Carretero, S., Ródenas, F., and Vivancos, M. (2010b) "The care of the informal caregiver's burden by the Spanish public system of social welfare: A review." *Archives of Gerontology and Geriatrics*, 50(3): 250–253.

Garcés, J., Ródenas, F., and Hammar, T. (2013) "Converging methods to link social and health care systems and informal care – Confronting Nordic and Mediterranean approaches." In K. Leichsenring, J. Bilings, and H. Nies (eds), *Long-term Care in Europe*, Basingstoke and New York: Palgrave Macmillan.

Garcés, J., Ródenas, F., and Sanjosé, V. (2003) "Towards a new welfare state: The social sustainability principle and health care strategies." *Health Policy*, 65: 201–215.

Garcés, J., Ródenas, F., and Sanjosé, V. (2004) "Care needs among the dependent population in Spain: An empirical approach." *Health Social Care Community*, 12(6): 466–474.

Garcés, J., Ródenas, F., and Sanjosé, V. (2006) "Suitability of the health and social care resources for persons requiring long-term care in Spain: An empirical approach." *Health Policy*, 76: 121–130.

García-Armesto, S., Abadía-Taira, M.B., Durán, A., Hernández-Quevedo, C., and Bernal-Delgado, E. (2011) *Spain: Health system review. Health Systems in Transition*, Copenhagen: World Health Organization.

Geels, F.W. (2002) *Understanding the Dynamics of Technological Transitions: A co-evolutionary and socio-technical analysis*, Enschede: Twente University Press.

Geels, F.W. (2004) "From sectoral systems of innovation to socio-technical systems: Insight about dynamics and change from sociology and institutional theory." *Research Policy*, 33(6): 897–920.

Geels, F.W. (2005) *Technological Transitions and System Innovations: A co-evolutionary and socio-technical analysis*, Cheltenham: Edward Elgar.

Geels, F.W. (2006) "The hygienic transition from cesspools to sewer systems (1840–1930): The dynamics of regime transformation." *Research Policy*, 35(7): 1069–1082.

Geels, F.W., and Raven, R.P.J.M. (2006) "Non-linearity and expectations in niche-development trajectories: Ups and downs in Dutch biogas development (1973–2003)." *Technology Analysis and Strategic Management*, 18(3/4): 375–392.

Geeels, F.W., and Schot, J. (2007) "Typology of sociotechnical transition pathways." *Research Policy*, 36(3): 399–417.

Geels, F.W., and Schot, J. (2010) "The dynamics of transitions: A sociotechnical perspective." In J. Grin, J. Rotmans, and J. Schot (eds), *Transitions to Sustainable Development: New directions in the study of long-term change*, New York: Routledge, pp. 9–101.

Geels, F.W., Hekkert, M., and Jacobsson, S. (2008) "The dynamics of sustainable innovation journeys." *Technology Analysis and Strategic Management*, 20(5): 521–536.

Geels, F.W., Kemp, R., Dudley, G., and Lyons, G. (eds) (2012) *Automobility in Transition? A socio-technical analysis of sustainable transport*, New York: Routledge.

Generalitat Valenciana (2004) *Plan para la mejora de la atención domiciliaria en la Comunidad Valenciana (IMAD), 2004–2007*, Valencia: Generalitat Valenciana, Conselleria de Sanitat.

George, V., and Miller, S. (1994) "The Thatcherite attempt to square the circle." In V. George and S. Miller (eds), *Social Policy Towards 2000: Squaring the welfare circle*, London, Routledge.

Gezondheidsraad (2010) *New and needed. Medical products that make life better*, The Hague: Gezondheidsraad (Health Council of the Netherlands).

Giddens, A. (1984) *The Constitution of Society: Outline of the theory of structuration*, Cambridge: Polity Press.

Giddens, A. (1991) *Modernity and Self-identity: Self and society in the late modern age*, Stanford, CA: Stanford University Press.

Gielen, A-J., and Grin, J. (2010) "De betekenissen van 'evidence based handelen' en de aard van 'evidence': Lessen rond rugscholen en radicalisering." In D. Verlet and C. Devos (eds), *Efficiëntie en effectiviteit van de publieke sector in de weegschaal*, Brussels: Studiedienst van de Vlaamse Regering, pp. 59–78.

Gilbert, N., and Terrell, P. (2004) *Dimensions of Social Welfare Policy* (6th edn), New York: Allyn & Bacon.

Glaser, B.G., and Strauss, A.L. (1967) *The Discovery of Grounded Theory: Strategies for qualitative research*, Chicago, IL: Aldine.

Glaser, E.M., Abelson, H.H., and Garrison, K.N. (1983) *Putting Knowledge to Use*, San Francisco, CA: Jossey-Bass.

Godman, B., Malmström, R.E., Diogene, E., Gray, A., Jayathissa, S., Timoney, A., Acurcio, F., Alkan, A., Brzezinska, A., Bucsics, A., and Campbell, S.M. (2015) "Are new models needed to optimize the utilization of new medicines to sustain healthcare systems?" *Expert Review of Clinical Pharmacology*, 8(1): 77–94.

Goffmann, E. (1961) *Asylums. Essays on the social situation of mental patients and other inmates*, New York: Doubleday Anchor.

Graetz, B. (1993) "Health consequences of employment and unemployment: Longitudinal evidence for young men and women." *Social Science and Medicine*, 36(6): 715–724.

Grant-Pearce, C., Miles, I., and Hills, P. (1998) *Mismatches in Priorities for Health Research between Professionals and Consumers: Manchester*, Manchester: Manchester University Press.

Greenwood, D.J., and Levin, M. (1998) *Introduction to Action Research: Social research for social change*, Thousand Oaks, CA: Sage.

Grimaldo, F., Orduna, J.M., Lozano, M., Ródenas, F., and Garcés, J. (2014) "Towards a simulator of integrated long-term care systems for elderly people." *International Journal on Artificial Intelligence Tools*, 23(1): 1440005.

Grimaldo, F., Ródenas, F., Lozano, M., Carretero, S., Orduña, J.M., Garcés, J., Duato, J., and Fatas, E. (2013) "Design of an ICT tool for decision making in social and health policies." In M.M. Cruz-Cunha, I.M. Miranda, and P. Gonçalves (eds), *Handbook of Research on ICTs for Human-centered Healthcare and Social Care Services*, Hershey, PA: IGI Global Publications, pp. 802–819.

Grin, J. (2000) "Vision assessment to support shaping 21st century society? Techno-logy assessment as a tool for political judgement." In J. Grin and A. Grunwald (eds), *Vision Assessment: Shaping technology in 21st century society. Towards a repertoire for technology assessment*, Heidelberg: Springer Verlag, pp. 9–30.

Grin, J. (2004) "Health technology assessment between our health care system and our health: Exploring the potential of reflexive HTA." *Poiesis and Praxis: International Journal of Technology*, 2(2–3): 157–174.

Grin, J. (2006) "Reflexive modernization as a governance issue – or: Designing and shaping re-structuration." In J.P. Voß, D. Bauknecht, and R. Kemp (eds), *Reflexive Governance for Sustainable Development*, Cheltenham: Edward Elgar, pp. 57–81.

Grin, J. (2008) "The multi-level perspective and the design of system innovations." In J.C.J.M. Van den Bergh and F. Bruinsma (eds), *Managing the Transition to Renewable Energy: Theory and practice from local, regional and macro perspectives*, Cheltenham: Edward Elgar, pp. 74–80.

Grin, J. (2010) "Understanding transitions from a governance perspective." In J. Grin, J. Rotmans, and J. Schot (eds), *Transitions to Sustainable Development: New directions in the study of long-term change*, New York: Routledge, pp. 221–319.

Grin, J. (2012a) "The governance of transitions and its politics. Conceptual lessons from the earlier agricultural transition and implications for transition management." *International Journal of Sustainable Development*, 15(1–2): 72–89.

Grin, J. (2012b) "Changing government, kitchens, supermarkets, firms and farms: The governance of transitions between societal practices and supply systems." In G. Spaargaren, A. Loeber, and P. Oosterveer (eds), *Food Practices in Transition. Changing food consumption, retail and production in the age of reflexive modernity*, New York and Oxford: Routledge, pp. 35–56.

Grin, J. (forthcoming) "Recognizing and understanding patient agency as a key pre-requisite for health care transitions in contemporary welfare states: A transition strategy focusing on transforming medical knowledge and technology development." *Technological Forecasting and Social Change*.

Grin, J., Felix, F., Bos, B., and Spoelstra, S. (2004) "Practices for reflexive design: Lessons from a Dutch programme on sustainable agriculture." *International Journal of Foresight and Innovation Policy*, 1(1–2): 126–149.

Grin, J., and Loeber, A. (2007) "Theories of policy learning: Agency, structure and change." In F. Fischer, G.J. Miller, and M.S. Sidney (eds), *Handbook of Public Policy Analysis. Theory, Politics, and Methods*, Abingdon: CRC Press/Taylor & Francis Group, pp. 201–219.

Grin, J., Rotmans, J., and Schot, J. (eds) (2010) *Transitions Toward Sustainable Development: New directions in the study of long-term change*, New York: Routledge.

Grin, J., Schot, J., and Rotmans, R. (2011) "On patterns and agency in transition dynamics: Some key insights from the KSI programme." *Environmental Innovation and Societal Transitions*, 1(1): 76–81.

Grin, J., ter Haar-van Twillert, E., and Stevens, P. (2008) *Kwalitatieve rapportage van de monitor zorg-op-afstand, zorg-op-afstand: altijd aanwezig en juist dichtbij*, Utrecht: Actiz.

Grin, J., and Van de Graaf, H. (1996) "Technology assessment as learning." *Science, Technology and Human Values*, 21(1): 72–99.

Grin, J., and Van Staveren, A. (2007) *Werken aan systeeminnovaties; Lessen uit de praktijk van InnovatieNetwerk*, Assen: Koninklijke Van Gorcum.

Grin, J., and Weterings, R. (2005) "Reflexive monitoring of system innovative projects: Strategic nature and relevant competences." *Sixth Open Meeting of the Human Dimensions of Global Environmental Change Research Community*, Bonn: University of Bonn.

Gröne, O., and Garcia-Barbero, M. (2002) *Trends in Integrated Care – Reflections on conceptual issues*, Copenhagen: World Health Organization.

Grundy, E., and Glaser, K. (2000) "Socio-demographic differences in the onset and progression of disability in early old age: A longitudinal study." *Age Ageing*, 29: 149–157.

Gurwitz, J.H., and Goldberg, R.J. (2011) "Age-based exclusions from cardiovascular clinical trials: Implications for elderly individuals (and for all of us)." *Archives of Internal Medicine*, 171(6): 557–558.

Guyatt, G., Rennie, D., Meade, M., and Cook, D. (2008) *Users' Guides to the Medical Literature: A manual for evidence-based clinical practice* (2nd edn), New York: McGraw-Hill.

Guyatt, G., Cairns, J., Churchill, D., Cook, D., and Haynes, B. (1992) "Evidence-based medicine: A new approach to teaching the practice of medicine." *The Journal of the American Medical Association*, 268(17): 2420–2425.

Gwatkin, D.R. (2001) "The need for equity oriented health sector reforms." *International Journal of Epidemiology*, 30: 720–723.

Hall, P. (1993) "Policy paradigms, social learning and the state: The case of economic policy making." *Comparative Politics*, 25: 275–296.

Hall, P., and Thelen, K. (2006) *Institutional Change in Varieties of Capitalism*. Paper presented at the Europeanists Conference, Chicago, IL.

Hanley, B., Bradburn, J., Barnes, M., Evans, C., Goodare, H., Kelson, M., Kent, A., Oliver, S., Thomas, S., and Wallcraft, J. (2004) *Involving the Public in NHS, Public Health, and Social Care Research: Briefing notes for researchers*, INVOLVE.

Hanney, S.R. and Gonzalez Block, M.A. (2006) "Building health research systems to achieve better health." *Health Research Policy Systems*, 4: 10.

Hanson, A. (2007) *Workplace Health Promotion: A salutogenic approach*, Bloomington, VA: Author House.

Hardon, A., and Van Haastrecht, E. (2005) "Socio-cultural and political factors which facilitate and constrain representation and analysis of diversity in clinical research." In N.F. Wieringa, A.P. Hardon, K. Stronks, and A. M'charek (eds), *Diversity among Patients in Medical Practice: Challenges and implications for clinical research*, Amsterdam: University of Amsterdam.

Harrison, M.I. (2004) *Implementing Change in Health Systems*, London: Sage.

Harrison, S., and Pollitt, C. (1994) *Controlling Health Professionals: The future of work and organization in the National Health Service*, State of Health Series, Philadelphia: Open University Press.

Havens, B. (1999) *Home-based and Long-term Care*, Geneva: World Health Organization.

Hébert, R. (2002) *Integrated Service Delivery for Frail Elderly People. The Canadian experience*, Valencia: Valencia Forum Spain.

Helderman, J.K., Schut, F.T., Van der Grinten, T.E.D., and Van de Ven, W.P.M.M. (2005) "Market-oriented health care reforms and policy learning in the Netherlands." *Journal of Health Politics, Policy and Law*, 30(1–2): 189–210.

Hendriks, C.M. (2008) "On inclusion and network governance: The democratic disconnect of Dutch energy transitions." *Public Administration*, 86(4): 1009–1031.

Hendriks, C.M., and Grin, J. (2007) "Contextualizing reflexive governance: The politics of Dutch transitions to sustainability." *Journal of Environmental Policy and Planning*, 9(3–4): 333–350.

Hendrix, H., Konings, J., Doesburg, J., and Groot., M.D. (1991) *Functionele samenwerking. Werkboek voor samenwerkingsverbanden in de zorgsector*, Baarn: H. Nelissen BV.

Henneman, P. (2008) *Watermerk. 1e Zeeuwse transitieagenda*. Rotterdam: DRIFT.

Hessels, L. (2010) *Science and the Struggle of Relevance*, Oisterwijk: Uitgeverij BOXpress.

Hewlett, S., De Wit, M.D., Richards, P., Quest, E., Hughes, R., Heiberg, T., and Kirwan, J. (2006) "Patients and professionals as research partners: Challenges, practicalities, and benefits." *Arthritis and Rheumatism-Arthritis Care and Research*, 55(4): 676–680.

Hirdes, J.P., Ljunggren, G., Morris, J.N., Frijters, D.H., Finne Soveri, H., and Gray, L. (2008) "Reliability of the interRAI suite of assessment instruments: A 12-country study of an integrated health information system." *BMC Health Services Research*, 8: 277.

Hisschemöller, M., and Hoppe, R. (1995) "Coping with intractable controversies: The case for problem structuring in policy design and analysis." *Knowledge, Technology and Policy*, 8(4): 40–60.

Hisschemöller, M., Hoppe, R., Dunn, W.N., and Ravetz, J. (2001) "Knowledge, power and participation in environmental policy analysis." *Policy Studies Review Annual, Volume 12*, New Brunswick: Transaction Publishers.

Hoes, A.C., Beekman, V., Regeer, B.J., and Bunders, J.F.G. (2011) "Unravelling the dynamics of adopting novel technologies: An account of how the closed greenhouse opened-up." *International Journal of Foresight and Innovation Policy*, 8(1): 37–59.

Hoeven-Mulder, H.B., Leerlooijer, J.N., and Van Hattem, M. (2014) *Evaluatie Pilot Buurtzorg Jong in Putten*, Putten: Gemeente Putten.

Hoey, J. (2000) "Time for a new Canada Health Act." *Canadian Medical Association Journal*, 163: 6.

Hoffman, J. (2013) "Theorizing power in transition studies: The role of creativity and novel practices in structural change." *Policy Sciences*, 46(3): 257–275.

Hoffman, J., and Loeber, A.M.C. (2016) "Exploring the micro-politics in transitions from a practice perspective: The case of greenhouse innovations in the Netherlands." *Journal of Environmental Policy and Planning*, 18(5): 692–711.

Hoogendoorn, D. (1978) "De relatie tussen de hoogte van de perinatale sterfte en de plaats van bevalling: Thuis, dan wel in het ziekenhuis." *Nederlands Tijdschrift Voor Geneeskunde*, 122: 1171–1178.

Hoogma, R. (2000) *Exploiting Technological Niches: Strategies for experimental introduction of electric vehicles*, PhD thesis, Enschede: Twente University Press.

Hoogma, R., Kemp, R., Schot, J., and Truffer, B. (2002) *Experimenting for Sustainable Transport: The approach of strategic niche management*, London: Spon Press.

Horton, R. (2013) "Non-communicable diseases: 2015 to 2025." *The Lancet*, 381(9866): 509–510.

Hotta, S. (2014) *Comprehensive Community Care in the Netherlands: Enhancing care provision system and securing care workers*, JILPT Research Report No. 167, Tokyo.

Houtman, I.L.D. (1997) *Trends in arbeid en gezondheid*, Amsterdam: NIA/TNO.

Houwaart, E.S. (1991) *De hygiënisten: Artsen, staat and volksgezondheid*, Groningen: Historische Uitgeverij Groningen.

Houwaart, E.S. (1996) *Het ziekenhuis: De ontwikkeling van het ziekenhuis in de moderne tijd*, Heerlen: Open Universiteit.

Howell, J.D. (1995) *Technology in the Hospital: Transforming patient care in the early twentieth century*, Baltimore, MD, and London: Johns Hopkins University Press.

Huber, M., Knottnerus, J.A., Green, L., Van der Horst, H., Jadad, A.R., Kromhout, D., Leonard, B., Lorig, K., Loureiro, M.I., Van der Meer, J.W.M., Schnabel, P., Smith, R., Van Weel, C., and Smid, H. (2011) "How should we define health?" *British Medical Journal*, 343(6): d4163.

Illich, I. (1975) *Het medisch bedrijf, een bedreiging voor de gezondheid?* Baarn: Het Wereldvenster.

Illich, I. (1976) *Limits to Medicine; Medical nemesis: The expropriation of health*, New York: Pantheon Books.

Ilmarinen, J. (2009) "Work ability: A comprehensive concept for occupational health research and prevention." *Scandinavian Journal of Work, Environment and Health*: 1–5.

ILO (2000) *Mental Health and Work: Impact, issues and good practices*, Geneva: ILO.

Institute of Medicine (2011) *Allied Health Workforce and Services – Workshop summary*. Institute of Medicine.

Instituto Nacional de Estadística (2012) *Cifras de Población y Censos Demográficos*, Madrid.

Jackson, R., and Howe, N. (2003) *The Aging Vulnerability Index. An assessment of the capacity of twelve developed countries to meet the aging challenge*, Washington, DC: Center for Strategic and International Studies and Watson Wyatt Worldwide.

Jacobson, N., Butterill D., and Goering, P. (2004) "Organizational factors that influence university-based researchers' engagement in knowledge transfer activities." *Science Communication*, 25(3): 246–259.

Jameton, A., and McGuire, C. (2002) "Toward sustainable health-care services: Principles, challenges, and a process." *International Journal of Sustainability in Higher Education*, 3(2): 113–127.

Jankauskienė, D., and Jankauskaitė, I. (2011) "Access and quality of health care system by opinion of patients in ten European countries." *Management in Health*, 15(3): 31–39.

Jansen, M.W.J., De Vries, N.K., Kok, G., and Van Oers, H.A. (2008) "Collaboration between practice, policy and research in local public health in the Netherlands." *Health Policy*, 86(2–3): 295–307.

Jones, M., and Basser, L.E. (1999) *Disability, Divers-ability, and Legal Change*, The Hague: Martinus Nijhoff.

Jordan, A., McCall, J., Moore, W., Reid, H., and Steward, D. (2006) *Health Systems in Transition: The Northern Ireland (NI) Report*, Copenhagen: WHO Regional Office for Europe, European Observatory on Health Systems and Policies.

Jordan, J., Dowswell, T., Harrison, S., Lilford, R.J., and Mort, M. (1998) "Health needs assessment: Whose priorities? Listening to users and the public." *British Medical Journal*, 316(7145): 1668–1670.

Kane, R.L., Chen, Q., Finch, M., Blewett, L., Burns, R., and Moskowitz, M. (2000) "The optimal outcomes of post-hospital care under Medicare." *Health Services Research*, 35(3): 615–661.

Kappen, T., and Van Dulmen, S., (2008) "General practitioners' responses to the initial presentation of medically unexplained symptoms: A quantitative analysis." *BioPsychoSocial Medicine*, 2: 22.

Keizer, B., and Bless, R. (2010) *Pilot Study on the Position of Health Consumer and Patients' Organisations in Seven EU Countries*, The Hague: ZonMw.

Kemp, R., Geels, F.W., and Dudley, G. (2012) "Introduction: Sustainability trans-ition in the automobility regime and the need for a new perspective." In F.W. Geels, R. Kemp, G. Dudley, and G. Lyons (eds), *Automobility in Transition? A socio-technical analysis of sustainable transport*, New York: Routledge, pp. 3–28.

Kemp, R., and Loorbach, D. (2003) *Governance for Sustainability through Transition Management*, unpublished manuscript.

Kemp, R., Loorbach, D., and Rotmans, J. (2007) "Transition management as a model for managing processes of co-evolution." *The International Journal of Sustainable Development and World Ecology*, 14: 78–91.

Kemp, R., and Rotmans, J. (2005) "The management of the co-evolution of technical, environmental and social systems." In M. Weber and J. Hemmelskamp, *Towards Environmental Innovation Systems*, Berlin and Heidelberg: Springer.

Kemp, R., Schot, J., and Hoogma, R. (1998) "Regime shifts to sustainability through processes of niche formation. The approach of strategic niche management." *Technology Analysis and Strategic Management*, 10(2): 175–195.

Kerkhoff, A.H.M. (1994) *Honderd jaar gemeentelijke geneeskundige en gezondheidsdiensten*, Bussum: Coutinho.

Kern, F., and Smith, A. (2008) "Restructuring energy systems for sustainability? Energy transition policy in the Netherlands." *Energy Policy*, 36(11): 4093–4103.

Kingo, L. (2010) "Corporate responsibility as a driver of innovation in healthcare." In J.E.W. Broerse and J.F.G. Bunders (eds), *Transitions in Health Systems: Dealing with persistent problems*, Amsterdam: VU University Press, pp. 129–168.

Kirkpatrick, D.L. (1994) *Evaluating Training Programs: The four levels*, San Francisco, CA: Berrett-Koehler.

Kirwan, J.R., Hewlett, S.E., Heiberg, T., Hughes, R.A., and Carr, M. (2005) "Incorporating the patient perspective into outcome assessment in rheumatoid arthritis – Progress at OMERACT 7." *Journal of Rheumatology*, 32: 2250–2256.

Kirwan, J.R., Newman, S., Tugwell, P.S., Wells, G.A., and Hewlett, S. (2009) "Progress on incorporating the patient perspective in outcome assessment in rheumatology and the emergence of life impact measures at OMERACT 9." *Journal of Rheumatology*, 36(9): 2071–2076.

Kjeken, I., Ziegler, C., Skrolsvik, J., Bagge, J., and Smedslund, G. (2010) "How to develop patient-centered research: Some perspectives based on surveys among people with rheumatic diseases in Scandinavia." *Physical Therapy*, 90(3): 450–460.

Knapp, M.R.J., Hardy, B., and Forder, J. (2001) "Commissioning for quality: Ten years of social care markets in England." *Journal of Social Policy*, 30(2): 283–306.

Knepper, S. (2007) "Achthonderd meter in één uur tien." *AMC Magazine*: 61.

Knoop, A., and Schuiringa, K. (1998) *Door allen voor allen, een heerlijk streven! Een kleine geschiedenis van het kruiswerk in Nederland*, Nederlands: Openluchtmuseum.

Kodner, D.L., and Spreeuwenberg, C. (2002) "Integrated care: Meaning, logic, applications, and implications – a discussion paper." *International Journal of Integrated Care*, 2(4). DOI: http://doi.org/10.5334/ijic.67.

Koelen, M.A., and Van den Ban, A.W. (2004) *Health education and health promotion*, Wageningen: Wageningen Academic Publishers.

Koelen, M.A., Vaandrager, L., and Wagemakers, A. (2008) "What is needed for coordinated action for health?" *Family Practice*, 25(Suppl.1): i25–i31.

Kompier, M., and Cooper, C.L. (1999) *Preventing Stress, Improving Productivity: European case studies in the workplace*, London: Routledge.

Kotlikoff, L., and Hagist, C. (2005) *Who's Going Broke?* Cambridge: National Bureau of Economic Research.

Krol, L. (1985) *De consument als leidend voorwerp in de gezondheidszorg*, Amsterdam: University of Amsterdam.

Kukk, P., Moors, E.H.M., and Hekkert, M.P. (forthcoming) "Institutional power play in innovation systems: The case of Herceptin." *Resarch Policy*.

Lalonde, M. (1974) *A New Perspective on the Health of Canadians: A working document*, Ottawa: Government of Canada.

La Revue Prescrire (2005) "Innovation en panne et prises de risques." *La Revue Prescrire*, 25(258): 139–148.

Lauridsen, E.H., and Jørgensen, U. (2010) "Sustainable transition of electronic products through waste policy." *Research Policy*, 39(4): 486–494.

Lavis, J.N., Robertson, D., Woodside, J.M., McLeod, C.B., and Abelson, J. (2003) "How can research organizations more effectively transfer research knowledge to decision makers?" *Milbank Quarterly*, 81(2): 221.

Leenen, H.J.J. (1991) "De verdeling van de schaarse middelen in de gezondheidszorg." *Nederlands Tijdschrift Voor Geneeskunde*: 904–908.

Le Fanu, J. (1999) "The fall of medicine." *Prospect Magazine*, July 20.

Le Fanu, J. (2000) *The Rise and Fall of Modern Medicine*, London: Abacus.

Leichsenring, K., and Alaszewski, A. (eds) (2004) *Providing Integrated Health and Social Care Services to Older Persons. A European overview of issues at stake*, Aldershot: Ashgate.

Leichsenring, K., Billings, J., and Nies, H. (eds) (2013) *Long-term Care in Europe: Improving policy and practice*, Basingstoke and New York: Palgrave Macmillan.

Levy, S.B., and Marshall, B. (2004) "Antibacterial resistance worldwide: Causes, challenges and responses." *National Medicine*, 10(12 Suppl): S122–S129.

Liberati, A. (1997) "Consumer participation in research and health care." *British Medical Journal*, 315(7107): 499.

Lieburg, M.J., Snelders, H.A.M., Palm, L.C., Visser, R.P.W., and Juch, A. (1997) *De medisch specialisten in de Nederlandsche gezondheidszorg: Hun manifestatie en consolidatie 1890–1941*, Rotterdam: Erasmus Publishing.

Lindblom, C.E. (1979) "Still muddling, not yet through." *Public Administration Review*, 39: 517–526.

Lindenmeyer, A., Hearnshaw, H., Sturt, J., Ormerod, R., and Aitchison, G. (2007) "Assessment of the benefits of user involvement in health research from the Warwick Diabetes Care Research User Group: A qualitative case study." *Health Expectations*, 10(3): 268–277.

Lissandrello, E., and Grin, J. (2011) "Reflexive planning as design and work: Lessons from the Port of Amsterdam." *Planning Theory and Practice*, 12(2): 223–248.

LOC (2009) *Waardevolle zorg. over de toekomst van de gezondheidszorg 2010–2050*, Utrecht: Landelijk Overleg Cliëntenraden.

Lodenstein E., Dieleman, M., Gerretsen, B., and Broerse, J.E.W. (2013) "A realist synthesis of the effect of social accountability interventions on health service providers' and policymakers' responsiveness." *Systematic Reviews*, 2: 98.

Loeber, A. (2004) *Practical Wisdom in the Risk Society. Methods and practice of interpretive analysis on questions of sustainable development*, PhD thesis, University of Amsterdam.

Loeber, A., Van Mierlo, B., Grin, J., and Leeuwis, C. (2007) "The practical value of theory: Conceptualising learning in pursuit of a sustainable development." In A.E.J. Wals (ed.), *Social Learning towards a Sustainable World*, Wageningen: Wageningen Academic Publishers.

Logdon, R.G., Gibbons, L.E., McCurry, S.M., and Teri, L. (1999) "Quality of life in Alzheimer's disease: Patient and caregiver reports." *Gerontologist*, 5: 21–32.

Lomas, J. (2000) "Connecting research and policy." *Canadian Journal of Policy Research*, 1(1): 140–144.

Lomas, J. (2007) "The in-between world of knowledge brokering." *British Medical Journal*, 334: 129–132.

Longley, M. (2004) *Health Systems in Transition: The Welsh Report*, Copenhagen: European Observatory on Health Systems and Policies.

Loorbach, D. (2002) "Transition management: Governance for sustainability." Paper presented at the International Dimensions of Human Change, Berlin.

Loorbach, D. (2007) *Transition Management: New mode of governance for sustainable development*, Utrecht: International Books.

Loorbach, D., and Rotmans, J. (2006) "Managing transitions for sustainable development." In X. Olshoorn and A.J. Wieczorek (eds), *Understanding Industrial Transformation. Views from different disciplines*, Dordrecht: Springer, pp. 187–206.

Loorbach, D., and Rotmans, J. (2010) "Part II: Towards a better understanding of transitions and their governance: A systemic and reflexive approach." In J. Grin, J. Rotmans, and J. Schot (eds), *Transitions to Sustainable Development: New directions in the study of long-term change*, New York: Routledge.

Lotgering, F.K. (2003) *Verloskunde anno 2003. Authority based, evidence biased*, Nijmegen: SUN.

Luhmann, N. (1984) *Soziale systemen*, Frankfurt am Main: Suhrkampf.

Maarse, J.A.M. (2001) "De hervorming van de gezondheidszorg. Enkele politieke aspecten." *Bestuurskunde*, 10: 186–196.

Macinko, J., Starfield, B., and Shi, L. (2003) "The contribution of primary care systems to health outcomes within Organization for Economic Cooperation and Development (OECD) countries, 1970–1998." *Health Services Research*, 38: 831–865.

Mangham, L.J., and Hanson, K. (2010) "Scaling up in international health: What are the key issues?" *Health Policy and Planning*, 25: 85–96.

Marland, H. (2001) "Smooth, speedy, painless, and still midwife delivered? The Dutch midwife and childbirth technology in the early twentieth century." In A. Hardy and L. Conrad (eds), *Women and Modern Medicine*, Amsterdam: Atlanta, pp. 173–194.

Marsh, D. (2010) "Meta-theoretical issues." In D. Marsh and G. Stoker (eds), *Theory and Methods in Political Science*, Basingstoke: Palgrave, pp. 212–231.

Martineau, T.B.A., and Buchan, J (2000) "Human resource and the success of health sector reform." *Resources for Health Development Journal*, 3(4): 8–15.

McCusker, J., and Verdon, J. (2006) "Do geriatric interventions reduce emergency department visits? A systematic review." *Journals of Gerontol Series A Biological Sciences Medical Sciences.*, 61: 53–62.

McGuire, P., and Fulmer, T. (1997) "Elder abuse." In C.K. Cassel, H.J. Cohen, E.B. Larson, D.E. Meier, N.M. Resnick, L.Z. Rubenstein, and L.B. Sorenson (eds), *Geriatric Medicine*, New York: Springer.

Medawar, C., and Hardon, A.P. (2004) *Medicines Out of Control? Antidepressants and the conspiracy of goodwill*, Amsterdam: Aksant.

Medlin, C.A., Chowdhury, M., Jamison, D.T., and Measham, A.R. (2006) "Improving the health of populations: Lessons of experience." In D.T. Jamison, J.G. Breman, and A.R. Measham (eds), *Disease Control Priorities in Developing Countries* (2nd edn), New York: Oxford University Press.

Meier, V., and Werding, M. (2010) *Ageing and the Welfare State: Securing sustainability*, Munich: Center for Economic Studies and Ifo Institute for Economic Research.

Mills, A.J., and Ranson, M.K. (2012) "The design of health systems." In M.H. Merson, R.B. Black, and A. Mills, *Global Health: Diseases, programs, systems and policies*, Sudbury: Jones and Bartlett Publishers.

Ministerie van Sociale Zaken en Volksgezondheid (1966) *Volksgezondheidsnota*.

Ministerie van Volksgezondheid en Milieuhygiëne (1974) *Structuurnota Gezondheidszorg*.

Ministerie van Volksgezondheid en Milieuhygiëne (1977) *Financieel Overzicht Zorg*.

Ministerie van Volksgezondheid en Milieuhygiëne (1979) *Het beleid ter zake van de gezondheidszorg met het oog op de kostenontwikkeling*.

Ministerie van Volksgezondheid en Milieuhygiëne (1980) *Schets van de eerstelijnsgezondheidszorg*.

Ministerie van Welzijn, Volksgezondheid en Cultuur (1984) *Volksgezondheidsbeleid bij beperkte middelen*.

Mockus Parks, S., and Novielli, K.D. (2000) "A practical guide to caring for caregivers." *American Family Physician*, 15: 2215–2219.

Moens, D.P. (2010) *Aspects that Form Researchers' Attitude on Patient Involvement in Health Research*, Amsterdam: VU University Amsterdam.

Mokyr, J. (1990) *The Lever of Riches: Technological creativity and economic progress*, Oxford: Oxford University Press.

Mol, A.M. (2008) *The Logic of Care: Health and the problem of patient choice*, London: Routledge.

Mol, A.M., and Van Lieshout, P. (1989) *Ziek is het woord niet. Medicalisering, normalisering en de veranderende taal van huisartsgeneeskunde en geestelijke gezondheidszorg, 1945–1985*, Nijmegen: SUN.

Monsen, K.A., and De Blok, J. (2013) "Buurtzorg: Nurse-led community care." *Creative Nursing*, 19(3): 122–127.

Mooij, A. (1999) *De polsslag van de stad: 350 jaar academische geneeskunde in Amsterdam*, Amsterdam: De Arbeiderspers.

More, T. (1516) *Utopia*.

Moret-Hartman, M., Van der Wilt, G.J., and Grin, J. (2007) "Health technology assessment and ill-structured problems: A case study concerning the drug mebeverine." *International Journal of Technology Assessment in Health Care*, 23(3): 316–323.

Morgan, S.G., Bassett, K.L., Wright, J.M., Evans, R.G., Barer, M.L., and Caetano, P.A. (2005) "'Breakthrough' drugs and growth in expenditure on prescription drugs in Canada." *British Medical Journal*, 331(7520): 815–816.

Mosconi, P., Colombo, C., Satolli, R., and Liberati, A. (2007) "PartecipaSalute, an Italian project to involve lay people, patients' associations and scientific-medical representatives in the health debate." *Health Expectations*, 10(2): 194–204.

Mossialos, E., Dixon, A., Figueras, J., and Kutzin, J. (eds) (2002) *Funding Health Care: Options for Europe*, Buckingham: Open University Press.

Mot, E., and Windmeijer, F. (2002) "De invloed van promotie door de farmaceutische industrie op het voorschrijfgedrag." In A. Van den Berg-Jeths and G.W.M. Peters-Volleberg (eds), *Geneesmiddelen en medische hulpmiddelen. Trends en dilemma's*, Houten: Bohn Stafleu Van Loghum.

Moynihan, R., and Cassels, A. (2005) *Selling Sickness: How the world's biggest pharmaceutical companies are turning us all into patients*, New York: Nation Books.

MTAS (2005) *Libro Blanco de la Dependencia*, Madrid: IMSERSO, Ministerio de Trabajo y Asuntos Sociales.

Mulder, C.L., and Kroon, H. (2005) *Assertive Community Treatment*, Amsterdam: Boom.

Murray, C.L., and Evans, D.B. (2003) *Health Systems Performance Assessment: Debates, methods and empiricism*, Geneva: World Health Organization.

Muszynska, M.M., and Rau, R. (2012) "The old-age healthy dependency ratio in Europe." *Journal of Population Ageing*, 5: 151–162.

Naaldenberg, J., Vaandrager, L., Koelen, M., Wagemakers, A., Saan, H., and De Hoog, K. (2009) "Elaborating on systems thinking in health promotion practice." *Global Health Promotion*, 16(1): 39–47.

Naiditch, M., Triantafillou, J., Di Santo, P., Carretero, S., and Durrett, E.H. (2013) "User perspectives in long-term care and the role of informal carers." In K. Leichsenring, J. Billings, and H. Nies (eds), *Long-term Care in Europe: Improving policy and practice*, Basingstoke and New York: Palgrave Macmillan, pp. 45–80.

National Alliance for Caregiving, and AARP (1997) *Family Caregiving in the U.S.: Findings from a national survey*, Washington, DC: National Alliance for Caregiving and AARP.

Nelson, R.R. (1994) "The co-evolution of technology, industrial structure, and supporting institutions." *Industrial and Corporate Change*, 3: 47–63.

Netherlands Court of Audit (2004) *Opvang zwerfjongeren*, The Hague: Netherlands Court of Audit.

Neuteboom, J., Van Raak, R., and Rotmans, J. (eds) (2009) *Mensenzorg – een transitiebeweging*, Rotterdam: DRIFT.

Newhouse, J.P. (1970) "Towards a theory of non-profit institutions. An economic model of the hospital." *American Economic Review*, 60: 64–74.

Newman, J., and Tonkens, E. (2011) *Participation, Responsibility and Choice: Summoning the active citizen in Western European welfare states*, Amsterdam: Amsterdam University Press.

Nierse, C.J., and Abma, T.A. (2011) "Developing voice and empowerment: The first step towards a broad consultation in research agenda setting." *Journal of Intellectual Disability Research*, 55: 411–421.

Nierse, C., Abma, T., Haker, F., Broerse, J., Caron-Flinterman, F., Houdijk, N., and Widdershoven, G. (2006) "Engaging people with intellectual disabilities in health research agenda setting." *Journal of Applied Research in Intellectual Disabilities*, 19(3): 260.

Nies, H., Leichsenring, K., and Mak, S. (2013) "The emerging identity of long-term care systems." In K. Leichsenring, J. Billings, and H. Nies (eds), *Long-term Care in Europe: Improving policy and practice*, Basingstoke and New York: Palgrave Macmillan, pp. 19–41.

Nordin, I. (2000) "Expert and non-expert knowledge in medical practice." *Medical Health Care and Philosophy*, 3(3): 297–304.

Northern Ireland Department of Health, Social Services and Public Safety (2001) *Best Practice, Best Care*, Belfast: Department of Health, Social Services and Public Safety.

Northern Ireland Department of Health, Social Services and Public Safety (2002a) *Investing for Health*, Belfast: Department of Health, Social Services and Public Safety.

Northern Ireland Department of Health, Social Services and Public Safety (2002b) *Developing Better Services. Modernising hospitals and reforming structures*, Belfast: Department of Health, Social Services and Public Safety.

Nouws, H. (2008) *Klant in Beeld*, Utrecht: Actiz.

Novilla, M.L.B., Barnes, M.D., De La Cruz, N.G., Williams, P.N., and Rogers, J. (2006) "Public health perspectives on the family: An ecological approach to promoting health in the family and community." *Family and Community Health*, 29(1): 28–42.

Nowotny, H., Scott, P., and Gibbons, M.T. (2001) *Re-thinking Science: Knowledge and the public in an age of uncertainty*, Cambridge: Blackwell.

Nutbeam, D., and Harris, E. (1999) *Theory in a Nutshell: A guide to health promotion theory*, Sydney: McGraw-Hill.

Nutley, S., Walter, I., and Davies, H.T.O. (2007) *Using Evidence: How research can inform public services*, Bristol: Policy Press.

O'Connell, D., and Mosconi, P. (2006) "An active role for patients in clinical research?" *Drug Development Research*, 67(3): 188–192.

OECD (1998) *The Future of Female-dominated Occupations*, Paris: OECD Publishing.

OECD (2005) *The OECD Health Project: Long-term care for older people*, Paris: OECD Publishing.

OECD (2007) *Health at a Glance*, Paris: OECD Publishing.

OECD (2011) *Health: Spending continues to outpace economic growth in most OECD countries*, Paris: OECD Publishing.

OECD (2012) *Health at a Glance: Europe 2012*, Paris: OECD Publishing.

Oldenziel, R., and Hård, M. (2013) *Consumers, Tinkerers, Rebels: The people who shaped Europe*, New York: Palgrave Macmillan.

Oliver, S.R., Rees, R.W., Clarke-Jones, L., Milne, R., Oakley, A.R., Gabbay, J., Stein, K., Buchanan, P., and Gyte, G. (2008) "A multidimensional conceptual framework for analyzing public involvement in health services research." *Health Expectations*, 11(1): 72–84.

Olson, L.K. (ed.) (1994) *The Graying of the World: Who will care for the frail elderly?* Binghamton, NY: Haworth Press.

Owen, J., Cooke, J., and Wilson, A. (2002) "Research and development at the health and social care interface in primary care. A scoping exercise in one National Health Service region." *Health Social Care Community*, 10(6): 435–444.

Pandolfini, C., and Bonati, M. (2005) "A literature review on off-label drug use in children." *European Journal of Pediatrics*, 164(9): 552–558.

Pang, T., Sadana, R., Hanney, S., Bhutta, Z.A., Hyder, A.A., and Simon, J. (2003) "Knowledge for better health: A conceptual framework and foundation for health research systems." *Bulletin of the World Health Organization*, 81: 815–820.

Patel, K., and Rushefsky, M.E. (1999) *Health Care Politics and Policy in America*, Armonk, NY, and London: ME Sharpe.

Pawson, R. (2002a) "Evidence-based policy: In search of a method." *Evaluation*, 8(2): 157–181.

Pawson, R. (2002b) "Evidence-based policy: The promise of realist synthesis." *Evaluation*, 8(3): 340–358.

Pawson, R. (2006) *Evidence-based Policy: A realist perspective*, London: Sage.

Payne, J., D'Antoine, H.A., France, K.E., McKenzie, A.E., and Henley, N. (2011) "Collaborating with consumer and community representatives in health and medical research in Australia: Results from an evaluation." *Health Research Policy and Systems*, 9(1): 18.

Peeters, J.M., Francke, A.L., and Bos, J.T. (2007) *Monitor videonetwerken*, Utrecht: Nivel.

Peeters, J.M., Francke, A.L., and De Veer, A.J.L. (2009) *Monitor zorg op afstand*, Utrecht: Nivel.

Peeters, J.M., Wiegers, T.A., and Friele, R.D. (2013) "How technology in care at home affects patient self-care and self-management: A scoping review." *International Journal of Environmental Research and Public Health*, 10(11), pp. 5541–5564.

Pel, B., Avelino, F.R., and Jhagroe, S.S. (2016) "Critical approaches to transition theory." In H.G. Brauch, U.O. Spring, J. Grin, and J. Scheffran (eds), *Sustainability Transition and Sustainable Peace Handbook*, Hexagon Series on Human and Environmental Security and Peace 10, Heidelberg, New York, Dordrecht, and London: Springer.

Perehudoff, S.K., Laing, R.O., and Hogerzeil, H.V. (2010) "Access to essential medicines in national constitutions." *Bulletin of the World Health Organization*, 88(11): 800.

Perez, C. (1983) "Structural change and the assimilation of new technologies in the economic and social system." *Futures*, 15: 357–375.

Petit-Zeman, S., Firkins, L., and Scadding, J.W. (2010) "The James Lind Alliance: Tackling research mismatches." *The Lancet*, 376(9742): 667–669.

Phelps, C. (2007) "25 years of excellence: The Journal of Health Economics in retrospective." *The Journal of Health Economics*, 26: 1075–1080.

Pickett, K.E., and Wilkinson, R.G. (2015) "Income inequality and health: A causal review." *Social Science and Medicine*, 128: 316–326.

Pierson, P. (2004) *Politics in Time: History, institutions and social analysis*, Princeton, NJ: Princeton University Press.

Pittens, C.A.C.M., Elberse, J.E., Visse, M., Abma, T.A., and Broerse, J.E.W. (2014) "Research agendas involving patients: Factors that facilitate or impede translation of patients' perspectives in programming and implementation." *Science and Public Policy*. doi: 10.1093/scipol/scu010.

Pittens, C.A.C.M., Elberse, J.E., Tax, S., Van Leeuwen-Stok, A.E., Schrieks, M., Jonker, M., and Broerse, J.E.W. (2012) "34 patients' perceptions on breast cancer clinical trials." *European Journal of Cancer*, 48: S50.

Ploumen, L. (1987) *Het imago van de farmaceutische industrie: Een historische schets van de interactie tussen samenleving en onderneming*, Rotterdam: Erasmus University Press.

Plsek, P.E., and Greenhalgh, R. (2001) "The challenge of complexity in healthcare." *British Medical Journal*, 10(323): 625.

PMPRB (2004) *2003 Annual Report*, Ottawa: Patented Medicine Prices Review Board.

Pollmann, T. (1976) "De dure valium en de goedkope valium." *Vrij Nederland*, February 14.

Pollock, A. (2005) "The Private Finance Initiative: A policy built on sand." *Science in Parliament*, 62(4): 25(1).

Pols, B. (1990) "Longtransplantaties betaald uit veilingen en loterijen." *NRC*, December 27.

Popay, J., Williams, G., Thomas, C., and Gatrell, T. (1998) "Theorising inequalities in health: The place of lay knowledge." *Sociology of Health and Illness*, 20(5): 619–644.

Postl, B. (2011) "Building capacity for change: Examples from the Winnipeg Regional Health Authority." In T. Sullivan and J. Denis (eds), *Building Better Healthcare for Canada*, Toronto: McGill-Queen's University.

Pronk, E.J. (2007) "Meer dan een ExcuusTruus: Patiëntenparticipatie in wetenschap is nuttig maar niet eenvoudig." *Medisch Contact*, 62(14): 610–613.

Purves, D. (1997) *Neuroscience*, Sunderland, MA: Sinauer Associates.

Querido, A. (1965) *Een eeuw staatstoezicht op de volksgezondheid*, 's-Gravenhage: Staatsuitgeverij.

Raaijmakers, T., Baart, P., Evers, H., and Van Capelleveen, C. (2009) *Gezond management. De meerwaarde van gezondheidsmanagement voor de bedrijfsvoering*, Amsterdam: WEKA.

Rachlis, M., Evans, R.G., Lewis, P., and Barer, M.L. (2001) *Revitalizing Medicare: Shared problems, public solutions*, Vancouver: Tommy Douglas Research Institute.

Raven, R.P.J.M. (2005) *Strategic Niche Management for Biomass*, Eindhoven: Technische Universiteit Eindhoven.

Raven, R.P.J.M. (2012) "Analyzing emerging sustainable energy niches in Europe: A strategic niche management perspective." In G. Verbong and D. Loorbach (eds), *Governing the Energy Transition: Reality, illusion or necessity?*, New York: Routledge, pp. 125–150.

Raven, R.P.J.M., and Geels, F.W. (2010) "Socio-cognitive evolution in niche development: Comparative analysis of biogas development in Denmark and the Netherlands (1973–2004)." *Technovation*, 30: 87–99.

Raven, R.P.J.M., Van der Bosch, S., and Weterings, R. (2010) "Transitions and strategic niche management: Towards a competence kit for practitioners." *International Journal of Technology Management*, 51(1): 57–74.

Ready, P.D. (2010) "Leishmaniasis emergence in Europe." *Euro Surveill*, 15(10), article 5.

Reiser, S.J. (1984) "The machine at the bedside: Technological transformations of practices and values." In S.J. Reiser and M. Anbar (eds), *The Machine at the Bedside. Strategies for using technology in patient care*, Cambridge: Cambridge University Press, pp. 3–19.

RGO (2006) *Advies Onderzoeksagenda Medische Biotechnologie*, The Hague: Raad van Gezondheidsonderzoek.

RGO (2007) *Patiëntenparticipatie in gezondheidsonderzoek*, The Hague: Raad van Gezondheidsonderzoek.

Rhenen, W., Blonk, R.B., Schaufeli, W., and Dijk, F.H. (2007) "Can sickness absence be reduced by stress reduction programs: On the effectiveness of two approaches." *International Archives of Occupational and Environmental Health*, 80(6): 505–515.

Rip, A., and Kemp, R. (1998) "Technological change." In S. Rayner and E.L. Malone (eds), *Human Choice and Climate Change*, Columbus, OH: Battelle Press.

Riper, H., Smit, F., Van der Zanden, R., Conijn, B., Kramer, J., and Mutsaers, K. (2007) *E-Mental Health*, Utrecht: Trimbos.

Rittel, H.W.J., and Webber, M.M. (1973) "Dilemmas in a general theory of planning." *Policy Sciences*, 4(2): 155–169.

RIVM (2010) *Nationaal Kompas Volksgezondheid*, Bilthoven: RIVM.

Robert, E., Ridde, V., Marchal, B., and Fournier, P. (2012) "Protocol: A realist review of user fee exemption policies for health services in Africa." *BMJ Open*, 2: 1–7.

Roberts, M.J., Hsiao, W., Berman, P., and Reich, M.R. (2004) *Getting Health Reform Right: A guide to improving performance and equity*, New York: Oxford University Press.

Robinson, J. (2001) *Prescription Games*, London: Simon and Schuster.

Robinson, R., and Dixon, A. (1999) *Health Systems in Transition. United Kingdom. The United Kingdom Health System*, Copenhagen: European Observatory on Health Systems and Policies.

Ródenas, F., Garcés, J., Carretero, S., and Megía, M.J. (2008) "Case management method applied to older adults in the primary care centres in Burjassot (Valencian Region, Spain)." *European Journal of Ageing*, 5: 57–66.

Ródenas, F., Garcés, J., and Doñate-Martínez, A. (2013) "Innovation in the management of patients at risk of hospital readmissions: New technological solutions to promote quality of life in older people." *The International Journal of Interdisciplinary Social Sciences*, 7(2): 31–39.

Roelofsen, A., Broerse, J.E.W., De Cock-Buning, T.J., and Bunders, J.F.G. (2008) "Exploring the future of ecological genomics: Integrating CTA with vision assessment." *Technological Forecasting and Social Change*, 75(3): 334–355.

Roep, D., Van der Ploeg, J.D., and Wiskerke, J.S.C. (2003) "Managing technical-institutional design processes: Some strategic lessons from environmental co-operatives in the Netherlands." *Netherlands Journal of Agrarian Studies*, 51(1–2): 195–217.

Rogers, E.M. (1995) *Diffusion of Innovations*, New York: The Free Press.

Röling, N. (2002) "Beyond the aggregation of individual preferences. Moving from multiple to distributed cognition in resource dilemmas." In C. Leeuwis and R. Pyburn (eds), *Wheelbarrows Full of Frogs. Social learning in rural resource management*, Assen: Van Gorcum.

Romanow, R.J. (2003) *Building on Values: The future of health care in Canada*, Final Report, Saskatoon: Commission on the Future of Health Care in Canada.

Roscam Abbing, H.D.C. (1991) "Kiezen en delen; Rapport van de commissie Keuzen in de zorg (Commissie-Dunning)." *Nederlands Tijdschrift Voor Geneeskunde*.

Rotmans, J. (2003) *Transitiemanagement: Sleutel voor een duurzame samenleving*, Assen: Van Gorcum.

Rotmans, J. (2005) *Societal Innovation: Between dream and reality lies complexity*, Inaugural Address, Rotterdam: Erasmus University Rotterdam.

Rotmans, J., Grin, J., Schot, J., and Smits, R. (2004) *Multi-, Inter- and Transdisciplinary Research Program into Transitions and System Innovations*, Maastricht.

Rotmans, J., Kemp, R., and Van Asselt, M. (2001) "More evolution than revolution: Transition management in public policy." *Foresight*, 3(1): 1–17.

Rotmans, J., and Loorbach, D. (2001) "Transitiemanagement: een nieuw sturingsmodel." *Arena/Het Dossier*, 6: 5–8.

Rotmans, J., and Loorbach, D. (2006) "Transition management: Reflexive steering of societal complexity through searching, learning and experimenting." In J.C.J.M. Van den Bergh and F.R. Bruinsma (eds), *The Transition to Renewable Energy: Theory and practice*, Cheltenham: Edward Elgar.

Rotmans, J., and Loorbach, D. (2010) "Towards a better understanding of transitions and their governance: A systemic and reflexive approach." In J. Grin, J. Rotmans, and J. Schot (eds), *Transitions to Sustainable Development. New directions in the study of long term transformative change*, London: Routledge.

Roy, A.D., Cantin, S., and Rivard, S. (2011) "The EXTRA experience in Montérégie." In T. Sullivan and J. Denis (eds), *Building Better Healthcare for Canada: Implementing evidence*, Montreal: McGill-Queen's University Press, pp. 167–177.

Rubenstein, L.Z., Stuck, A.E., Siu, A.L., and Wieland, D. (1991) "Impacts of geriatric evaluation and management programs on defined outcomes: Overview of the evidence." *Journal of the American Geriatric Society*, 39(9Pt2): 8S–18S.

Rycroft-Malone, J., Seers, K., Titchen, A., Harvey, G., Kitson, A., and McCormack, B. (2004) "What counts as evidence in evidence-based practice?" *Journal of Advanced Nursing*, 47(1): 81–90.

Sackett, D.L., Rosenberg, W.M., Gray, J.A., Haynes, R.B., and Richardson, W.S. (1996) "Evidence based medicine: What it is and what it isn't." *British Medical Journal*, 13, 312(7023): 71–72.

Saunders, C., and Girgis, A. (2010) "Status, challenges and facilitators of consumer involvement in Australian health and medical research." *Health Research Policy and Systems*, 8(1): 34.

Scharlach, A.E., Giunta, N.Y., and Mills-Dick, K. (2001) *Case Management in Long-term Care Integration: An Overview of Current Programs and Evaluations*, Center for the Advanced Study of Aging Services, Berkeley: University of California Press.

Scheirer, M.A., and Dearing, J.W. (2011) "An agenda for research on the sustainability of public health programs." *American Journal of Public Health*, 101(11): 2059–2076.

Schipper, K. (2012) *Patient Participation and Knowledge*, Amsterdam: VU University Press.

Schippers, E.I. (2016) "Visie op geneesmiddelen: Nieuwe geneesmiddelen snel bij de patient tegen aanvaardbare kosten." Brief aan de Voorzitter van de Tweede Kamer der Staten-Generaal, January 29, The Hague: Ministerie van Volksgezondheid, Welzijn en Sport.

Schnabel, P. (1995) "Overheid tussen overlaten en overhalen. Een eeuw van wisselende verhoudingen in de zorg voor ziekte en gezondheid." In R.B.M. Rigter (ed.), *Overheid en gezondheidszorg in de twintigste eeuw*, Rotterdam: Erasmus Publishing, pp. 9–29.

Schön, D.A. (1983) *The Reflective Practitioner: How professionals think in action*, New York: Basic Books.

Schön, D.A., and Rein, M. (1994) *Frame Reflection: Towards the resolution of intractable policy controversies*, Cambridge, MA: The MIT press.

Schot, J.W. (1998) "The usefulness of evolutionary models for explaining innovation: The case of the Netherlands in the nineteenth century." *History of Technology*, 14: 173–200.

Schot, J.W., and Geels, F.W. (2007) "Niches in evolutionary theories of technical change – A critical survey of the literature." *Journal of Evolutionary Economics*, 17(5): 605–622.

Schouten, B. (2013) *De nieuwe Thuiszorg: naar wijkgerichte en zelfsturende teams. Evaluatie uit de eerste teams bij Thuiszorg Amstelring*, Zeist: MoVida.

Schouwstra, C.P. (1995) "Over de invloed van wet- en regelgeving op de ontwikkeling van de huisartsgeneeskunde." In B.J.M. Aulbers and G.J. Bremer (eds), *De Huisarts van Toen*, Rotterdam: Erasmus Publishing.

Schrijvers, A.J.P. (ed.) (1997) *Health and Health Care in the Netherlands, A critical self assessment by Dutch experts in the medical and health sciences*, Utrecht: De Tijdstroom.

Schrijvers, G. (2008) "Lessons from the past: Integrated prevention is successful." *International Journal of Integrated Care*, 8: e70.

Schuitmaker, T.J. (2010) "Persistent problems in the Dutch healthcare system: An instrument for analyzing system deficits." In J.E.W. Broerse and J.F.G. Bunders (eds), *Transitions in Health Systems: Dealing with persistent problems*, Amsterdam: VU University Press, pp. 21–18.

Schuitmaker, T.J. (2012) "Identifying and unraveling persistent problems." *Technological Forecasting and Social Change*, 79(6): 1021–1031.

Schuitmaker, T.J. (2013) *Persistent Problems in the Dutch Healthcare System: Learning from novel practices for a transition in healthcare with the UPP framework*, Amsterdam: Faculty of Social and Behavioural Sciences, University of Amsterdam.

Schut, J. (1970) *Van dolhuys tot psychiatrisch centrum: Ontwikkeling en functie*, Haarlem: De Toorts.

Scott, J. (1998) *Seeing Like a State: How certain schemes to improve the human condition have failed*, New Haven, CT: Yale University Press.

Shain, M., and Kramer, D.M. (2004) "Health promotion in the workplace: Framing the concepts; reviewing the evidence." *Occupational and Environmental Medicine*, 61(7): 643–648.

Shea, B., Santesso, N., Qualman, A., Heiberg, T., Leong, A., Judd, M., Robinson, V., Wells, G., and Tugwell, P. (2005) "Consumer-driven health care: Building partnerships in research." *Health Expectations*, 8(4): 352–359.

Sheller, M. (2012) "The emergence of new cultures of mobility: Stability, openings and prospects." In F.W. Geels, R. Kemp, G. Dudley, and G. Lyons (eds), *Automobility in Transition? A Socio-technical Analysis of Sustainable Transport*, New York: Routledge, pp. 180–202.

Shepperd, S., Lewin, S., Straus, S., Clarke, M., Eccles, M.P., Fitzpatrick, R., Wong, G., and Sheikh, A. (2009) "Can we systematically review studies that evaluate complex interventions?" *PLoS Medicine*, 6: 1–8.

Simmons, R., Fajans, P., and Ghiron, L. (eds) (2007) *Scaling up Health Service Delivery: From Pilot Innovations to Policies and Programmes*, Geneva: WHO.

Simons, J.L. (ed.) (1995) *The State of Humanity*, Oxford and Cambridge: Blackwell.

Singh, D. (2005) *Transforming Chronic Care. Evidence about improving care for people with long-term conditions*, Birmingham: NHS Institute for Innovation and Improvement.

Skinner, B., and Rovere, M. (2011) *Canada's Medicare Bubble: Is government health spending sustainable without user-based funding?*, Vancouver: The Fraser Institute.

Skocpol, T. (2008) "Bringing the state back in: Retrospect and prospect." *Scandinavian Political Studies*, 31(2): 9–24.

Smit, C. (2009) *"Het verhaal van...", Negen verhalen over patientenparticipatie in geneesmiddelenonderzoek*, Badhoevedorp: Drukkerij De Adelaar.

Smith, A. (2007) "Translating sustainabilities between green niches and socio-technical regimes." *Technology Analysis and Strategic Management*, 19(4): 427–450.

Smith, A., and Raven, R. (2012) "What is protective space? Reconsidering niches in transitions to sustainability." *Research Policy*, 41(6): 1025–1036.

Smith, A., and Stirling, A. (2007) "Moving outside or inside? Objectification and reflexivity in the governance of socio-technical systems." *Journal of Environmental Policy and Planning*, 9(3–4): 351–373.

Smith, A., Voß, J.P., and Grin, J. (2010) "Innovation studies and sustainability transitions: The allure of the multi-level perspective and its challenges." *Research Policy*, 39(4): 435–448.

Smith, R. (2001) "Measuring the social impact of research." *British Medical Journal*, 323: 528.

Smith, R. (2003) "Limits to medicine. Medical nemesis: The expropriation of health." *Journal of Epidemiology and Community Health*, 57: 928.

Smith, V.K., Des Jardins, T., and Peterson, K.A. (2000) *Exemplary Practices in Primary Care Case Management*, Centre for Health Care Strategies, Inc., The Robert Wood Johnson Foundation.

Snelders, S., and Meijman, F. (2009) *De mondige patiënt. Historische kijk op een mythe*, Amsterdam: Bert Bakker.

Soroka, S.N. (2011) *Public Perceptions and Media Coverage of the Canadian Healthcare System*, Toronto: Canadian Health Services Research Foundation.

Sowada, B.J. (2003) *Call to Be Whole: The Fundamentals of Health Care Reform*, Westport, CT: Praeger Publishers.

Spaargaren, G., Oosterveer, P., and Loeber, A. (eds) (2012) *Food Practices in Transition: Changing food consumption, retail and production in the age of reflexive modernity*, New York: Routledge.

Stambolovic, V. (2003) "Epidemic of health care reforms." *European Journal of Public Health*, 13: 77–79.

Staniszewska, S., Herron-Marx, S., and Mockford, C. (2008) "Measuring the impact of patient and public involvement: The need for an evidence base." *International Journal for Quality in Health Care*, 20(6): 373–374.

Stanton, J. (1999) "Making sense of technologies in medicine." *Social History of Medicine*, 12(3): 437–448.

Starfield, B. (1998) *Primary Care: Balancing health needs, services, and technology*, New York: Oxford University Press.

Stevens, P. (2005) *Monitor videonetwerken voor zorg-thuis, Beweegredenen, Proces en Ervaringen*, Utrecht: Actiz.

Stevens, T., Wilde, D., Hunt, J., and Ahmedzai, S.H. (2003) "Overcoming the challenges to consumer involvement in cancer research." *Health Expectations*, 6(1): 81–88.

Steward, F., and Wibberley, G. (1980) "Drug innovation: What's slowing it down?" *Nature*, 284: 118–120.

Stewart, R.J., Caird, J., Oliver, K., and Oliver, S. (2011) "Patients' and clinicians' research priorities." *Health Expectations*, 14(4): 439–448.

Stirman, S.W., Kimberly, J., Cook, N., Calloway, A., Castro, F., and Charns, M. (2012) "The sustainability of new programs and innovations: A review of the empirical literature and recommendations for future research." *Implementation Science*, 7: 17.

Stones, R. (2005) *Structuration Theory*, Basingstoke: Palgrave Macmillan.

Stooker, R. (2001) "Costs of the last year of life in the Netherlands." *Springer*, 38(1): 73–80.

Stuck, A.E., Siu, A.L., Wieland, G.D., Adams, J., and Rubenstein, L.Z. (1993) "Comprehensive geriatric assessment: A meta-analysis of controlled trials." *The Lancet*, 342: 1032–1036.

Sullivan, T., and Denis, J. (eds) (2011) *Building Better Healthcare for Canada: Implementing evidence*, Montreal: McGill-Queen's University Press.

Swaans, K., Broerse, J., Meincke, M., Mudhara, M., and Bunders, J. (2009) "Promoting food security and well-being among poor and HIV/AIDS affected households: Lessons from an interactive and integrated approach." *Evaluation and Program Planning*, 32(1): 31–42.

Swilling, M., Musango, J., and Wakeford, J. (2016) "Developmental states and sustainability transitions: Prospects of a just transition in South Africa." In J. Grin, S. Jhagroe, and B. Pel, B., Special Issue on the Politics of Transitions. *Journal of Environmental Policy and Planning*, 18(5): 650–672.

Switzer, A., Bertolini, L., and Grin, J. (2013) "Transitions of mobility systems in urban regions: A heuristic framework." *Journal of Environmental Policy and Planning*, 15(2): 141–160.

Szasz, T. (1961) *The Myth of Mental Illness: Foundations of a theory of personal conduct*, New York: Harper & Row.

Taanman, M. (2014) *Looking for Transitions: Monitoring approach for sustainable transition programmes*, Rotterdam: Erasmus University Rotterdam.

Tallon, D., Chard, J., and Dieppe, P. (2000) "Relation between agendas of the research community and the research consumer." *The Lancet*, 355(9220): 2037–2040.

Telford, R., Beverley, C.A., Cooper, C.L., and Boote, J.D. (2002) "Consumer involvement in health research: Fact or fiction?" *British Journal of Clinical Governance*, 7(2): 92–103.

Ten Doesschate, G. (ed.) (1949) *Gedenkboek der Koninklijke Nederlandsche Maatschappij tot bevordering der geneeskunst ter gelegenheid van haar honderd-jarig bestaan, 1849–1949*, Amsterdam.

Termeer, C.J.A.M., and Dewulf, A. (2012) "Towards theoretical multiplicity for the governance of transitions: The energy-producing greenhouse case." *International Journal of Sustainable Development*, 15(1/2): 37–53.

Terraza Núñez, R., Vargas Lorenzo, I., and Vázquez Navarrete, M. (2006) "La coordinación entre niveles asistenciales: una sistematización de sus instrumentos y medidas." *Gac Sanit*, 20(6): 485–495.

Teunissen, G.J., Visse, M.A., Laan, D., De Boer, W.I., Rutgers, M., and Abma, T.A. (2013) "Patient involvement in lung foundation research: A seven year longitudinal case study." *Health*, 5(suppl2A): 320–330.

't Hoen, E.F., Hogerzeil, H.V., Quick, J.D., and Sillo, H.B. (2014) "A quiet revolution in global public health: The World Health Organization's prequalification of medicines programme." *Journal of Public Health Policy*, 35(2): 137–161.

Thornhill, J., Judd, M., and Clements, D. (2009) "(Re)introducing the self assessment tool that is helping decision-makers assess their organization's capacity to use research." *Healthcare Quarterly*, 12(1): 22–24.

Thornicroft, G., Alem, A., Antunes Dos Santos, R., Barley, E., and Drake, R.E. (2010) "WPA guidance on steps, obstacles and mistakes to avoid in the implementation of community mental healthcare." *World Psychiatry*, 9(2): 67–77.

Timmermans, S., and Berg, M. (2003) *The Gold Standard: The challenge of evidence-based medicine and standardization in health care*, Philadelphia, PA: Temple University Press.

Timmermans, J., Van der Heiden, S., and Born, M.Ph. (2014) "Policy entrepreneurs in sustainability transitions: Their personality and leadership profiles assessed." *Environmental Innovation and Societal Transitions*, 13: 96–108.

Titmuss, R. (1968) *Commitment to Welfare*, London: Allen & Unwin.

Toebes, B.C.A. (1999) *The Right to Health as a Human Right in International Law*, Antwerp: Intersentia.

Tonkens, E. (1999) *Het zelfontplooiingsregime. De actualiteit van Dennendal en de jaren zestig*, Amsterdam: Bert Bakker.

Tonkens, E. (2008) *Mondige burgers, getemde professionals. Marktwerking en professionaliteit in de publieke sector*, Amsterdam: Van Gennep.

Tonkens, E. (2013) "Keuzevrijheid of keuzedwang: burgers en de zorg." In C. Bakker and G. van Overbeeke (eds), *Het burgerperspectief in het toezicht*, Utrecht: Inspectie voor de Gezondheidszorg.

Toulmin, S. (2001) *Return to Reason*, Cambridge, MA: Harvard University Press.

Transition Arena Long-term Care (2009) *Human Care: A transition movement*, Rotterdam: DRIFT.

Transition Programme in the Care (2008) Flyer.

Traulsen, J.M., and Noerreslet, M. (2004) "The new consumer of medicine – The pharmacy technicians' perspective." *Pharmacy World and Science*, 26(4): 203–207.

Triantafillou, J., Naiditch, M., Repkova, K., Stiehr, K., and Carretero, S. (2010) *Informal Care in the Long-term Care System*, European Overview Paper, European Centre for Social Welfare Policy and Research.

Trimbos, K. (1975) *Anti-psychiatrie. Een overzicht*, Deventer: Van Loghum Slaterus.

Truffer, B., Voß, J.P., and Konrad, K. (2008) "Mapping expectations for system transformations. Lessons from sustainability foresight in German utility sectors." *Technological Forecasting and Social Change*, 75: 1360–1372.

Tuohy, C.H. (1999) *Accidental Logics: The dynamics of change in the health care arena in the United States, Britain, and Canada*, New York: Oxford University Press.

Tuohy, C.H., and Wolfson, A.D. (1977) "The political economy of professionalism: A perspective." In M.J. Rebilcock (ed.), *Four Aspects of Professionalism*, Ottowa: Consumer Research Council, Department of Consumer and Corporate Affairs, Government of Canada.

Ulmanen, J. (2013) *Exploring Policy Protection and Biofuel Niche Development. A policy and strategic niche management analysis of Dutch and Swedish biofuel development, 1970–2010*, Eindhoven: TU Eindhoven.

Vaandrager, L., and Koelen, M. (2013) "Salutogenesis in the workplace: Building general resistance resources and sense of coherence." In G.F. Bauer and G.J. Jenny (eds), *Salutogenic Organizations and Change: The Concepts Behind Organizational Health Intervention Research*, Dordrecht: Springer.

Vaandrager, L., Koelen, M.A., Baart, P., and Raaijmakers, T. (2006) *System Innovation for Workplace Health Promotion: Project proposal for the KSI research programme System Innovations and Transitions in Health Care*, Wageningen: Wageningen University.

Van Bijsterveldt, M., and Van Mechelen, P. (2011) "ZonMW-directeur Henk Smid langs de meetlat." *Mediator*, 22(1): 33–35.

Van Bokhoven, M.A., Koch, H., Van der Weijden, T., Grol, R.P.T.M., and Kester, A.D. (2009) "Influence of watchful waiting on satisfaction and anxiety among patients seeking care for unexplained complaints." *Annals of Family Medicine*, 7(2): 112–120.

Van Bokhoven, M.A., Koch, H., Van Der Weijden, T., Grol, R.P.T.M., Bindels, P.J.E., and Dinant, G.J. (2006) "Blood test ordering for unexplained complaints in general practice: The VAMPIRE randomised clinical trial protocol", *BMC Family Practice*, 7: 20.

Van de Bovenkamp, H.M., Trappenburg, M.J., and Grit, K.J. (2010) "Patient participation in collective healthcare decision making: The Dutch model." *Health Expectations*, 13(1): 73–85.

Van den Berg Jeths, A., and Peters-Volleberg, G. (2002) *Geneesmiddelen en medische hulpmiddelen: Trends en dilemma's*, Bilthoven: Rijksinstituut voor Volksgezondheid en Milieu.

Van den Bosch, S. (2010) *Transition Experiments. Exploring societal changes towards sustainability*, PhD thesis, Erasmus University, Rotterdam.

Van den Bosch, S., and Rotmans, J. (2008) *Deepening, Broadening and Scaling Up: A framework for steering transition experiments*, Essay 02, Delft/Rotterdam, Knowledge Centre for Sustainable System Innovations and Transitions (KCT).

Van den Bosch, S., and Taanman, M. (2006) "How innovation impacts society. Patterns and mechanisms through which innovation projects contribute to transitions." Paper presented at the Innovation Pressure Conference, March 15-17, Tampere, Finland.

Van der Grinten, T., and Kasdorp, J. (1999) *25 jaar sturing in de gezondheidszorg: Van verstatelijking naar ondernemerschap*, The Hague: Sociaal en Cultureel Planbureau.

Van der Ham, A.J., Shields, L.S., and Broerse, J.E.W. (2013) "Towards integration of service user knowledge in mental healthcare in low-income countries: Insights from transition theory." *Knowledge Management for Development*, 9(2): 125–139.

Van der Heyden, J.T.M. (1994) *Het ziekenhuis door de eeuwen: Over geld, macht en mensen*, Rotterdam: Erasmus Publishing.

Van der Klink, J.J.L., Blonk, R.W.B., Schene, A.H., and Van Dijk, F.J.H. (2003) "Reducing long term sickness absence by an activating intervention in adjustment disorders: A cluster randomised controlled design." *Occupational and Environmental Medicine*, 60(6): 429–437.

Van der Maesen, L. (1987) *Transformatie van de gezondheidszorg in Nederland tussen 1974 en 1987*, Rotterdam: Erasmus University Rotterdam.

Van der Wilt, G.J. (1995) "Alternative ways of framing Parkinson's Disease: Implications for priorities in health care and biomedical research." *Industrial and Environmental Crisis Quarterly*, 9(1): 13–48.

Van Dieren, Q. (2007) "Overzichtsartikel – Medisch onverklaarde somatische symptomen zijn geen onverklaarbare, onbegrepen of vage lichamelijke klachten." *Tijdschrift voor psychiatrie*, 49(11): 823–834.

Van Dijk, B., Versteeg, L., Roosenschoon, B.J., and Bogaards, M. (2006) *Het ACT-jeugd team. Rapportage van een pilotstudy naar Assertive Community Treatment (ACT) voor jongeren in Rotterdam*, internal document, Rotterdam: Bavo RNO Groep.

Van Dijk, J.A.G.M. (1999) "The one-dimensional network society of Manuel Castells." *New Media and Society*, 1(1): 127–138.

Van Doorn-De Leeuw, M. (1982) "Wie gaat de gezondheidszorg beheersen?" In J.A.A. Van Doorn and C.J.M. Schuyt (eds), *De Stagnerende Verzorgingsstaat*, Meppel/Amsterdam: Boom.

Van Driel, H., and Schot, J. (2005) "Radical innovation as a multi-level process: Introducing floating grain elevators in the port of Rotterdam." *Technology and Culture*, 46(1): 51–76.

Van Erp, B. (2008) "Bel de ambulance maar. Reportage thuisbevallen in Nederland." *De Volkskrant*, May 31.

Van Fulpen, A. (2008) *Strategische checklist zorg op afstand*, Utrecht: Actiz.

Van Lieburg, M.J. (1995) "Overheid, medisch beroep en instellingswezen. De contouren van de overheidsbemocienis met de infrastructuur van de gezondheidszorg in deze eeuw." In R.B.M. Rigter (ed.), *Overheid en gezondheidszorg in de twintigste eeuw*, Rotterdam: Erasmus Publishing.

Van Meurs, R. (1976) "De fraude met geneesmiddelen gaat nog steeds door." *Vrij Nederland*, December 6.

Van Meurs, R. (1978) "Bonussen, kortingen, cheques, belastingvoordeel en bootreisjes: Wie schrijft de meeste antibiotica voor?" *Vrij Nederland*, April 8.

Van Raak, R. (2010) "The transition (management) perspective on long-term change in healthcare." In J.E.W. Broerse and J.F.G. Bunders, *Transitions in Health Systems: Dealing with persistent problems*, Amsterdam: VU University Press, pp. 49–86.

Van Sas, N.C.F. (2005) *De metamorfose van Nederland: Van oude orde naar moderniteit*, Amsterdam: Amsterdam University Press.

Verbong, G., and Loorbach, D. (eds) (2012) *Governing the Energy Transition. Reality, illusion or necessity?*, New York: Routledge.

Verhaak, P.F.M., Meijer, S.A., Visser, A.P., and Wolters, G. (2006) "Persistent presentation of medically unexplained symptoms in general practice." *Family Practice*, 23(4): 414–420.

Vermeulen, M. (2008) "'Kerngezond', maar wel in een rolstoel." *de Volkskrant*, October 1.

Vijselaar, J. (1982) *Krankzinnigen gesticht: Psychiatrische inrichtingen in Nederland, 1880–1910*, Fibula: Van Dishoeck.

Vololona, R. (2003) "The struggle against neuromuscular diseases in France and the emergence of the 'partnership model' of patient organisation." *Social Science and Medicine*, 57(11): 2127–2136.

Voß, J.P. (2007) "Innovation processes in governance: The development of 'emissions trading' as a new policy instrument." *Science and Public Policy*, 34(5): 329–343.

Voß, J.P., Bauknecht, D., and Kemp, R. (eds) (2006) *Reflexive Governance for Sustainable Development*, Cheltenham: Edward Elgar.

VWS (2006) *Niet van later zorg*, The Hague: VWS.

VZG (1996) *15 jaar VZB = VZG, 1981–1996*, Utrecht: VZG.

Walsh, E.G., and Clark, W.D. (2002) "Managed care and dually eligible beneficiaries: Challenges in coordination." *Health Care Finance Review*, 24(1): 63–82.

Walshe, K., and Rundall, T.G. (2001) "Evidence-based management: From theory to practice in health care." *The Millbank Quarterly*, 79(3): 429–457.

Ward, P.R., Thompson, J., Barber, R., Armitage, C.J., Boote, J.D., Cooper, C.L., and Jones, G.L. (2010) "Critical perspectives on 'consumer involvement' in health research: Epistemological dissonance and the know–do gap." *Journal of Sociology*, 46(1): 63–82.

Wells, P., Nieuwenhuis, P., and Orsato, R.J. (2012) "The nature and causes of inertia in the automotive industry: Regime stability and non-change." In F.W. Geels, R. Kemp, and G. Lyons (eds), *Automobility in Transition? A socio-technical analysis of sustainable transport*, New York: Routledge, pp. 123–139.

Whitehead, M., Dahlgren, G., and Evans, T. (2001) "Equity and health sector reform: Can low income countries escape the medical poverty trap?" *The Lancet*, 358: 833–836.

Whitstock, M.T. (2003) "Seeking evidence from medical research consumers as part of the medical research process could improve the uptake of research evidence." *Journal of Evaluation in Clinical Practice*, 9(2): 213–224.

WHO (1946) *Preamble to the Constitution of the World Health Organization as Adopted by the International Health Conference*, New York, 19–22 June, Geneva: World Health Organization.

WHO (1978) *Primary Healthcare: Report of the International Conference Primary Healthcare*, Geneva: World Health Organization.

WHO (1986) *Ottawa Charter of Health Promotion*, Copenhagen: World Health Organization.

WHO (1989) *Constitution*, reprinted from basic documents, Geneva: World Health Organization.

WHO (2000) *The World Health Report 2000 – Health systems: Improving performance*, Geneva: World Health Organization.

WHO (2002a) *Current and Future Long-term Care Needs: An analysis based on the 1990 WHO study The Global Burden Disease and the International Classification of the Functioning, Disability and Health*, Collection on Long-Term Care, Geneva: World Health Organization.

WHO (2002b) *Lessons for Long-term Care Policy. The cross-cluster initiative on long-term care*, Geneva: World Health Organization.

WHO (2002c) *Reducing Risks, Promoting Healthy Life*, Geneva: World Health Organization.

WHO (2008) *Primary Healthcare, More Than Ever. The world health report 2008*, Geneva: World Health Organization.

WHO (2011) *World Report on Disability*, Geneva: World Health Organization.

Whyte, W.F. (1991) *Participatory action research*, Newbury Park, CA: Sage.

Wieringa, N., Hardon, A., Stronks, K., and M'charek, A. (eds) (2005) *Diversity among Patients in Medical Practice: Challenges and implications for clinical research*, Amsterdam: UvA-AMC.

Wilkinson, R.G., and Pickett, K.E. (2006) "Income inequality and population health: A review and explanation of the evidence." *Social Science and Medicine*, 62: 1768–1784.

Willems, D.L. (1995) *Tools of Care. Explorations into the semiotics of medical technology*, Maastricht: Maastricht University.

Williamson, C. (2008) "The patient movement as an emancipation movement." *Health Expectations*, 11(2): 102–112.

Williamson, C. (2010) *Towards the Emancipation of Patients. Patients' experiences and the patient movement*, Bristol: Policy Press.

Wilson, H.J. (2000) "The myth of objectivity: Is medicine moving towards a social constructivist medical paradigm?" *Family Practice*, 17(2): 203–209.

Wladimiroff, J.W. (2002) "Honderd jaar Gezondheidsraad. III Ziekenhuiszorg en onderzoek." *Nederlands Tijdschrift Voor Geneeskunde*, 1895–1896.

WNT (1998) *Woordenboek der Nederlandse Taal*.

Wolleswinkel-Van den Bosch, J. (1998) *The Epidemiological Transition in the Netherlands*, Rotterdam: Erasmus University Rotterdam.

Woolhandler, S., Campbell, T., and Himmelstein, D.U. (2003) "Costs of health care administration in the United States and Canada." *New England Journal of Medicine*, 349: 768–775.

WRR (2004) *Bewijzen van goede dienstverlening*, Amsterdam: Wetenschappelijke Raad voor Regeringsbeleid.

Wyatt, K., Carter, M., Mahtani, V., Barnard, A., Hawton, A., and Britten, N. (2008) "The impact of consumer involvement in research: An evaluation of consumer involvement in the London Primary Care Studies Programme." *Family Practice*, 25(3): 154–161.

Wyngaarden, J.B. (1979) "The clinical investigator as an endangered species." *New England Journal of Medicine*, 301: 1254–1259.

Yanow, D. (2004) "Translating local knowledge at organizational peripheries." *British Medical Journal*, 15(1): 15–29.

Zarit, S.H. (1998) *Dementia: Caregivers and stress. Community paper series: Paper 8*, Centre on Aging, Victoria, BC: University of Victoria.

Zarit, S.H. (2002) "Caregiver's burden." In S. Andrieu and J.P. Aquino (eds), *Family and Professional Carers: Findings lead to action*, Paris: Serdi Edition y Fondation Médéric Alzheimer, pp. 20–24.

Ziekenfondsraad (1983) *Grenzen aan de groei van het verstrekkingenpakket*, Amstelveen: Ziekenfondsraad.

Zimmermann, R. (2004) *PGA-Jeugd in netwerkverband. Plan van aanpak*, Internal document, Rotterdam: GGZ Groep Europoort.

Zollman, C., and Vickers, A. (1999), "What is complementary medicine?" ABC of complementary medicine, *British Medical Journal*, 391(7211): 693–696.

ZonMW, and VSBfonds (2009) *Programmavoorstel Patiëntenparticipatie in onderzoek, kwaliteit en beleid*, The Hague: ZonMW.

Zwetsloot, G., Gründemann, R., and Vaandrager, L. (2003) *Integraal Gezondheids Management (IGM). Eindrapportage*, Hoofddorp: TNO.

Zwetsloot, G., and Pot, F. (2004) "The business value of health management." *Journal of Business Ethics*, 55(2): 115–124.

Zwols, G. (1985) *Het ontstaan en de ontwikkeling van het beroep verpleegkundige*, Lochem: De Tijdstroom.

Index

Page numbers in *italics* denote tables, those in **bold** denote figures.